Statistics for Biology and Health

Series Editors

Mitchell Gail, Division of Cancer Epidemiology and Genetics, National Cancer Institute, Rockville, MD, USA

Jonathan M. Samet, Department of Environmental & Occupational Health, University of Colorado Denver - Anschutz Medical Campus, Aurora, CO, USA

Statistics for Biology and Health (SBH) includes monographs and advanced textbooks on statistical topics relating to biostatistics, epidemiology, biology, and ecology.

Daniel Zelterman

Applied Multivariate Statistics with R

Second Edition

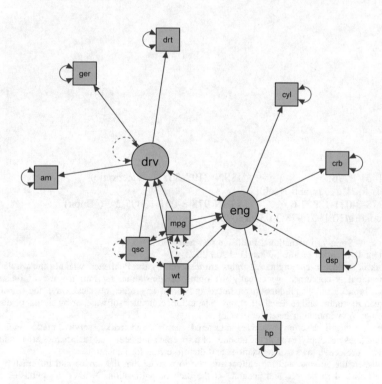

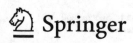 Springer

Daniel Zelterman
School of Public Health
Yale University
New Haven, CT, USA

ISSN 1431-8776   ISSN 2197-5671   (electronic)
Statistics for Biology and Health
ISBN 978-3-031-13007-6   ISBN 978-3-031-13005-2   (eBook)
https://doi.org/10.1007/978-3-031-13005-2

This Springer imprint is published by the registered company Springer Nature Switzerland AG
The registered company address is: Gewerbestrasse 11, 6330 Cham, Switzerland

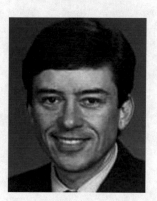

Barry H Margolin
1943–2009
Teacher, mentor, and friend

Permissions

R is Copyright ©2014 The R Foundation for Statistical Computing. R Core Team (2014). R: A Language and Environment for Statistical Computing. R Foundation for Statistical Computing Vienna, Austria. URL: http://www.R-project.org/.

We are grateful for the use of data sets, used with permission as follows:

Public domain data in Table 1.4 was obtained from the U.S. Cancer Statistics Working Group. *United States Cancer Statistics: 1999–2007 Incidence and Mortality Web-based Report.* Atlanta: U.S. Department of Health and Human Services, Centers for Disease Control and Prevention and National Cancer Institute; 2010. Available online at: www.cdc.gov/uscs.

The data of Table 7.1 is used with permission of S&P Dow Jones.

The data of Table 7.4 was collected from www.fatsecret.com and used with permission. The idea for this table was suggested by the article originally appearing in The Daily Beast, available online, at

http://www.thedailybeast.com/galleries/2010/06/17/40-unhealthiest-burgers.html

The data in Table 7.5 is used with permission of S&P Dow Jones Indices.

The data in Table 7.4 was gathered from www.fatsectret.com and used with permission. The idea for this table was suggested by the article originally appearing in The Daily Beast, available online at

http://www.thedailybeast.com/galleries/2010/10/18/halloween-candy.html

The data in Table 7.5 was obtained from https://health.data.ny.gov/.

The data in Table 8.2 is used with permission of Dr. Deepak Nayaran, Yale University School of Medicine.

The data in Table 8.4 was reported by the National Vital Statistics System (NVSS): http://www.cdc.gov/nchs/deaths.htm

The data in Table 9.3 was generated as part of the Medicare Current Beneficiary Survey: http://www.cms.gov/mcbs/ and available on the cdc.gov website.

The data in Table 9.4 was collected by the United States Department of Labor, Mine Safety and Health Administration. This data is available online at

http://www.msha.gov/stats/centurystats/coalstats.asp

The data of Table 9.6 is used with permission of StreetAuthority and David Sterman.

The data in Table 11.1 is adapted from: Statistics Canada (2009) "Health Care Professionals and Official-Language Minorities in Canada 2001 and 2006," Catalog no. 91-550-X, Text Table 1.1, appearing on page 13.

The data source in Table 11.5 is copyright 2010, Morningstar, Inc., Morningstar Bond Market Commentary September, 2010. All Rights Reserved. Used with permission.

The data in Table 11.6 is cited from US Department of Health and Human Services, Administration on Aging. The data is available, online, at

`http://www.aoa.gov/AoARoot/Aging\_Statistics/index.aspx`

The website `http://www.gastonsanchez.com` provided some of the code appearing in Output 11.1.

Global climate data appearing in Table 13.2 is used with permission: *Climate Charts & Graphs*, courtesy of Kelly O'Day.

Tables 14.1 and 14.10 are reprinted from Stigler (1994) and used with permission of the Institute of Mathematical Statistics.

Table 14.11 is data collected by the US Federal Election Committee and reposted by the NYTimes on Aug. 2, 2019.

In Addition

Several data sets referenced and used as examples were obtained from the UCI Machine Learning Repository [`http://archive.ics.uci.edu/ml`]. Irvine, CA: University of California, School of Information and Computer Science. (Bache and Lichman, 2013). Additional sources of cited data were obtained from DASL [`https://dasl.datadescription.com/`].

Grant Support

The author acknowledges support from grants from the National Institute Of Mental Health, the National Cancer Institute, and the National Institute of Environmental Health Sciences. The content is solely the responsibility of the author and does not necessarily represent the official views of the National Institutes of Health.

Preface to the Second Edition

The popularity of the first edition and new developments have motivated this second edition, over 25% larger. With this second edition, newly added is the material in Chap. 11 on Gaussian mixture models, the EM algorithm, nearest neighbor clustering, and DBscan. The chapter on factor methods has been expanded to include structural equations, latent growth modeling, and confirmatory factor analysis. I added penalized likelihood methods for both linear models and logistic regression. A section is included on image processing showing how data may appear when we least expect it. Also added is an introduction to methods for longitudinal data. I discuss causal inference including mediation and counterfactuals. Section 14.6 on overdispersion diagnostics has been added, including the convexity plot and heterogeneity residuals.

Throughout, I continue to make extensive use of real examples, **R** code, and graphical illustrations, important features of the first edition. New examples include Table 14.11 on fundraising by political candidates and Exercise 14.9 measuring the highest rates of COVID-19.

Special thanks go out to many readers of the first edition who pointed out innumerable errors.

The dedication to Barry Margolin continues with this second edition. If he were alive today, I would like to think this is the book he would have written.

New Haven, USA

Daniel Zelterman

Preface to the First Edition

MULTIVARIATE STATISTICS is a mature field with many different methods. Many of these are mathematical. Fortunately, these methods have been programmed so you should be able to run these on your computer without much difficulty.

This book is targeted at a graduate-level practitioner who may need to use these methods but does not necessarily know about the mathematical derivations. For example, we use the sample average of the multivariate distribution to estimate the population mean but do not need to prove the optimal properties of such an estimator when sampled from a normal parent population. Readers may want to analyze their data, motivated by discipline-specific questions. They will discover ways to get at some important results without a degree in statistics. Similarly, those well-trained in statistics will likely be familiar with many of the univariate topics covered here, but now can learn about new methods.

Readers should have taken at least one course in statistics previously and have some familiarity with such topics as t-test, degrees of freedom (df), p-values, statistical significance, and the chi-squared test of independence in a 2×2 table. They should also know the basic rules of probability such as independence and conditional probability. The reader should have some basic computing skills including data editing. It is not necessary to have experience with **R** or with programming languages although these are good skills to develop.

We will assume the reader has a rudimentary acquaintance of the univariate normal distribution. We begin a discussion of multivariate models with an introduction to the bivariate normal distribution in Chapter 6. These are used to make the leap from the scalar notation to the use of vectors and matrices used in Chapter 7 on the multivariate normal distribution. A brief review of linear algebra appears in Chapter 4, including the corresponding computations in **R**. Other multivariate distributions include models for extremes, described in Section 14.5.

We frequently include the necessary software to run the programs in **R**, because we need to be able to perform these methods with real data. In some cases, we need to manipulate the data in order to get it to fit into the proper format. Readers may want to produce some of the graphical displays given in Chapter 3 for their own data. For these readers, the full programs to produce the figures are listed.

The field of statistics has developed many useful methods for analyzing data and many of these methods are already programmed for you and readily available in **R**. What's more, **R** is free, widely available, open source, flexible, and the current fashion in statistical computing. Authors of new statistical methods are regularly contributing to the many libraries in **R** so many new results are included as well.

As befitting the Springer series in Life Sciences, Medicine, and Health, a large portion of the examples given here are health-related or biologically oriented. There are also a large number of examples from other disciplines. There are several reasons for this, including the abundance of good examples available. Examples from other disciplines do a good job of illustrating the method without a great deal of background knowledge of the data.

For example, Chapter 9 on multivariable linear regression methods begins with an example of data for different car models. Because the measurements on the cars are readily understood by the reader with little or no additional explanation, we can concentrate on the statistical methods rather than spending time on the example details. In contrast, the second example, presented in Section 9.3, is about a large health survey and requires a longer introduction for the reader to appreciate the data. But in Chapter 9, we should already be familiar with the statistical tools and can address issues raised by the survey data.

New Haven, CT, USA   Daniel Zelterman

Acknowledgments

Special thanks are due to Michael Kane and Forrest Crawford who together taught me enough **R** to fill a book. Also thanks to Rob Muirhead, who taught multivariate statistics using TW Anderson's text (Anderson 2003).[1]

Long talks with Alan Izenman provided large doses of encouragement. Steve Schwager, first suggested writing this book and gave me the initial Table of Contents. Ben Kedem read and provided useful comments on Chap. 13. Chang Yu provided many comments on the technical material. Thanks to Beth Nichols whose careful reading and red pencil provided many editorial improvements to the manuscript. Thanks also to many teachers, students, and colleagues who taught me much. Many thanks to caring and supportive friends and family who encouraged and put up with me during the whole process.

The APL computer language and TW Anderson's book (Anderson 2003) on multivariate statistics provided me with the foundation for writing this book as a graduate student in the 1970s. I watched Frank Anscombe[2] working on his book (Anscombe 1981) and was both inspired and awed by the amount of effort involved.

June 2022   Daniel Zelterman

---

[1] Theodore Wilbur Anderson (1918–2016). American mathematician and statistician.

[2] Francis John Anscombe (1918–2001). British statistician. Founded the Statistics Department at Yale.

Contents

About the Author

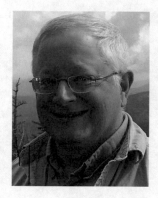

Daniel Zelterman, Ph.D. is Professor Emeritus in the Department of Biostatistics at Yale University. His research areas include computational statistics, models for discrete-valued data, and the design of small clinical trials in cancer studies. In his spare time, he plays oboe and bassoon in amateur orchestral groups and has backpacked hundreds of miles of the Appalachian Trail.

Other books by the author are as follows:

Models for Discrete Data, Oxford University Press. 1999.

Advanced Log-Linear Models Using SAS, SAS Institute. 2002.

Discrete Distributions: Application in the Health Sciences, J. Wiley. 2004.

Models for Discrete Data, Revised Edition, Oxford University Press. 2006.

Applied Linear Models with SAS, Cambridge University Press. 2010.

Applied Multivariate Statistics with R. Springer. 2015.

Regression for Health and Social Science: Applied Linear Models with R, Cambridge University Press. 2022.

Chapter 1
Introduction

W E ARE SURROUNDED by data. How is multivariate data analysis different from more familiar univariate methods? This chapter provides a summary of most of the major topics covered in this book. We also want to provide advocacy for the multivariate methods developed.

This chapter introduces some useful datasets and uses them to motivate the topics and basic principles and ideas of multivariate analysis. Why do we need multivariate methods? What are the shortcomings of the marginal approach, looking at variable measurements one at a time? In many scientific investigations, there are several variables of interest. Can they be examined one at a time? What can be lost by performing such univariate analysis?

1.1 Goals of Multivariate Statistical Techniques

Let us summarize the types of problems to be addressed in this book and briefly describe some of the methods to be introduced in subsequent chapters. As an example, consider the data given in Table 1.1. This table lists each of the 50 US states (plus DC) and several indications of the costs associated with living there. For each state, this table shows the population, average gross income, cost of living index relative to the US as a whole, median monthly apartment rentals, and then median housing price. Because the cost of living index is calculated on estimates of prices including housing costs, we quickly see there may be a strong relationship between measures in this table.

© Springer Nature Switzerland AG 2022
D. Zelterman, *Applied Multivariate Statistics with R*, Statistics for Biology and Health,
https://doi.org/10.1007/978-3-031-13005-2_1

Table 1.1 Costs of living in each of the 50 states

State	Median apartment rent in $	Median home value in $1,000	Cost of living index	2009 Population in 1,000s	Average gross income in $1,000
AK	949	237.8	133.2	698.47	68.60
AL	631	121.5	93.3	4708.71	36.11
AR	606	105.7	90.4	2889.45	34.03
⋮	⋮	⋮	⋮	⋮	⋮
WV	528	95.9	95.0	1819.78	33.88
WY	636	188.2	99.6	544.27	64.88

Source US Census, 2007 and 2009 data

As an example of a multivariate statistical analysis, let us create a 95% joint (simultaneous) confidence interval of both the mean rent and housing prices.[1] In Fig 1.1, we present both the marginal confidence intervals and the joint, bivariate confidence ellipsoid described more fully in Sect. 6.3.

The marginal confidence intervals treat each variable individually, and the resulting 95% confidence interval for the two means is pictured as a rectangle. The bivariate confidence ellipsoid takes into account the correlation between rents and housing prices resulting in an elongated elliptical shape oriented to reflect the positive correlation between these two prices.

The elliptical area and the rectangle overlap. There are also areas included in one figure but not the other. More importantly, notice the area of the ellipse is smaller than the area of the rectangle. This difference in area illustrates the benefit of using multivariate methods over the marginal approach. If we were using univariate methods and obtaining confidence intervals for each variable individually, then the resulting confidence region is larger than the region taking the bivariate relationship of rents and housing costs into account. This figure provides a graphical illustration of the benefits of using multivariate methods over the use of a series of univariate analyses.

1.2   Data Reduction or Structural Simplification

Which variables should be recorded when constructing a multivariate data set? We certainly want to include everything which might eventually turn out to be relevant, useful, and/or important. Much of these decisions require knowledge of the specific subject matter and cannot be adequately covered in a book on statistics. There is a

---

[1] The thoughtful reader might argue this exercise does not make sense because there are only 50 states, and this *census* represents the values of the complete population. In other words, there is no uncertainty associated with these data because there is no larger population of states for us to sample from.

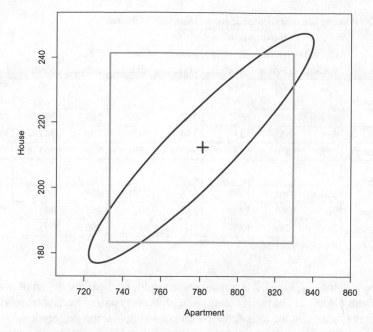

Figure 1.1 Joint 95% confidence ellipsoid for housing prices and monthly apartment rents. The box is formed from the marginal 95% confidence intervals. The sample averages are indicated in the center

trade-off between the fear of leaving out some information later proving to be critical. Similarly, it may be next to impossible to go back to record data not recorded earlier.

Hopefully, the subject matter experts have collected the most useful sets of measurements (with or without the aid of a statistician). The first task for the data analyst is to sort through it and determine those variables worthy of our attention. Similarly, much of the data collected may be redundant. A goal of data analysis is to sift through the data an identify what should be kept for further examination and what can safely be discarded.

Let us consider the data in Table 1.2 on the outcome of a standardized test of students taken in different countries (or economies) in 2009. The Program for International Student Assessment (PISA) is a triennial survey of academic achievements of 15-year-old students in each of 70 different countries.[2] The US is #17 on this list behind homogeneous populations of Finland, Korea, Hong Kong.

The overall reading score is broken down into five different subscales measuring specific skills. Mathematics and science are listed separately. How much is gained by providing the different subscales for reading? Is it possible to remove or combine some of these with little loss of detail?

---

[2] This survey is funded by The Organization for Economic Co-operation and Development (OECD).

Table 1.2   Reading and other academic scores from OECD nations

Nation	Overall reading	Reading subscales					Math	Science
		Access retrieve	Integrate interpret	Reflect eval.	Con- -tinuous	Non- contin.		
China: Shanghai	556	549	558	557	564	539	600	575
Korea	539	542	541	542	538	542	546	538
Finland	536	532	538	536	535	535	541	554
HongKong	533	530	530	540	538	522	555	549
⋮ ⋮		⋮		⋮		⋮		⋮
Peru	370	364	371	368	374	356	365	369
Azerbaijan	362	361	373	335	362	351	431	373
Kyrgyzstan	314	299	327	300	319	293	331	330

Source OECD PISA 2009 database

More specifically, Fig. 1.2 is a matrix scatterplot of the eight different academic scores from Table 1.2. The matrix scatterplot plots every pair of measurements against each other twice, with the axes reversed above and below the diagonal.

The immediate impression we get from this figure is how highly correlated all of the measurements are with each other. There are a few outliers and some pairs of measurements are more tightly correlated, of course, but it is clear any one academic measurement in the data could stand as a good representation for most of the others. A large amount of data simplification can be performed for these data without significant loss of information.

1.3   Grouping and Classifying Observations

In 2006, Pluto was demoted from the family of planets in our solar system and it is now classified as just one of many objects orbiting the sun. Part of the argument for Pluto's re-assignment consists of the large number of smaller and larger additional objects orbiting the sun at about the same distance. One group of these is referred to as the Kuiper Belt[3] extending from the orbit of Neptune at about 30AU out to about 55AU. (One astronomical unit (AU) is the distance to the earth from the sun.) The Kuiper Belt contains more than a thousand known objects, and there are estimates of many tens of thousands more yet to be discovered. Data on several of the largest of these appears in Table 1.3.

Albedo refers to the percentage of light reflected rather than absorbed. Snow, for example, appears very bright and has a high albedo. The absolute magnitude is a measure of apparent brightness, corrected for the distance of the object, measured on

---

[3] Named for Dutch astronomer Gerard Peter Kuiper (rhymes with viper) 1905–1973.

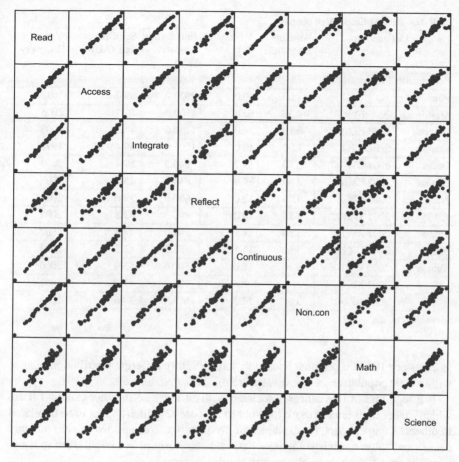

Figure 1.2 Matrix scatterplot of reading and academic scores of 15 year-old students in 2009 in OECT nations

a logarithmic scale. Higher absolute magnitude refers to dimmer objects. The semi-major axis is the orbit's greatest distance from the sun, measured in AU. Many of the values in this table are, at best, rough estimates for these distant, poorly understood objects.

Is Pluto a real standout object among the items in this list, or does it appear similar in character to the others? Does Pluto deserve to regain its former planet status or is it just one member of a larger club? In Sect. 8.1 we look at these data and see if there is a way to simplify it. Can this multivariate data can be summarized in a way retaining much of the useful information? Where does Pluto fall in this larger schema of things?

A comparison of the cancer rates in each of 50 states is another example to illustrate grouping. The data in Table 1.4 lists overall 2007 cancer rates for each of the 50 US states as well as for several of the most common cancers. These rates are reported

Table 1.3 Several Kuiper Belt objects

Designation		Absolute magnitude	Albedo (%)	Equatorial diameter (km)	Semi-major axis (AU)	Year of discovery
Permanent	Provisional					
Pluto		−1.00	60.0	2320.0	39.4	1930
Makemake	2005 FY9	−0.30	80.0	1500.0	45.7	2005
Haumea	2003 EL61	0.10	84.0	1150.0	43.3	2005
Charon	S/1978 P 1	1.00	40.0	1205.0	39.4	1978
Orcus	2004 DW	2.30	19.7	946.3	39.4	2004
Quaoar	2002 LM60	2.60	19.9	844.0	43.5	2002
Ixion	2001 KX76	3.20	12.0	650.0	39.6	2001
55636	2002 TX300	3.30	10.0	800.0	43.1	2002
55565	2002 AW197	3.30	11.7	734.6	47.4	2002
55637	2002 UX25	3.60	11.5	681.2	42.5	2002
Varuna	2000 WR106	3.70	16.0	500.0	43.0	2000
	2002 MS4	3.80	8.4	726.2	41.8	2002
	2003 AZ84	3.90	12.3	685.8	39.6	2003

Source Wikipedia

as cases per 100,000 persons. Each state has a slightly different distribution of ages within their populations so these rates are *age adjusted,* as well.

Is a high rate of one cancer associated with an increase in other cancers? If so, which cancer rates tend to move together in lock-step? Which appear to be unrelated to others? Lung cancers, for example, are frequently associated with environmental causes and colon cancers sometimes have a dietary origin. We might want to know how different cancer types cluster into similar patterns.

We can also ask about states clustering. Which states are comparable in their various rates? Do neighboring states have similar rates? Do the southern states group together with comparable cancer rates? How do Southern states differ from the Western states?

Perhaps the best summary is just group all of the data together. As an example, the "All cancers" rate is a sum of all cancer types, including the many diseases not listed here. Is this rate a reasonable summary of the rates for each state? Do the states clustering together also have comparable rates of their "all cancers"? Instead of a simple sum of all individual rates, would it be better to construct a weighted average, where some cancers receive more emphasis than others? Should rarer cancers (liver and cervix, for example) be given more or less weight than more common cancers?

Methods to answer these questions are described in Chaps. 10 and 11. Discrimination and classification are used to identify characteristics of groups of individuals, when group membership is known. Clustering assumes there are groups of individuals but their group membership is not known.

Table 1.4 Age adjusted cancer rates per 100,000 persons, combined for sexes and all races

State	All cancers	Lung	Colon	Melanoma	Female breast	Pancreas	Leukemia	Ovary	Cervix	Prostate	Liver
CT	584.1	54.4	52.4	27.9	133.9	16.2	13.7	12.1	6.5	172.8	9.8
ME	598.9	70.4	53.6	24.6	128.9	13.1	20.7	11.8	7.5	165.7	6.2
MA	571.0	62.6	50.7	26.0	131.7	13.3	16.0	11.8	5.3	166.9	10.9
				⋮	⋮	⋮	⋮				
OR	508.8	59.1	46.1	28.7	129.6	12.2	13.5	12.7	7.9	145.2	8.5
WA	525.3	56.6	45.9	27.5	124.0	13.0	17.1	12.5	5.9	155.1	10.1
US:	535.3	65.2	52.7	23.5	120.4	13.2	15.0	12.2	7.9	156.9	9.9

Source US Centers for Disease Control

1.4   Examination of Dependence Among Variables

Table 1.5 lists a survey of the recommended investment allocations from major financial management firms as of early 2011. The numbers represent percent allocations
for their "model portfolios" but they would usually make specific recommendations
for individual circumstances. Stocks and bonds are broken into three categories: US,
non-US industrialized countries, and developing nations. Alternative investments
include leases, oil and gas partnerships, real estate property, precious metals, and
similar investments. Cash includes short-term investments such as money-market,
bank deposits, and certificates of deposit.

At the time this table was created, the US was pulling out of a deep recession. It
was generally felt US stocks and bonds were the appropriate investments at the time,
so these two columns represent the largest entries in the table. Interest rates on cash
equivalents were very low so only small allocations appear there.

The numbers add up to 100% for each advisory firm. We should expect a small
overall negative mutual correlation of all of the percentages within each row because
of this restriction on these percentages. (The totals may be off by a small amount
due to rounding.)

Each of the investment firms hears the same economic news and reads each other's
published recommendations, so we should expect a small correlation between the
different rows of these data. As befits the conservative nature of this business, no firm
wants to be known for a consistently deviant recommendation, so there probably is an
attenuation of extreme opinions present as well. Within each firm's recommendations,
there are certain percentages allocated to traditional stocks and bonds. Each of these
is further broken down by firms specializing in domestic and foreign companies.

Another example of the data we might encounter appears in the nutritional data in
Table 1.6. This a collection of some of the highest calorie hamburgers served in chain
restaurants collected on the website `fatsecret.com`. Nutrition is an intrinsically
multivariate concept. We cannot talk about calories alone when discussing nutrition
but also need to include data on how much of the caloric value is derived from
fat. Amounts of sodium (salt) and protein are not part of calorie count and provide
different qualities to the total nutritional content.

The nutritional content was obtained from the individual restaurant's websites.
Each burger lists its calories and calories from fat, fat, saturated fat, sodium, carbohydrates, and protein content. The nutritional content of each menu item is not a
single measurement but expressed as these seven separate components. The seven
values are related to each other and must be taken as a whole. This is the fundamental
concept of multivariate data: each individual item is characterized by a set of several
related measurements on each.

The seven nutritional values are mutually correlated. Saturated fat and carbohydrates are related to the calories. Sodium is different from the other six. Perhaps we
want to create a "health index" constructed as a weighted average of the components
of each burger, thereby reducing the seven-dimensional data into a single number for
each. This is the aim of some multivariate methods such as factor analysis, described

Table 1.5 Recommended investment allocations (in %'s) by financial management firms at the beginning of 2011

Manager	Stocks			Bonds			Alternative	Cash
	US	Non-US	Dev.	US	Non-US	Dev.		
Alliance Bernstein	45	3	17	35	0	0	0	0
Atlantic Trust	28	6	9	30	3	0	24	0
Bank of America	53	9	3	28	1	1	0	5
BNY Mellon	26	9	10	30	0	0	25	0
Bessemer	19	9	3	20	4	5	34	6
Brown Advisory	29	13	12	19	3	0	20	4
Citi Private Bank	18	27	3	18	16	1	17	0
Constellation	20	10	10	25	5	0	30	0
Deutsche Bank	29	14	6	29	2	4	17	2
Fidelity	40	14	4	35	2	0	6	0
Fiduciary Trust	40	10	13	31	0	0	5	2
Fifth Third Bank	28	9	7	36	0	0	15	5
GenSpring	13	8	5	18	8	0	45	5
Glenmede	35	12	5	18	2	3	23	2
Harris Private Bank	54	10	4	18	0	0	15	0
Highmount Capital	25	5	10	40	5	0	15	0
Janney Montgomery	47	4	4	26	4	5	10	0
JPMorgan	20	9	5	22	3	0	38	3
Legg Mason	55	3	7	17	0	0	15	3
Northern Trust	24	8	5	31	0	0	32	0
PNC Asset Mgmt	40	8	2	30	0	0	20	0
Charles Schwab	29	20	5	29	1	0	11	5
SunTrust	26	6	3	25	7	0	30	3
UBS	32	10	7	27	6	0	17	2
US Bank	43	16	7	21	3	0	10	0
Wells Fargo	27	13	5	21	4	2	28	0
Wilmington Trust	27	11	4	31	1	0	27	0
Averages:	32.3	10.2	6.5	26.3	3.0	0.8	19.6	1.7

Used with permission Dow Jones

in Chap. 8. Another goal might be to creatively display all nutritional components simultaneously such as in Fig. 3.15 or 3.22.

1.5 Describing Relationships Between Groups of Variables

Let us go back to the data given in Table 1.1. How can we describe the differences in costs associated with living in each of the states? There are three measures of costs (rents, home prices, and cost of living index), and these three are mutually correlated.

Table 1.6 Some of the highest calorie hamburgers served in chain restaurants

Restaurant	Name of burger	Calories		Fat (g)	Sat. fat (g)	Sodium (mg)	Carbs. (g)	Protein (g)
		From fat	Total					
Chili's	Bacon Burger	612	1050	68	21	1750	53	55
Chili's	Big Mouth Bites	1197	2120	133	38	4200	139	65
Chili's	Southern Bacon	963	1610	107	36	4150	81	53
⋮	⋮	⋮	⋮	⋮	⋮	⋮	⋮	⋮
Sonic	Cheese w/ Mayo	573	999	64	24	1591	62	46
Sonic	Dbl Cheese-burger	730	1160	81	33	1580	44	63

Source www.fatsecret.com . Used with permission

Each of these measures of costs might separately be explained by populations and incomes. Perhaps more people living there, with higher incomes would drive up the prices relative to sparsely populated states with lower average incomes.

The three measures of costs are themselves related but the use of three separate regressions would lose these relationships. How much of the cost of living index can be explained by population and income, for example, and after correcting for these, how much of these differences across states can be attributed to housing costs? Chapter 9 covers the topic of multivariable regression and in Exercise 9.1 we will examine this example in detail.

1.6　Hypothesis Formulation and Testing

Interesting data sets are generated by a wide range of disciplines as new discoveries increasingly rely on statistical methods. Massive amounts of data are collected in genetics and astronomy, for example, where hypotheses are generated from within the discipline as well as on the basis of statistical analyses of the data.

Let us illustrate some data from astrostatistics, a relatively new field bringing together astronomy and statistics. In Fig. 1.3, we plot the visual magnitude of 3,858 galaxies in a portion of the sky. Locations in the sky are addressed in polar coordinates much as we identify places on the earth: right ascension is similar to longitude and declination is similar to latitude.

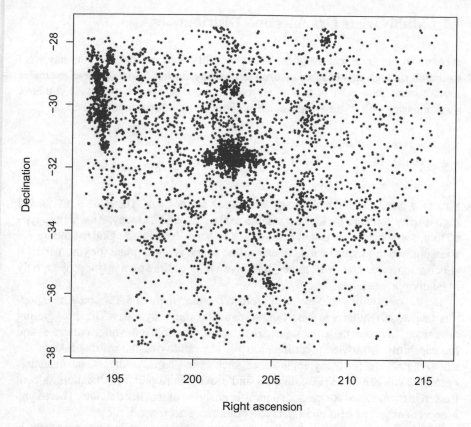

Figure 1.3 Visual magnitudes of 3858 galaxies in a portion of the sky. Brighter objects are plotted in red

Magnitude is visual brightness measured on an inverted log-scale: larger numbers are dimmer. Every increase in one unit is about 2.5 times dimmer. A magnitude of 6 is about the limit of the human eye, this is extended to about 10 with binoculars. Magnitude 27 is the approximate limit of the largest earth-bound telescopes, and the Hubble Space Telescope can detect magnitude 32. In Fig. 1.3, the brighter (and generally closer) galaxies are in red and dimmer ones are in blue.

The brighter galaxies in red appear to be distributed uniformly across this field, but the dimmer ones in blue seem to cluster in the upper left of this figure. It is well-known galaxies are not uniformly distributed across the universe, but rather, clustered much like the surface of bubbles, on curved walls, centered around vast, seemingly empty spaces.

Of course, this figure can only plot the objects known at the time the data was collected. Dimmer, as yet undetected galaxies are missing. There are many more objects to be plotted in blue in this figure at a future date as our technology improves.

1.7 Multivariate Graphics and Distributions

R offers strong graphical methods. These are illustrated in Chap. 3. You may want to thumb through this chapter before reading any further. Most of these examples require some knowledge of **R** in order to format the data appropriately. If you have no familiarity with **R**, then you can learn about its basic functions in Chap. 2.

1.8 Why **R**?

Finally, a word about the choice of **R** for the present book. There are a number of high-quality software packages available to the data analyst today. As with any type of tool, some are better suited for the task at hand than others. Understanding the strengths and limitations will help determine which is appropriate for your needs. It is better to decide this early, rather than invest a lot of time on a major project, only to be disappointed later.

Let us begin with a side-by-side (Table 1.7) comparison of SAS[4] and **R**, two popular languages regularly in use by the statistical community today. The most glaring differences between these packages are the capability to handle huge databases and the capability to provide a certification for the validity of the results. SAS is the standard package for many applications such as in pharmaceuticals and financials because it can handle massive datasets and provide third-party certification. In contrast, **R** is more suited for quick and nimble analyses of smaller datasets. There is no independent review of **R** and errors can continue, uncorrected, for years.

SAS is also more suitable for sharing programs and data, as in a business setting. SAS encourages the development of large programs through the use of its powerful *macro*[5] language. The macro program writes code which is expanded before the interpreter reads it and is then converted into computer instructions. In contrast, **R** has limited macro capabilities.

R was chosen as the software tool for the present book because of its extensive libraries to perform the relevant analyses and more flexible graphics capability. The author also teaches, regularly uses, and has written books using SAS. **R** is widely available as a free download from the Internet[6] Follow the instructions: It should not be too difficult to download **R** and install it on your computer. **R** is open-source, meaning in many cases, you can examine the source code and see exactly what action is being performed. Further, if you don't like the way it performs a task, then you can rewrite the code to have it do what *you* want it to do. Of course, this is a dangerous

---

[4] SAS is copyright © SAS Institute, Cary, NC.

[5] Briefly, a macro is a program to write a program.

[6] http://cran.r-project.org/ .

Table 1.7 A side-by-side comparison of SAS and **R**

SAS	R
Good for examining huge datasets	Not suitable for massive datasets
Good for shared projects	Better for individual work
Limited graphical presentation	Strong and flexible graphics
Difficult for custom analyses	Encourages customized analysis
Few independently written modules	Large 3-rd party software library
"Black box" code is hidden	Often open source
Iterative Matrix Language (IML)	Facilitates matrix operations
Powerful macro facility	Limited macro capabilities
Difficult to write new functions	Easy to write new functions
Point and click analyses	No hand-holding
Certified and verified	No promises made
Easy to produce tables with labels	More difficult to produce tables
Expensive for non-academics	Free
Fewer independently written references	Many independent reference books

capability if you are just a novice, but it does point out a more useful property: Anybody can contribute to it. As a result, there are hundreds of user-written packages available to you. These range from specialized programs for different analyses, both statistical and discipline specific, as well as collections of data.

The learning curve for **R** is not terribly steep. Most users are up and running quickly, performing many useful actions. **R** provides a nice graphical interface encouraging visual displays of information as well as mathematical calculation. Once you get comfortable with **R**, you will probably want to learn more.

It is highly recommended users of **R** work in `Rstudio`, an interface providing both assistance for novices as well as productivity tools for experienced users. The `Rstudio` opens four windows: one for editing code, a window for the console to execute **R** code, one to keep track of the variables defined in the workspace, and a fourth to display graphical images.

1.9 Additional Readings

There are many excellent introductory books on the capabilities of **R**, multivariate statistics, and the intersection of these two subjects.

An excellent introduction to **R** is Krause and Olson (1997). This book describes S and S-PLUS, the predecessors of **R**, and is light on statistical methods. Everitt and Hothorn (2011) also has a limited number of statistical topics and is more about **R** computing than statistical inference. Kabacoff (2011) describes **R** and statistical diagnostics but less statistical methodology. Venables and Ripley (2010) has a mix of statistical theory and **R**. Johnson and Wichern (2007) is more theoretical and does not incorporate software. Izenman (2008) is also theoretical, addresses current issues of mining large databases, references many relevant datasets, but does not emphasize computing. Mardia, Kent, and Bibby (1979) also offer a lot of theory. Anderson (2003) is the most theoretical of the books listed here.

Chapter 2
Elements of R

T HE SOFTWARE PACKAGE **R** has become very popular over the past decade for good reason. It has *open source,* meaning you can examine exactly what steps the program is performing. Compare this to the "black box" approach adopted by so many other software packages whose authors hope you will just push the `Enter` button and accept the results. Another feature of open software is if you identify a problem, you can fix it, or at least, publicize the error until it gets fixed. Finally, once you become proficient at **R** you can contribute to it. One of the great features of **R** is the availability of packages of programs written by **R** users for other **R** users. Best of all, **R** is free for the asking and easy to install on your computer.

On the downside, there is no certifying authority verifying the answers **R** gives you are actually correct. Errors are only judged in the court of popular opinion and may remain uncorrected for years. *Caveat emptor.*

Because **R** is so widely used, there are a number of good introductory books about its capabilities. While this chapter can't go over everything you can do in **R**, we can cover enough material to get you started with the computing needed to perform the statistical analyses described in this book.

Despite its many strengths, **R** does lack the capability to produce a nicely formatted output for a report. If your goal is to produce a formatted document then you will need to output graphics from **R** as a `.pdf` (or similar format) file and incorporate this into a word processing program such as LATEX. That is how this book was produced.

At the time of this writing, the **R** source can be found at

```
http://cran.r-project.org/
```

Simply follow the instructions on downloading the most recent package from any of the many mirror sites. There are versions of **R** for Mac, Linux, and Windows, so there should be a version for almost everybody.

© Springer Nature Switzerland AG 2022

D. Zelterman, *Applied Multivariate Statistics with R*, Statistics for Biology and Health,
https://doi.org/10.1007/978-3-031-13005-2_2

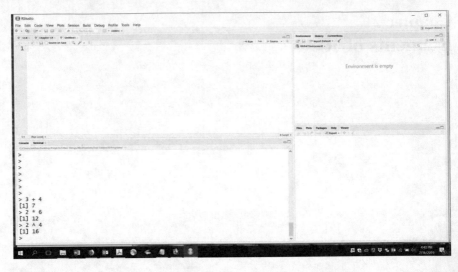

Figure 2.1   Screenshot of an R Studio session

While you are downloading software, the R studio [1] of is also a good environment to do your **R** work. You can find this at

```
https://www.rstudio.com/
```

and, yes, it is also free for most academic users.

Figure 2.1 is a screenshot of a session in R studio. The screen is divided into four windows: You type things in the left half and **R** tells you things about your session on the right. The lower left is a scratchpad where you can type and **R** will print numerical results. These are generally not saved when you are done.

The upper-left window is a text editor where you can cut and paste, search and replace, and similar things you would expect of a text editor. Everything you do in this window is saved in a text file. There are also tabs where you can jump from one file to another.

The right side of a R Studio session is for information about your environment. The upper-right window contains a list of all data and functions you have defined so far. The lower-right window contains any graphics you have created and also displays any help you have requested.

---

[1] RStudio is a registered trademark RStudio.

2.1 Getting Started in R

A nice feature of **R** is that it is interactive. You type something, and the computer types something in response. Try out the examples illustrated here, as they have been designed to ease your introduction to **R**.

2.1.1 R as a Calculator

Let's give **R** a try. Click on the **R** icon. It will open a window, and print some introductory text. Finally, you will see a line with a greater sign: > meaning you can now type something. In RStudio, this will happen in the lower-left window.

A typical session might go like this:

```
> 3 + 4

[1] 7

> 2 * 6

[1] 12

> 2 ^ 4

[1] 16

>
```

Information you enter appears on the lines beginning with >. For many operations, **R** produces lines beginning with a number in braces, (e.g., [1]). The numbers in braces will help find locations when there is a lot of output. This brief example shows **R** can be used as a calculator, but of course, it is much more than this.

We can assign a value to a name using the paired symbols < −.

```
> radius <- 3
> radius

[1]  3

> circum <- 2 * pi * radius
> circum

[1]  18.84956
```

In this brief dialog, we assign the value 3 to the variable called radius. Typing the name displays its value. We can then combine arithmetic with this named variable. We assign the result of a mathematical computation to yet another variable called circum but don't see the result unless we specifically ask for it.

The name `pi` has the value of $\pi = 3.14159\ldots$ and it would be a good idea not to change this. Another good idea is to use variable names having meaning to us rather than a name such as x conveying little information concerning its use. If you lose track of the variables used and their names, the `ls()` or `objects()` commands will provide a list of everything in the workspace.

You quit **R** with the `q()` command. You will be prompted if you want to save the workspace. It is a good idea to always check the YES button to save your results for a later session. If you end the **R** session in this manner, the variables `radius` and `circum` are still available after you close **R**, turn off your computer, and then restart it at a later time.

A variable, once created, is always available until you specifically ask for it to be deleted. To explicitly remove a variable, we use the `rm()` command as in

```
> radius

[1] 3

> rm(radius)
> radius

Error: object 'radius' not found
```

As you work in **R**, your workspace will soon become cluttered with a large number of intermediate results and data from various projects. You should make generous use of the `rm` function in order to keep your workspace free of litter. There is also a way to break up your **R** activities into different workspaces. These are described in Sect. 2.8.

2.1.2   Vectors in **R**

Vectors are a natural feature of **R** and can be constructed using the c (concatenate) function:

```
> evens <- c(2, 4, 6, 8, 10)
> evens

[1] 2   4   6   8 10
```

and then multiply the vector by a scalar:

```
> 2 * evens

[1] 4   8 12 16 20
```

The `rep( , )` function takes two arguments and is used to make multiple copies of the first argument. The first argument may be either a vector or a scalar. The `each`

= option makes copies of individual elements of the list. Here are examples of its use:

```
> c(1, rep(2, 3), 4)

[1] 1 2 2 2 4

> rep( c(1, 2), 4)

[1] 1 2 1 2 1 2 1 2

> rep( c(3, 5), each = 4)

[1] 3 3 3 3 5 5 5 5
```

The colon (:) operator produces an increasing or decreasing sequence of integers as in these two examples:

```
> 3 : 10

[1]  3  4  5  6  7  8  9 10

> 12 : 5

[1] 12 11 10  9  8  7  6  5
```

These can be combined in arithmetical expressions giving

```
> 4 : 8 / 4

[1] 1.00 1.25 1.50 1.75 2.00
```

so we are not restricted to working only with integer sequences.

In this last example, we see the sequence operation is given precedence over division. That is, the sequence operator in 4 : 8 / 4 is evaluated first, then the division. You should use parentheses to force the order if you are uncertain about which operation takes precedence.

We can combine arithmetic operations, sequences, and concatenation as in

```
> evens

[1]  2  4  6  8 10

> (evens <- c(evens, 2 * (6 : 10)))

[1]  2  4  6  8 10 12 14 16 18 20
```

Here we see an example where the name `evens` appears on both sides of the $< -$ operation. It is better to think of the $< -$ operation as *replacing* an existing value rather than *assigning* a value. In the last line here, we see an assignment contained in parenthesis will also print the resulting value for us.

Another good habit is to leave a *space* before and after the $< -$ symbols. This will avoid any ambiguity, (e.g., if you meant to write x < -3 instead of x < -3). This habit also makes your **R** code easier to read. It is generally a good idea to leave spaces before and after *any* operation symbols. We also leave a space after the coma in lists, as in `c(1, 2, 3)`. A larger set of operators is given in Table 2.1.

It is possible to address individual elements in a vector using square brackets `[ ]`. As examples, we have

```
> evens
[1]   2   4   6   8 10 12 14 16 18 20
> evens[4 : 7]
[1]   8 10 12 14
> evens[ c(1, 5, 6) ]
[1]   2 10 12
```

A negative subscript omits the corresponding element. If we want to omit the third element of a vector, for example, we can write

```
> evens
[1]   2   4   6   8 10 12 14 16 18 20
> evens[-3]
[1]   2   4   8 10 12 14 16 18 20
```

When subscripts are out of range or invalid, **R** is defined in an unintuitive manner. See Exercise 2.12 for some examples of these.

The `length()` function tells us the length of a vector:

```
> evens
[1]   2   4   6   8 10 12 14 16 18 20
> length(evens)
[1] 10
```

Suppose we wanted a subset of only those vector elements with values larger than 9. To accomplish this, we combine logical (true/false) values with a subscript as in the following:

```
> evens > 9
[1] FALSE FALSE FALSE FALSE  TRUE  TRUE  TRUE  TRUE  TRUE  TRUE
```

Table 2.1 A list of logical operators in **R**

==	Equal to	!	Not, negate
&&	And, element-wise	&	And, pairwise
||	Or, element-wise	|	Or, pairwise
>	Greater than	<	Less than
>=	Greater than or equal to	<=	Less than or equal to

```
> evens[evens > 9]

[1] 10 12 14 16 18 20
```

The evens > 9 script yields a list of logical TRUE and FALSE values indicating whether or not the corresponding vector element is greater than 9. If we use this list of logical values in the subscript brackets, then only values associated with TRUE are selected. A list of logical operators in **R** is given in Table 2.1. Finally, we can assign TRUE and FALSE as values to variables and abbreviate these as T and F.

Sometimes we want to find a member in a list of items. The %in% operator returns a logical value indicating whether or not an item is in the list. Here are examples:

```
> 3 %in% ( 1 : 5 )

[1] TRUE

> 8 %in% ( 1 : 5 )

[1] FALSE
```

The match() function allows us to find the location of specific elements in a vector. The match() function takes two arguments and finds the index of occurrences of the first argument in the second. So

```
> match( 3 : 4,  2 : 12)

[1] 2 3
```

shows the numbers 3 and 4 are located at positions 2 and 3 of the sequence 2:12. The match function is used in the production of Fig. 3.10, for example, in order to identify the index of unusual data points.

The which function is similar to match() except it works on logical values. So, for example,

```
> which( ( 2 : 5 ) > 3)

[1] 3 4
```

2.1.3   Printing in **R**

The last functions we will describe in this introduction control the output of results. The simplest way to see the value is to type the variable name. We also display the value of a variable using the print command. The digits = option in print() can be used to format the data by controlling the number of significant digits to be printed. Here is an example:

```
> x <- 1 / (6 : 7)
> print(x)

[1] 0.1666667 0.1428571

> print(x, digits = 2)

[1] 0.17 0.14
```

If you try to mix text and numbers in print, the whole result is converted into text strings but the result may look awkward. It is better to use the cat() function which concatenates the output.

```
> print(c("x is", x))

[1] "x is"              "0.166666666666667" "0.142857142857143"

> cat(c("x is", x))

x is 0.166666666666667 0.142857142857143
```

Similar results can be obtained using the noquote() command or the quote = FALSE option in print(). Notice cat() produces output without the leading subscript [1].

The format() command can be used with cat() to combine text and numbers printed to a specified number of significant digits:

```
> cat(c("x is", format(x, digits = 3)))

x is 0.167 0.143
```

To end this section, let us point out the extensive help available to the user of **R**. The help is most useful if you have a reasonably good idea of the procedure you want to perform and want to learn more.

If you have a general idea about what you want, the help button in the console window will open a set of **R** manuals. Many of these have search options allowing you to look for functions to perform the task you want. A search for *variance*, for example, returns a large number of operations containing this keyword in their help file including the var() function. If you want to know more about the var() function, typing help(var) will open a web page with a complete reference on this function. The web page will contain complete details about this function, examples of its use in **R**, along with names of several closely related functions, and some references on the relevant subjects. This web page also describes how missing values are treated, how a weighted variance estimate could be obtained, links to functions to calculate tests and confidence intervals for variances, as well as nonparametric procedures for these methods. Keep in mind **R** is user-supported, so not every help entry will be this extensive, complete, useful, or even correct. Sometimes the **R** function may have been written as part of a published book, and the help entry will be minimal in an attempt to boost sales.

2.2 Simulation and Simple Statistics

R allows us to generate random data. Statistical scientists will frequently use this important capability to test theories and to learn about the properties of procedures when the behavior of the data is known.

The rnorm() function generates observations from a standard normal distribution with mean zero and unit variance:

```
> rnorm(3)

[1] 0.3645054 1.1591904 1.7222996

> rnorm(4)

[1]  0.4007988 -0.6369772  0.8908059  0.2781956
```

Notice how the values are different every time this function is called. Your values will also be different from these when you try it. Let us illustrate this feature in a brief example of a *simulation*. We frequently perform a computer simulation to answer difficult questions not otherwise be answerable. The following question has a simple solution (see Exercise 2.4), and knowledge of the exact answer allows us to confirm the simulation method is working correctly.

Question: Suppose X is a standard normal variate. What is the probability X^2 is between 0.5 and 1.2?

To simulate a solution to this question in **R**, we can write

```
> nsim <- 500
> x <- rnorm(nsim)
> x <- x ^ 2
> sum(.5 < x  &  x < 1.2) / nsim

[1] 0.192
```

Table 2.2 Some continuous distributions and related functions available in **R**. These are found in the MASS, MCMCpack, and mvtnorm libraries

Distribution	Density function	Cumulative distribution	Quantile function	Generate random variables
Normal	dnorm	pnorm	qnorm	rnorm
Uniform	dunif	punif	qunif	runif
Student t	dt	pt	qt	rt
Central and noncentral chi-squared	dchisq	pchisq	qchisq	rchisq
Gamma	dgamma	pgamma	qgamma	rgamma
Multivariate				
Normal	dmvnorm	pmvnorm		rmvnorm
Multivariate				
Student t	dmvt	pmvt	qmvt	rmvt
Exponential	dexp	pexp	qexp	rexp
Cauchy	dcauchy	pcauchy	qcauchy	rcauchy
Wishart	dwish			rwish

At this point, it would be a good idea to type this text into the upper-left window of RStudio where you can edit and save the code. In the first line of this set of code, we define the number of replicates so it will be easier to change if we want to perform this simulation again later with a different sample size. In the next two lines of this sequence of **R** commands, we use rnorm to generate 500 standard normal values and then square these. The expression $(x > .5 \& x < 1.2)$ returns a set of 500 TRUE and FALSE values depending on whether these conditions are met for each of the components of x. We can sum over these logical values (TRUE is 1 and FALSE is 0) to see how many of the 500 values meet our criteria. Keep in mind your result will be slightly different every time you repeat this simulation. The exact answer is 0.206 so this simulation is not too far off the mark. A random sample much larger than 500 would likely produce a closer estimate to the true value, of course. See Exercise 2.4 for more information. In Sect. 2.5, we perform a larger simulation to describe the behavior of the correlation coefficient.

There are many continuous statistical distributions already programmed in **R**. A brief list of these is given in Table 2.2. The general pattern for the names of these functions is density functions begin with a d, cumulative distributions with a p, the quantile function begins with a q, and the random number generator with an r.

As an example of several simple statistical functions useful in data analysis, the code in Output 2.1 generates 10 uniform variates, sorts these, and finds their minimum, maximum, mean, standard deviation, and variance.

In each of these operations, we see the arguments for the **R** functions are vectors of arbitrary length. Such *vector-valued arguments* for functions are convenient for us. The mean function returns a scalar-valued average of the vector values, but the sort function returns a sorted vector of the same length. Notice the original values are not replaced by their sorted values unless we assign these, as in x < −sort(x).

Another useful **R** function is hist(), a function to produce a histogram. As an example, hist(rnorm(75)) produces Fig. 2.2 from 75 random, standard normal variates.

Output 2.1   **R** code to generate uniform random values, sort these, and generate simple statistics

```
> x <- runif(10)
> x


[1] 0.5330116 0.2722369 0.5743971 0.3922796 0.2738410 0.1701639
[7] 0.8477313 0.5537144 0.1998406 0.7271472


> sort(x)


[1] 0.1701639 0.1998406 0.2722369 0.2738410 0.3922796 0.5330116
[7] 0.5537144 0.5743971 0.7271472 0.8477313


> min(x)


[1] 0.1701639


> max(x)


[1] 0.8477313


> mean(x)


[1] 0.4544364


> sd(x)


[1] 0.2296803


> var(x)


[1] 0.05275305
```

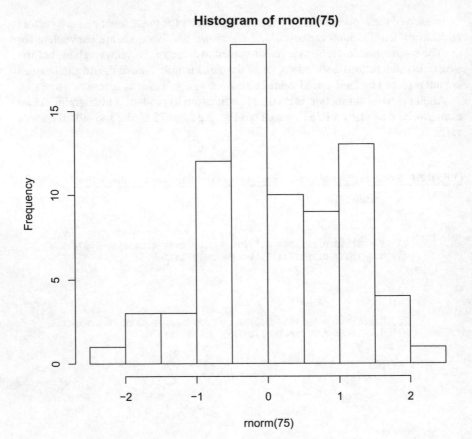

Figure 2.2 Histogram of randomly distributed normal variates

This figure will be a little different from yours, of course, and will also differ every time you run it. In RStudio, the typing is done on the left side and graphical figures will appear in the window at the lower right. We will discuss other graphical methods in the following chapter. In Sect. 3.1, we discuss how to save graphical images as a .pdf file for inclusion in the document.

We have covered some examples of basic arithmetic, simple statistics, and random number generation in **R**, so let us move on to importing and manipulating data from external files. In Chap. 3, we describe the hist () command again, along with other graphical presentations of multivariate data.

2.3 Handling Data Sets

This section covers two topics: bringing your data into **R** from files and then constructing `data.frames`. You don't want to type in a large data set using only the `c()` command. Rather, we need a way to get your data into **R**. Once it is in **R**, the `data.frame` is a convenient way to structure it in a useful format with handy labels identifying the columns and/or rows. If you are familiar with other data processing languages such as SAS then you will already be comfortable with this data format.

The easiest way to get your data into **R** is to prepare a file whose contents follow a pattern such as this:

```
          Apartment    House
    AK       949       237.8
    AL       631       121.5
    AR       606       105.7
    AZ       866       229.2

              .  .  .

    WI       704       173.3
    WV       528        95.9
    WY       636       188.2
```

This file, `housing.txt`, appears on this book's website. It contains the average apartment rents and house prices in each of the 50 states.

Such a table is relatively easy to create if your data is already arranged as rows and columns in a spreadsheet program. Beginning with the data in Table 1.1, for example, we can select the columns we want, copy these to a separate worksheet, then save it as a file, or perhaps copy and paste the result into a word processing language to clean it up further.

The headings and labels clarify the meanings of the numerical values in the various rows and columns. In this example, the rows have labels for each of the states, and the columns for apartment rents and housing prices are clearly marked. These labels are a very helpful feature when you put **R** aside for a few days and forget what the columns of data values represent. Similarly, try to avoid headings with names like x which convey no meaning.

The `read.table()` function is very useful for reading such formatted data into **R**. This function can be used to read data sets along with row and column labels. As an example, we can read the data from the `housing.txt` file using

```
>housing <- read.table("housing.txt", header = TRUE, row.names = 1)
>housing

      Apartment House
AK       949 237.8
AL       631 121.5
AR       606 105.7
AZ       866 229.2
```

```
            . . .
    WA          874 308.1
    WI          704 173.3
    WV          528  95.9
    WY          636 188.2
```

The result of the read.table() is assigned to a variable called housing and printed here. The name of the external file (in the appropriate working directory) is listed in quotes. This directory may be different on your computer. Working directories are discussed in Sect. 2.8.

The header option in read.table indicates column headings are present. The row.names= value indicates which column contains the labels for each row. In this case, the abbreviations for the state names appear in the first column of the data.

In this example, the read.table function builds what is called a *data frame* in **R**. Individual columns of data can be referenced from the data frame using either of two methods illustrated here:

```
> housing$Apartment

 [1]  949  631  606  866 1135  848  970 1011  917  947  787 1298  607
[14]  690  811  670  654  578  698  991 1074  702  706  734  657  638
[27]  631  694  534  626  914 1068  668 1011  953  667  614  780  726
[40]  850  675  569  660  768  784  934  797  874  704  528  636

> housing[1]

    Apartment
AK        949
AL        631
AR        606
AZ        866
         . . .
WI        704
WV        528
WY        636
```

In the first method, housing$Apartment refers to the column of apartment rents which are given as a vector of values without labels. In the second method, housing[1] is listed as the rent values along with their corresponding state labels.

R also treats the data.frame as a matrix, with two subscripts separated by commas. The first subscript addresses rows, as in this example:

```
> housing[1 : 4, ]

    Apartment House
AK        949 237.8
AL        631 121.5
AR        606 105.7
AZ        866 229.2
```

listing the first four rows.

The second subscript addresses columns, as in

```
housing[,1]

 [1]  949  631  606  866 1135  848  970 1011  917  947  787 1298  607  690  811
[16]  670  654  578  698  991 1074  702  706  734  657  638  631  694  534  626
[31]  914 1068  668 1011  953  667  614  780  726  850  675  569  660  768  784
[46]  934  797  874  704  528  636
```

We can use this property to subset the data as in this example

```
housing[ housing$Apartment > 1000 , ]

     Apartment House
CA      1135 467.0
DC      1011 474.1
HI      1298 560.2
MD      1074 341.2
NJ      1068 364.1
NV      1011 271.5
```

in which we select only those observations whose average monthly apartment rents exceed $1,000.

We can also create subsets of subsets as in

```
> housing[ housing$Apartment > 1000, ] [-3,]
     Apartment House
CA      1135 467.0
DC      1011 474.1
MD      1074 341.2
NJ      1068 364.1
NV      1011 271.5
```

using a −3 in a second set of subscripts to omit the third item (HI) from the list.

R recognizes the labels as such so it is valid to take the log of these values as either

```
> log( housing[1] )

     Apartment
AK   6.855409
AL   6.447306
AR   6.406880
   .   .   .
```

or else as

```
> log(housing$Apartment)

 [1] 6.855409 6.447306 6.406880 6.763885 7.034388 6.742881 6.877296 6.918695
   .   .   .
```

with no confusion about accidentally trying to take the logarithm of character values. Notice how **R** includes row labels in the first example, but not the second.

If you get tired of writing `housing$Apartment` and just want to refer to the data by the column names, the `attach()` command allows **R** to understand you are always referring to data frame of interest:

```
> attach(housing)
> Apartment

  [1]  949  631  606  866 1135  848  970 1011  917  947  787 1298  607  690
 [15]  811  670  654  578  698  991 1074  702  706  734  657  638  631  694
 [29]  534  626  914 1068  668 1011  953  667  614  780  726  850  675  569
 [43]  660  768  784  934  797  874  704  528  636
```

The `cbind` command works to add columns to data frames the way the `c()` command works to append to vectors. So the example

```
> lh <- cbind( housing, log(housing[1] ))
> lh[1 : 5, ]

   Apartment House Apartment
AK       949 237.8  6.855409
AL       631 121.5  6.447306
AR       606 105.7  6.406880
AZ       866 229.2  6.763885
CA      1135 467.0  7.034388
```

appends the log of apartment rents as another column onto the housing data frame.

We can fix the column heading using `colnames()` command. This command can either be used to print the column names, as in

```
> colnames(lh)

[1] "Apartment" "House"       "Apartment"
```

or else be used to assign a value, as in this example

```
> colnames (lh) [3] <- "Log Apt"
> lh[1 : 5, ]

   Apartment House  Log Apt
AK       949 237.8 6.855409
AL       631 121.5 6.447306
AR       606 105.7 6.406880
AZ       866 229.2 6.763885
CA      1135 467.0 7.034388
```

There is a similar command called `rbind()` adding rows to a `data.frame` and the function `row.names()` can be used to both query and manipulate the row names of a data frame.

There are several other **R** commands to read more diverse types of data in different formats. The `scan` function is very general and can be used to read numerical values from external files. The values read using `scan()` will appear as a single vector in **R**. You will need to format these appropriately into rows and columns using `matrix()` function and possibly use `t()` to transpose the matrix. The `data.frame()` command creates a data frame from a matrix and subsequently allows you to add row and column titles.

For reading different types of files, the `foreign` library contains **R** programs allowing you to read files from other data analysis programs such as SAS, S, Minitab, dBase, and Stata, to name a few. Programs such as Excel can export files where columns are separated by tab characters. In this case, you might have to use instructions such as

```
housing <- read.table("housing.txt", sep="\t",
    header=TRUE, row.names=1)
```

to indicate the separators (`sep=`) between columns are tab characters.

You can also use `read.table` to read from the *clipboard*. The familiar `copy` and `paste` operation involves highlighting a block of numbers or text in Excel or a word processing language. The `copy` operation is performed using a `Ctrl-C` command, which copies the highlighted material into a file called the `clipboard`. This material can be retrieved in **R** with the command

```
mydata <- read.table(file = "clipboard")
```

as though the `clipboard` were an actual file. This approach for reading data into **R** is best suited for small amounts of data.

2.4 Basic Data Manipulation and Statistics

R will sort your data. We sort a vector or a column in a `data.frame` using the `sort` command:

```
> sort(housing$Apartment)

 [1]  528  534  569  578  606  607  614  626  631  631  636  638  654  657
[15]  660  667  668  670  675  690  694  698  702  704  706  726  734  768
[29]  780  784  787  797  811  848  850  866  874  914  917  934  947  949
[43]  953  970  991 1011 1011 1068 1074 1135 1298
```

R can also rank the values:

```
> order(housing$Apartment)

 [1] 50 29 42 18  3 13 37 30  2 27 51 26 17 25 43 36 33 16 41 14 28 19 22
[24] 49 23 39 24 44 38 45 11 47 15  6 40  4 48 31  9 46 10  1 35  7 20  8
[47] 34 32 21  5 12
```

In a data.frame, we can sort on one column of data values and apply this ordering to all of the rows. Then

```
> housing [ order(housing$Apartment), ]
     Apartment House
WV         528  95.9
ND         534 112.5
SD         569 126.2
KY         578 118.4
       .   .   .
NJ        1068 364.1
MD        1074 341.2
CA        1135 467.0
HI        1298 560.2
```

rearranges all of the rows so the values in Apartment column are increasing.
For values decreasing in this column, we can sort on the *negative values*:

```
> housing [ order( -housing$Apartment), ]
     Apartment House
HI        1298 560.2
CA        1135 467.0
       .   .   .
ND         534 112.5
WV         528  95.9
```

and this provides the ordering from largest to smallest.
To calculate simple statistics on a data.frame, we can write

```
> colMeans(housing)

Apartment     House
 781.1765  212.3255
```

and this provides sample averages and column names for each of the columns.
The variance/covariance matrix is obtained

```
> var(housing)

             Apartment      House
Apartment    29391.83   16349.12
House        16349.12   10668.70
```

and the correlation matrix is

```
> cor(housing)

            Apartment      House
Apartment    1.000000   0.923263
House        0.923263   1.000000
```

Functions such as the mean and standard deviation are best applied to the columns of the `data.frame` using the `sapply` function. Examples of these are

```
> sapply(housing, mean)

Apartment      House
 781.1765   212.3255

> sapply(housing, sd)

Apartment      House
 171.4405   103.2894
```

R provides the capacity to *merge* data from two different data.frames. When working with large data sets, we frequently find the data is spread across more than one physical file. A merge is a process combining the files into one, by matching individual rows on the values in a specified column.

Let us illustrate the merge capabilities in **R** with a simple example. Suppose we have a data.frame with names and ages:

```
> first <- data.frame(
+     name = c("Charles", "Bill", "Amy", "Fred"),
+     age  = c(15, 25, NA, 22))
> first

    name age
1 Charles  15
2    Bill  25
3     Amy  NA
4    Fred  22
```

(Notice how **R** produces a + prompt because the unbalanced parenthesis expects a resolution in a subsequent line rather than another **R** command.)

Suppose a second data.frame containing names and heights:

```
> second <- data.frame(
+     handle = c("Charles", "George", "Amy", "Bill"),
+     height = c(61, 65, 60, 67))
> second

   handle height
1 Charles     61
2  George     65
3     Amy     60
4    Bill     67
```

There are a number of problems immediately appearing. Specifically, there are names in one data.frame absent from the other, and, further, the names occurring in both data.frames appear in different orders. Nevertheless, we want to produce a single file containing names, ages, and heights. Even so, there is some ambiguity as to how this should be accomplished, in light of the missing data.

In one version of the `merge` command, we can combine the two data.frames

```
> m1 <- merge(first, second, by.x = "name", by.y = "handle")
> m1

     name age height
1     Amy  NA     60
2    Bill  25     67
3 Charles  15     61
```

and recover only those names appearing in both data.frames.

The `merge` command in this example creates a new data.frame with the combined attributes (age and height) from the two separate data.frames. The `by.x=` and `by.y=` options specify the columns containing the data values we wish to merge on.

We can also combine all names, regardless of whether these appear in only one or both lists:

```
> m2 <- merge(first, second, by.x = "name", by.y = "handle", all=TRUE)
> m2

     name age height
1     Amy  NA     60
2    Bill  25     67
3 Charles  15     61
4    Fred  22     NA
5  George  NA     65
```

using the `all=TRUE` option.

In this last example, notice how the `merge` function fills in the missing values with NA's when the corresponding values are absent in one of the merged data.frames.

It is possible to clean your data and remove any records with missing values. This is especially useful for those procedures in **R** which will not perform analyses on missing (NA) values. These records need to be deleted for the procedure to work properly.

The easiest way to delete incomplete rows of data is through the `complete.cases` function. The `complete.cases` function identifies rows in a data.frame with no missing values. So, in the case of the merged data.frame m2, we have

```
> complete.cases(m2)

[1] FALSE  TRUE  TRUE FALSE FALSE
```

showing only lines 2 and 3 have no missing data values.

We can then build a data.frame with no missing data using

```
> m2[complete.cases(m2), ]

      name age height
2     Bill  25     67
3  Charles  15     61
```

After performing a merge, there may be several duplicated records. These can be identified using the duplicated function, which works on vectors as well as on data.frames.

As an example of its use,

```
> list <- c(1, 2, 5, 4, 2, 4, 5, 3)
> duplicated(list)

[1] FALSE FALSE FALSE FALSE  TRUE  TRUE  TRUE FALSE

> list[ !duplicated(list) ]

[1] 1 2 5 4 3
```

the duplicated items in this list are removed.

2.5 Programming and Writing Functions in **R**

A powerful feature of **R** is the capability to program your own functions, adding new and useful functionality within your work. We regularly use a number of **R** library functions, such as the square root (sqrt()). It is useful to write your own functions if you have some you use frequently or if you need to create long sequences of **R** commands. You can break these up into short procedures to be written and tested separately. This is especially useful when you want to tackle a large task. Break the task into component units to be sequentially built upon smaller segments.

To write a function in **R**, assign a variable the name function, followed by the arguments and then the definition. As an example, consider the function

```
> addA <- function(x) x + A
```

returning the sum of the argument (x) and the variable A.

To test it out, we have

```
> A <- 4
> addA(5)

[1] 9
```

```
> A <- 6
> addA(2)

[1] 8
```

Typing the name of the function, without an argument will print the definition:

```
> addA

function(x) x + A
```

If the function definition takes more than one line, put it in curved brackets: { }. A function can return more than one value if these are put into a vector. Results are returned when they are at the end of the function definition, as though we were printing the values in the interactive mode. We can also use the return statement.

As an example of a function spanning several lines and returning more than one value, we have

```
> addTwo <- function(x)
+ {
+    first <- x + A
+    second <- 2 * x
+    c( first, second)
+ }
> A <- 5
> addTwo(6)

[1] 11 12

> first

Error: object 'first' not found
```

As we work with functions, the *scope* limits where data values can be accessed. In the two examples given, notice the value of A is "known" inside the definition of the function. In the second example, we are unable to access the values first and second because these are considered local and only exist inside the definition of the function.

Here's another example of writing a larger function in **R**. Suppose we want to look at the statistical properties of *spacings*. Spacings are the differences between adjacent ordered data values. We might use a large number of small adjacent spacings as statistical evidence of an area of high density of observations, for example.

As a numerical example of spacings, suppose we start with the data values {8, 14, 3, 16}. Then the sorted data values are

$$3 \quad 8 \quad 14 \quad 16$$

and the corresponding set of spacings are

$$5\ \ 6\ \ 2\ .$$

Notice the spacings themselves are not sorted, and there is one fewer spacing than the data value.

Here is a function in **R** to calculate the spacings of any vector:

```
spacing <- function(x)
# Calculate spacings in vector x
{
    n <- length(x)
    if(n <= 1)return(NA)      # undefined if x is empty or scalar
    sortx <- sort(x)          # sorted values of x
    sortx[ -1 ]-sortx[ -n]    # return spacings
}
```

A value of NA is returned if we ask for the spacings of a scalar, whose length is 1. The NA symbol is a special value in **R**. It stands for "not available" and is useful to indicate a missing value. "Not a number" or NaN may be the result of an invalid computation resulting in an ambiguous or erroneous value such as division by zero. See Exercise 2.10 for more on these special codes for invalid numerical values.

We exit the function in the middle of the function's definition and return some value using the return() statement. In the present example, the return() statement is used to return NA to indicate invalid data was entered and an error has occurred. As a good programming habit, anticipate any errors a user might make and catch these before they cause unpredictable results. We can also write spacing in a much simpler fashion (see Exercise 2.11), but the present form illustrates useful features of functions in **R**.

In this function to calculate spacings, notice how we *document* or explain to the human reader what is going on. Anything written on a line in **R** following a pound sign (#) is treated as a comment by **R** and ignored. Such comments are extremely useful when you look at your program after a time and do not want to forget the role of the program code. If you share your program with others, then documentation is even more essential.

Don't try to write more than a few lines of **R** code directly in the console. It is much better to use the text editor in Rstudio. You could also use your favorite word processor and then copy and paste the code into the **R** window.

Let us generate some data and run the spacing program. For example,

```
> z <- sample(25,5)
> z

[1]  3 18 12 22 15

> spacing(z)

[1] 9 3 3 4
```

The `sample(25,5)` function generates five random integers between 1 and 25. Then the `spacing` program returns the four spacings of the five data values `sample(25,5)` sent to it, as required.

When writing your own program, you should check all of the various branches and paths it might take to ensure these are all working properly. In our spacings program, we should also verify

```
> spacing(5)

[1] NA
```

to see the error processing works correctly as well.

In the next section, we use these function writing techniques to perform a larger simulation study than the one presented in Sect. 2.2.

2.6   A Larger Simulation

A small simulation was introduced in Sect. 2.2. Let us next consider a more complicated example of a simulation in **R**. Suppose we want a program to help address the following:

Question: How can we describe the distribution of the correlation coefficient calculated from normally distributed samples?

We will need to generate several sets of (possibly correlated) paired normal random values and find the sample correlation of each set. In this way, we will have a random sample of correlation coefficients produced under specified conditions. Then we can draw a histogram of these correlations and calculate summary statistics, as well. This is the essence of a simulation study: Produce randomly distributed quantities (such as normals) whose behavior is well understood in order to study functions of these (such as the correlations) whose distributions are less well known to us.

We will also look at the correlation coefficient under the model of sampled independent normals as well as under a model in which the samples of the underlying paired normals are correlated. There are approximations to the behavior of the correlation coefficient (see Sect. 6.3), but in this simulation study, we do not want to use any approximations.

This process is an example of a simulation experiment. Statistical scientists frequently perform experiments on the computer in order to test theories about the behaviors of random processes.

To begin, we will generate correlated, normal random variables with the program `rmvnorm` in the `mvtnorm` library. For example,

```
> library(mvtnorm)
> rmvnorm(5, mean = c(0, 0), sigma = matrix(c(1,.8, .8, 1), 2, 2))
```

```
                [,1]              [,2]
    [1,]    1.03550508    0.06044561
    [2,]    0.53386104    1.03063539
    [3,]  -0.06674766   -0.41792785
    [4,]  -0.59569721   -0.54805093
    [5,]    0.96581969    0.61702999
```

This example generates five pairs of bivariate, random normals as a 5×2 matrix. The mean= option specifies the means of these pairs. The correlation measures association independently of location, so we can assume the population means are both zero.

The variance matrix is specified using sigma=. In the present example, the 2×2 matrix

```
>   matrix(c(1,-.8,  -.8,  1),  2,  2)

        [,1] [,2]
[1,]    1.0 -0.8
[2,]   -0.8  1.0
```

specifies unit marginal variances for each of the two components and a correlation (and covariance) of $-.8$. (We will discuss the covariance matrix again, in Chap. 7.)

Using the rmvnorm program, we can provide a visual check everything is working correctly. The code

```
plot(rmvnorm(2000, mean = c(0,0),
      sigma = matrix(c(1,  -.8,  -.8,  1),  2,2)), cex.lab = 1.25,
      xlab="x1", ylab="x2", pch = 16, col = "red")
```

generates 2,000 pairs of random bivariate normals and produces Fig. 2.3 giving us good visual evidence rmvnorm works as described. Many of the options in the plot function are described in Chap. 3.

Now we are able to generate bivariate, correlated normally distributed random values, we need to calculate the correlation of these pairs. The cor() function produces a matrix of correlation coefficients when its argument is a matrix, as is the case with the output of rmvnorm. In the case of paired data, the output of cor is a 2×2 matrix:

```
> z <- rmvnorm(5, mean=c(0,0), sigma =  matrix(c(1,.8,  .8, 1), 2,2,))
> z

            [,1]            [,2]
[1,]    0.5400575  -0.1341743
[2,]  -0.5003746  -0.3225571
[3,]    0.0657274   0.4185394
[4,]  -1.7284671  -2.0219641
[5,]    0.3055753   0.6599834
```

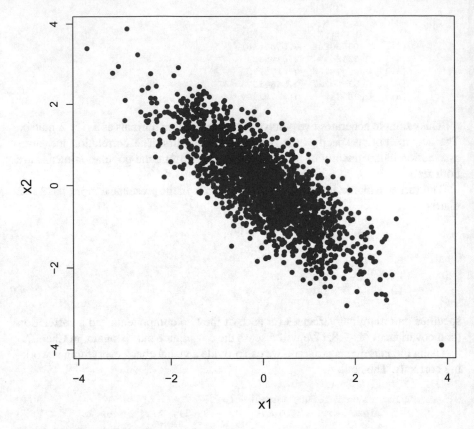

Figure 2.3 Simulated bivariate normals

```
> cor(z)

          [,1]      [,2]
[1,] 1.000000 0.903586
[2,] 0.903586 1.000000
```

We can address the specific matrix element

```
> cor(z) [1,2]

[1] 0.903586
```

in order to select the (scalar) value we want.

Now we have the tools to generate bivariate, correlated random normals and obtain their correlation, what parameters do we want to vary in our experiment? First, we need to decide how many correlation coefficients we want to generate. In the end, we will probably want to draw a histogram of their values in order to describe their distribution, so it makes sense to let this number vary in our program.

Let us denote the number of random correlation coefficients to be generated in our program by ncor. Each of these correlations will be based on a number of normally distributed pairs. Let us call the number of these pairs nnor in our program. In both of these parameters, let us use variables instead of fixed values. These variables will allow us greater flexibility. In both parameters, we choose names for the variables conveying meaning to their purpose.

Finally, we need a way to model the widest possible range of independence and dependence. We will examine a variety of correlated populations, so let us call this parameter rho.

The program called simcor to simulate the correlation is given in Output 2.2. Let us review several features of this program before we actually run it. A good feature of any program is to anticipate errors before these occur. Specifically, notice how the program checks the validity of the arguments ncor, nnor, and rho and will return NA's if these are not in the correct range. (Recall similar error checking in the program to calculate spacings, considered earlier in this section.)

We would not get an error message from **R** if ncor was a negative number, but it would be awkward for us to interpret the result. (See Exercise 2.6 for a discussion of this.) It is not clear how a negative value of nnor would be defined. The correlation coefficient needs at least two pairs of observed values in order to be defined. For this reason, we checked against these possibilities early in the program before **R** caught them, leading to unexpected results. To complete the error checking, notice how the program also checks the values of rho are in the valid range between −1 and +1.

The second feature of the simcor program is the use of the if() statement along with the corresponding else. The if() statement breaks up the order of

---

Output 2.2   **R** function to generate random correlation coefficients

```
simcor <- function(ncor, nnor, rho)

#  Simulate ncor random correlation coefficients based on nnor
#  pairs of bivariate normals with population correlation rho.
{

# Check validity of arguments:
   if( ncor < 1 || nnor < 2 || rho < -1 || rho > 1 )return(NA)
   library(mvtnorm)                   # access library

   vm <- matrix(c(1, rho, rho, 1),
                2, 2)                  # variance matrix
   simcor <- NULL                      # start a list of values
   for (i in 1 : ncor)                 # For every simulated correlation:
     {
       norv <- rmvnorm(nnor,           # generate normal pairs
         mean = c(0,0), sigma = vm )
       sc <-  cor(norv)[1, 2]          # correlation of these pairs
       simcor <- c(simcor, sc)         # add to list of values
     }
   simcor                              # Done
 }
```

instructions depending on whether or not the logical condition in the parenthesis is met. The statement following the `else` is executed if the logical condition evaluates to FALSE. See Table 2.1 for a list of comparisons resulting in logical TRUE or FALSE conditions.

If the logical condition in the `if()` is met, the next statement is executed. If the condition is not met, the program flows to the statement following the `else`. If we want several statements to be executed when the condition is met, then we can place those statements inside curly brackets.

The third feature of this program is called a *loop*. The loop is a powerful feature in programming getting the computer to repeat a series of instructions any number of times. All of the commands inside the code

```
for (i in 1:ncor)              # loop on the number of correlations
{
    ...                        # code lines to be repeated
}
```

will be repeated `ncor` times.

Inside this loop, the value of `i` will successively take on the values 1, 2, ..., `ncor`. Within each repeat of this loop, the program generates `nnor` pairs of correlated normal values and then finds their correlation, denoted by `sc`. These randomly generated correlation coefficients are accumulated in a vector with the same name as the function, `simcor`. These are returned at the completion of the function. It is not necessary to use the same name as the function for the returned values, but it can make it easier to remember.

The loop then repeats the process `ncor` times generating one random correlation coefficient with each repeat of the loop. We sometimes refer to each repeat as an *iteration*. Another habit good programmers have is to indent successive levels of brackets { }, making it easier to see the scope of the loop and where it begins and ends. Those with programming experience will already be familiar with the looping construct and the `if` and `else` conditional branching.

Let's try our new program. First verify the checks and error processing for invalid values of `ncor`, `nnor`, and `rho`, respectively:

```
> simcor(ncor = -1, nnor = 10, rho = 0)

[1] NA

> simcor(nco = 10, nnor = -1, rho = 0)

[1] NA

> simcor(ncor = 5, nnor = 15, rho = 1.8)

[1] NA

> simcor(ncor = 6, nnor = 12, rho = -1.2)

[1] NA
```

so the error checking appears to be working correctly.

Next, let's try the program using legitimate parameter values:

```
> simcor(ncor = 5, nnor = 15, rho = -.8)
[1] -0.7392940 -0.7368622 -0.8276200 -0.7509294 -0.8466513
```

using **R** to generate a set of ncor=5 simulated correlation coefficients, each from nnor pairs of normal variates. It is not necessary to identify the arguments (ncor, nnor, rho) by name, but including these names when invoking the function makes it easier to remember the roles of the three parameters, as opposed to having to recall their order in the list.

Now we can try the program at full strength with a large number of replicates:

```
> sim <- simcor(ncor = 2500, nnor = 15, rho = .8)
> mean(sim)
> hist(sim, main = " ", col = "blue")

[1] 0.7866204
```

generating 2,500 correlations, finding their mean, and producing the histogram given in Fig. 2.4.

The average of these values is reasonably close to the population value of 0.8. This provides some additional confirmation the program is doing what we expected it to do.

The histogram of these 2,500 values produced by simcor appears in Fig. 2.4. This histogram shows the distribution of the sample correlation coefficient is skewed with a longer tail to the left, as we would expect. The mean of these values is also reasonably close to where we expected it to be. Now we have the program to simulate correlation coefficients, we can use it for other purposes such as estimating statistical significance levels and approximating power for estimating the sample sizes of experiments. See Exercise 2.6 for an example of these uses.

Let us review the process to write the simulation program simcor and run it. We began with a clearly stated goal: To examine the behavior of the correlation coefficient. Then we identified the tools to generate bivariate normals and their correlations: mvnorm, matrix, cor. Next, we determined what variables we wanted to vary in the program: (ncor, nnor, rho).

In programming as well as simulation experiments, we need to go over similar steps: Define the task, then decide which factors are fixed and which will vary. This planning will save you from trouble later if you need to make revisions.

Be generous in placing comments inside your program. Experienced programmers will tell you there should be about one line of comments for every line of code. Such comments will help you if you put this project aside for a while and later come back to it. Sharing code with a colleague makes this documentation even more indispensable. Finally, avoid using abstract variable names such as x conveying no information about their role.

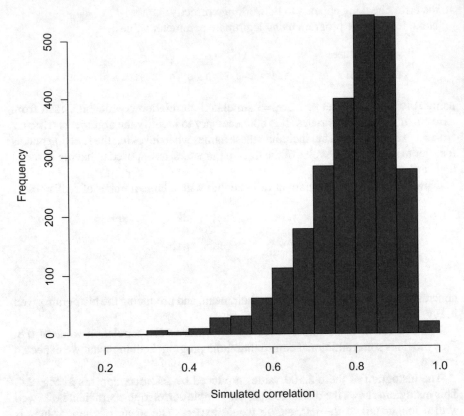

Figure 2.4 Histogram of 2500 simulated correlation coefficients

2.7 Advanced Numerical Operations

R allows for the numerical maximization and minimization of specified functions.
Beginning in Sect. 5.7, we see this process is an important tool in estimating model
parameters. Sometimes we can use calculus (and brute, mathematical force) to find
the maximum. But it is often easier to let the nlm (non-linear minimization) program
in **R** do this heavy lifting for us. This program requires that we write the objective
function and provide reasonably good starting values for the estimate of the location
of the minimum. In functions of many parameters, the choice of starting values can
often represent a large challenge, so be prepared to spend time on this.

The nlm() program will minimize a specified function of several variables. We
need to program the objective function to be minimized and provide a rough idea of
where the search for a minimum should begin. The output from nlm will include a list
of the parameter values minimizing the function and numerical estimates of the first
and second derivatives at the place the function is minimized. The first and second
derivatives are called the *gradient* and *Hessian*, respectively. These derivatives are

also estimated, numerically, by examining the change in the value of the objective function near the optimal parameter values. These estimates also help nlm in locating the minimum. Close to the true minimum, the objective function should behave approximately as a quadratic function, and **R** can numerically solve this equation for the next best place to look for a better estimate of the location of the minimum.

Unfortunately, nlm can get confused along the way. It can "wander off" and look for the minimum very far from where the minimum is located. In addition, it can give errors by looking in illegal or undefined places. This occurs when some parameter values are only defined for positive values, as a normal variance, for example. These problems will be illustrated in Sect. 5.7 and are often avoided by using good starting values. See Exercise 2.9 as an example.

We can also numerically evaluate integrals in **R**. This topic is often referred to as *numerical quadrature*. The integrate function will numerically approximate a one-dimensional integral, with possible infinite endpoints. Of course, if you are evaluating a function such as a cumulative distribution, then it is much better to use the specific function in **R** designed for the purpose, if available. There are routines in **R** to approximate multidimensional integrals as well, such as adaptIntegrate in the cubature library.

Finally, a wide variety of other mathematical computations can be obtained in **R** related to the matrix and linear algebra. These include determinants, solutions to linear equations, and eigenvectors, just to name a few. These are discussed in Chap. 4.

2.8 Housekeeping

In this section, we illustrate several additional **R** features worth knowing. Working directories allow you to better organize your workspace. Workspaces help organize your **R** work into separate folders for different projects. There is also a way to "take out the garbage" when it is time to clean up unused data within each project after these have outlived their usefulness. Finally, we show how to install new packages allowing you to take advantage of the many optional libraries of available programs.

After working with **R** for a while, your workspace can start to look like a very cluttered desk, containing many data sets from a variety of different projects. When you use the ls() or objects() commands to list all of the things in your workspace, you will see a huge number of variables (and maybe some programs) from a variety of different projects. The best way to organize your desk is to create a new *working directory* for each project.

Use getwd() to find the name of the current working directory and setwd() to change it. Don't forget to include the two parentheses on the getwd() command with no additional arguments. Typing getwd() on your computer might give

```
> getwd()

[1]"C:/Users/My Name/Desktop/"
```

This working directory probably points to some high level place on your computer. It would be much better to have a separate working directory specific to each project. In this case, we could change the working directory by typing something like

```
> setwd("C:/Users/My Name/Desktop/Projects/multivariate/data")
```

particular to your computer.

Changing the working directory will also be useful for reading data sets into **R** because a shorter address can be used. Specifically, commands such as `read.table()` or `scan()` will look for files in the current working directory. After we quit **R**, there will be an icon for the **R** program written into the working directory. Later, you can click on this icon from the directory and not have to change it again with a `setwd()` command. This process can be repeated, resulting in an **R** icon in each of the directories of each of your different projects. Each icon will open **R** in the corresponding directory. Finally, notice the address of the directory is delimited with a forward-leaning slash (/) and not the more commonly used backslash used in directory addresses.

As a final note on organizing your workspace, consider generous use of the `rm()` command to remove unused variables. A cluttered workspace will make it difficult to find important things at some future date, often with forgotten names.

A great feature of **R** is the huge amount of software written by other users. A list of the libraries used in this book is given in the Appendix. To take advantage of the many libraries available, you will need to install these packages on your computer. First you will need to learn the name of the specific package you want to install. (More on this, below.)

Let's say you want to install the `TeachingDemos` package which contains introductory tutorials in **R**. The **R** command to install packages is

```
install.packages("TeachingDemos")
```

This command will be followed by a prompt for you to select a mirror site[2] from which the packages are to be downloaded to your computer. After choosing a mirror site, you will be prompted for the name of the package. After a few seconds, you will receive a message when the package finishes loading. This command only needs to be done once for all of your working directories. The command `installed.packages()` provides a complete list of all packages installed, including many included as part of your original download of **R** to your computer.

To access the package in each working directory, interchangeably use either the `library` or `require` command, as in

```
library(TeachingDemos)
```

---

[2] There is some debate on how to choose a mirror site. There is a cloud option to pick a site for you. Picking a site geographically close to you will reduce web traffic. Conversely, a very distant site may offer faster service because most people on the other side of the earth are asleep.

or else as

```
require(TeachingDemos)
```

without the quote marks. Either of these is needed every time you begin a session in **R** to access the installed package.

After installing and loading the package, you can then type help(Teaching Demos) to learn more about the package and its contents.

How can you learn about the various packages and their contents? One approach is through **R** itself. The **R** help file frequently describes features available in packages not already installed on your computer. You will see help file entries with a notation of the form

faces{*TeachingDemos*}

indicating the name of the function and the package containing it.

A second way to learn about packages for **R** is on the web through your favorite search engine. There are a huge number of packages available, and the authors of these will frequently create websites publicizing their capabilities. There are packages written for specialized statistical methods as well as areas of application such as genetics, chemistry, psychology, or economics. Some packages complement a book, in which case the help may be minimal to encourage you to buy the book to learn more.

This completes an introduction to the important elements of **R**. Additional features will be introduced in subsequent chapters as needed. As with piano playing, the best way to learn **R** is not just by reading the book but by sitting at the keyboard, trying the exercises, and engaging in some creative experimentation.

2.9   Exercises

2.1 The seq command in **R** is similar to the colon : operator but allows for non-integer sequences. It takes three arguments: the starting value, the final value, and (optionally) the incremental value. Here are two examples of its use:

```
> seq(5, 9)

[1] 5 6 7 8 9

> seq(9.1, 8.3, -.1)

[1] 9.1 9.0 8.9 8.8 8.7 8.6 8.5 8.4 8.3
```

Use the seq and c functions to create a single vector of values from zero to one by 0.1 and then from 1 to 10 by 1. Be careful the value 1 is not included twice.

2.2 Write a program in **R** starting with a positive integer j and producing a vector of the form

$$1, \ 1, \ 2, \ 1, \ 2, \ 3, \ 1, \ 2, \ 3, \ 4, \ 1, \ 2, \ 3, \ 4, \ 5, \ \dots \,, 1, \ 2, \ \dots \,, j.$$

2.3 The mean absolute deviation of a set of values $x_1, x_2, \dots, x_n$ is the average absolute difference between the observations and their mean. Mathematically,

$$\text{mean absolute deviation}(x) = n^{-1} \sum_{i=1}^{n} |x_i - \bar{x}|$$

where $\bar{x}$ is the sample average of the x's. It is sometimes used instead of the standard deviation as a *robust* measure of the variability of the data values. Robust methods are insensitive to any extreme outliers present in the data.

a. Write a function in **R** to compute the mean absolute deviation of a vector of values. You may find the `mean()` and `abs()` functions useful in writing this program.
b. Discuss the pros and cons of using the median, as opposed to the mean $\bar{x}$ in this definition. Similarly, consider the median absolute deviation about the median value as a measure of variability in a sample.
c. One way we describe the robust properties of a statistical estimator is to introduce seemingly outlandish outliers into the data to see how these affect the final result. Perform an experiment comparing the change in the standard deviation with the mean absolute deviation for a sample of observations with increasingly distorted outliers. Which statistic is more robust?

2.4 If X behaves as a standard normal, then X^2 behaves as chi-squared with 1 df. The cumulative chi-squared distribution can be found in **R** using the function `pchisq(y,d)` where y is the ordinate and d is the degree of freedom. Use this function to find the probability of a 1 df chi-squared variate taking values between 0.5 and 1.2.

2.5 Look at the academic score data in Table 1.2. The various scores in this table have been standardized across countries to adjust for cultural differences.

a. Are the standard deviations of the different scores comparable? Consider using the `bartlett.test()` test for equality of variances. Other tests of equality of variances available in R are `var.test()`, `flinger.test()`, `ansari.test()`, and `mood.test()`. Use the `help()` file to read about these tests.
b. Examine the correlation matrix of these data using the the `cor` function. Describe what you see. See also Exercise 8.7.

2.6 Explore properties of the `simcor` program to simulate statistical significance of the correlation coefficient.

  a. What would happen if we allowed the `ncor` parameter to be negative? Remove the error check for this condition and explain how the new program behaves for `ncor` < 0.
  b. Generate a large sample (m) of correlation coefficients from pairs of normal variates for a specified sample size and zero correlation. Estimate the 95% confidence interval covering these, for a fixed size of the (normal) sample n. Do this by sorting the many simulated correlations and finding their 2.5- and 97.5-percentiles.
  c. Propose a more efficient method for estimating the 95% confidence interval of the correlation coefficient using the symmetry of the distribution.
  d. One of the most important questions asked of statisticians concerns the sample size (n) necessary to conduct a research project. Write a program with iterations and convergence criteria to achieve a small 95% confidence interval of the correlation coefficient. How fast does the size of this interval shrink as a function of the sample size n? Draw a graph of this relationship.
  e. Suppose the data is sampled from a population with a correlation coefficient of ρ. Use the `simcor` program to estimate the value of ρ needed so 80% of the sampled correlations are not included in the interval you found in part b. This sample size (n) will have 80% power to detect this value of ρ at statistical significance .05.

2.7 How useful is the histogram to detect normally distributed data?

  a. Use `runif(50)` to generate a set of 50 random values, distributed uniformly between zero and one. Draw the histogram of these using `hist()`. Do these look normally distributed?
  b. Generate 50 random values, each the sum of 3 uniforms, and plot the histogram. Do these look normally distributed? Suppose we looked at the histogram of the sum of 20 uniforms. How many uniform random values do we need to add together to produce a "normal-looking" histogram?
  c. As a comparison, look at a histogram of 50 normal random values generated using `rnorm()`. How normal does this histogram appear?

2.8 Consider the function
$$f(x) = \frac{1}{2 + \sin(5\pi x)}$$

for values of $0 \le x \le 1$.

  a. Plot the function f in **R**. (See Sect. 3.1 for an example of how to do this.)
  b. Find the area under this curve using numerical quadrature with `integrate()`.
  c. Identify maximums and minimums of this function in **R** using `nlm()`. Show how the results depend on the starting values.

2.9 Use `nlm` to find the minimum of the function:

$$f(x, y, z) = 100 - \sum_{i=1}^{5} \exp\{-5(x-i)^2\}/i + \exp\{-5(y-i)^2\}/i + \exp\{-5(z-i)^2\}/i.$$

The true minimum of f occurs at $x = y = z = 1$ but there are several other local minimums. Show by varying the starting values for `nlm`, we can converge on any of these other local minimums.

2.10 As you work in **R**, you will notice a variety of symbolic values in addition to numerical values. A list of these and tests for their values are given in Table 2.3.

a. What happens when we use `Inf` in arithmetical statements? For example,

```
> x <- Inf
> is.infinite(x)

[1] TRUE
```

will assign and test an infinite value. How does **R** define `-x`? What is the result when we multiply x by -1 or by zero? Can we test $-\text{Inf} < 0$?

b. How does **R** work with `NULL` in arithmetic? How does `NULL` differ from `NaN`? For example, suppose we assign

```
x <- c( 1, 2, NULL, 4)
```

What is the `length` of x? What is the `sum` of x?
Similarly, suppose we assign

```
y <- c(1, 2, NaN, 4) ?
```

What is the length and sum of y?

c. Give examples of arithmetic operations yielding `NaN` and `Inf`. How are these results different? Which are accompanied with an error message?

d. Build a table of the resulting symbols when two of these symbols are used in arithmetic operations. For example, what does the sum of `NA` and `NaN` yield? What is the product of zero and `NULL`?

Table 2.3 Non-numeric, symbolic values in **R**

Symbol	Description	**R** test
NULL	No value	`is.null()`
NA	Not available, missing	`is.na()`
NaN	Not a number	`is.nan()`
Inf	+Infinity	`is.infinite()`
-Inf	−Infinity	`is.infinite()`

2.11 a. Can we access the values of `sortx` outside the `spacing` function given in Sect. 2.5? Explain.

b. Write a one line `function` in **R** to calculate the spacings of any set of numbers using the `diff()` function. The `diff(x)` function calculates the difference of adjacent observations in a vector `x`.

2.12 What does **R** do when we try to access subscripts out of range? Suppose we start with

```
>  x <- 1:3
```

a. A negative subscript such as `x[-2]` will omit the second element of the vector. What does `x[-5]` yield in this example?

b. What does `x[0]` give us? Can you explain this outcome?

c. Suppose we try to assign a value to an invalid element of the vector, such as in x[7] < −9. What does this produce?

d. Is an empty subscript `x[]` different from x with no subscript at all? As an example, how is x[] < −3 different from x < −3?

Chapter 3
Graphical Displays

You can observe a lot by just watching.

Yogi Berra

T HERE ARE MANY GRAPHICAL METHODS to be demonstrated
with little or no explanation. You are likely familiar with histograms and
scatterplots. Many options in **R** have improved on these in interesting and
useful ways. The ability to produce statistical graphics is a clear strength of **R**.
Graphics commands can produce files of a variety of file formats. All of the figures
in this book were produced in this manner, for example. We begin with a discussion
of the basics. Later sections of this chapter demonstrate a variety of more complex
procedures available to us.

3.1 Graphics in **R**

The plot function is a general-purpose routine with many options. The basic form
is plot(x,y) which produces a scatterplot of the values in x and y. The plot
function sets the frame and limits of the axes for you. There are many options
including printing titles along the axes and changing colors to be illustrated in this
chapter.

Let us illustrate the use of the plot function in drawing the densities of the
chi-squared distribution. A very basic figure can be drawn using

```
x <- (0 : 120) / 10
plot (x, dchisq(x, 4), type = "l")
lines(x, dchisq(x, 5))
lines(x, dchisq(x, 6))
lines(x, dchisq(x, 7))
lines(x, dchisq(x, 8))
```

© Springer Nature Switzerland AG 2022
D. Zelterman, *Applied Multivariate Statistics with R*, Statistics for Biology and Health,
https://doi.org/10.1007/978-3-031-13005-2_3

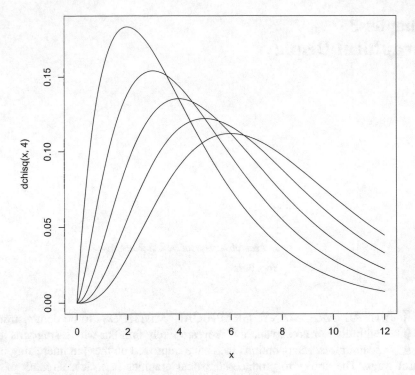

Figure 3.1 Basic chi-squared density plots

which produces Fig. 3.1 in a graphics window.

The **R** code begins by creating 121 evenly spaced values for x of 0, .1, .2, ..., 12. The dchisq(x,4) evaluates the chi-squared density function with 4 df at each value of x. The plot statement opens the graphics window and sets the limits of the horizontal and vertical axes. The type="l" option specifies lines that will be used to connect adjacent points. Omitting this option would produce a series of disconnected dots. The labels of the plot axes are copied from those of the plot statement. We will show how to replace these with more useful labels in the next example. (As a helpful hint introduced in Sect. 2.5, whenever we have several lines of code to enter into **R**, it is best to write these out in a word processor first and then copy them into the **R** command window.)

The lines command is like the plot except it produces lines between observations and plots these on top of the existing plot. These do not adjust for values running outside the bounds set earlier by the plot command. It is best to plan ahead and use the plot command first with the widest and tallest of values your figure is going to contain. It is possible to specify these limits manually, as we will see in the following section.

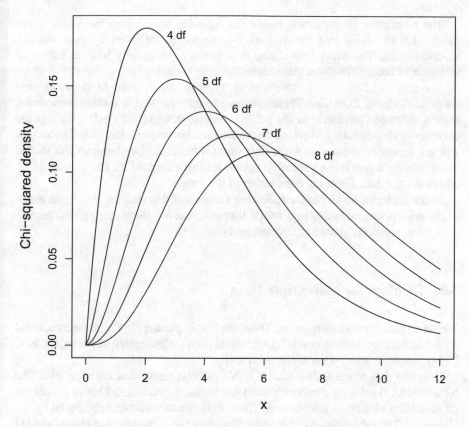

Figure 3.2 Chi-squared density functions for 4–8 df

We can spruce up this figure and make it more presentable for publication. Figure 3.2 adds labels and prints a useful y−axis. This figure was produced using the code

```
pdf(file = "chisquared2.pdf")
x <- (0 : 120) / 10
plot(x, dchisq(x, 4), type = "l",
    ylab = "Chi-squared density")
lines(x, dchisq(x, 5))
lines(x, dchisq(x, 6))
lines(x, dchisq(x, 7))
lines(x, dchisq(x, 8))

text( c(3, 4.2, 5.2, 6.2, 8), c(.18, .153, .137, .123, .11),
    labels = c("4 df", "5 df", "6 df", "7 df", "8 df"))
dev.off()
```

The placement of the labels inside the figure is done using the text statement. This statement lists the desired x-coordinates followed by those for the y-coordinates. The exact positioning is not tricky but usually takes a little trial and error in order to position these correctly.

The pdf(file= ...) statement is optional and is used to direct graphic images to external PDF files. These can later be incorporated into other documents. Unless addressed otherwise in the pdf() statement, these files will appear in the current working directory. Working directories are described in Sect. 2.8. The images will not appear on the screen while the output is directed elsewhere, so you should make sure the figure is correct before saving it to an external file. The dev.off() closes the graphics file at the completion of the image.

Other examples appear in the following sections of this chapter. We demonstrate additional options including how to add text and manipulate other graphical parameters such as colors, plotted characters, and size.

3.2 Displays for Univariate Data

We are all familiar with histograms. These are the simple display for one-dimensional data. The basic command in **R** is hist(x) to obtain a histogram of the values in x. Let us introduce some other methods as well.

Consider data on the CD4 counts in HIV+ patients enrolled in a clinical trial. The beneficial CD4 cells are a critical part of our immune system, and lower counts are an indication of disease progression. These cells are attacked and destroyed by the HIV virus. The cd4 data set in the boot library presents the baseline counts of CD4 cells of patients at the time of enrollment in the clinical trial and again after one year of treatment. The CD4 values are given in 100's. The critical value of 200 (or lower) is an AIDS-defining event.

A useful univariate display for small amounts of data is the *stem and leaf plot*. The stem and leaf plot is a useful improvement over the usual histogram because the data values are used as plotting characters, rather than the same character for every observation as used in the histogram.

As an example, the baseline CD4 counts are obtained

```
> require(boot)

Loading required package: boot

> cd4

    baseline oneyear
  1     2.12    2.47
  2     4.35    4.61
        .    .    .
 19     2.66    4.37
 20     3.00    2.40
```

Output 3.1 Back-to-back stem and leaf plots

```
> library(aplpack)
> stem.leaf.backback ( cd4$baseline, cd4$oneyear )
```

```
          1 | 2: represents 1.2, leaf unit: 0.1
            cd4$baseline          cd4$oneyear

                     |  1* |
            1      8| 1.  |
            3     41| 2*  |44             2
            7   9655| 2.  |58             4
           (6) 333300| 3*  |022            7
            7     75| 3.  |89             9
            5   3110| 4*  |0233          (4)
                     | 4.  |678            7
            1      1| 5*  |2              4
                     | 5.  |59             3
                     | 6*  |3              1
                     | 6.  |
                     | 7*  |

    n:           20            20
```

The corresponding stem and leaf plot is

```
> stem(cd4$baseline)

  The decimal point is at the |

  1 | 9
  2 | 15567
  3 | 000444468
  4 | 0123
  5 | 1
```

The stem and leaf display the actual data values, and we can recover the original data from the histogram. The vertical line | serves as the decimal point so we can read the data values directly from this plot as 1.9, 2.1, 2.5, 2.5, and so on. The originators of this display method saw the vertical line as the stem of a plant and the numbers to the right as leaves, hence the name.

There is also a back-to-back stem and leaf display in the aplpack library allowing us to compare two sets of data values. An example appears in Output 3.1. The frequency of the median category is identified in parenthesis. In this display, we can see the population of one-year CD4 values is larger and more variable than the baseline values.

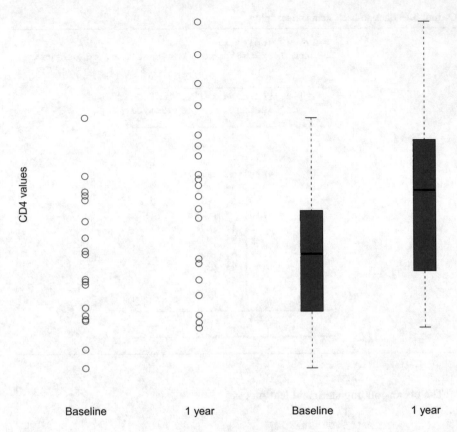

Figure 3.3 Univariate scatter plots and boxplots of CD4 counts

The stem and leaf use the actual data values to display the data. This may not be a useful method if the data set is very large. At the other extreme from the stem and leaf plot is the *boxplot* which reduces the histogram to a few summary statistics and then plots these.

The boxplots of the CD4 counts are given in Fig. 3.3. The dark central horizontal line is the location of the median, and the box identifies the quartiles. (The quartiles are located 25% in from both ends of the observed values.) The *whiskers* extend out from the central box. Sometimes extreme outliers are also identified by the boxplot. The pair of boxplots in Fig. 3.3 is easier to compare than the raw data values also given in this figure. Unlike a stem and leaf plot of the raw data, the boxplot does not become overwhelming when the sample size is large.

The **R** code to draw Fig. 3.3 is

```
library(boot)
data(cd4)
n <- length(cd4$baseline)                    # sample size
pdf(file = "boxplot.pdf")
op <- par(mfrow = c(1, 4), cex.lab = 1.5) # four plots, large labels
plot(rep(.5, n), cd4$baseline, axes = FALSE, xlab = "Baseline",
       xlim = c(0, 1), ylim = range(cd4), col = "red",
       ylab = "CD4 values", cex.lab = 1.5, cex = 2)
plot(rep(.5, n), cd4$oneyear, axes = FALSE, xlab = "1 year",
       xlim = c(0, 1), ylim = range(cd4), col = "red",
       yaxt = "n", ylab = "", cex.lab = 1.5, cex = 2)
text(c(0, 1), c(0, 0),
        c(boxplot(cd4$baseline, xlab = "Baseline", col = "red",
             ylim = range(cd4),axes = FALSE),
          boxplot(cd4$oneyear, xlab = "1 year", col = "red",
             ylim = range(cd4), axes = FALSE)))
par(op)
dev.off()
```

The par() statement specifies there will be four figures, side-by-side, in the
graphics window and increases the font size of the labels in the margins. The
par(op) statement resets this back to one figure in the window. Parameters with
cex = and cex.lab = specify character expansions to increase font sizes. There
are more sophisticated versions on the boxplot called *violin plots*. These are described
in Exercise 3.4.

Let us return to the histogram as the display tool. The **R** code

```
library(boot)                 # the data is in this library
op <- par(mfrow = c(1, 2))    # side by side plots on one
                                     page
hist(cd4$baseline, main = "", xlab = "At baseline")
hist(cd4$oneyear, main = "", xlab = "At 1 year")
par(op)                       # reset graphical parameters
```

produces the side-by-side histograms in Fig. 3.4.

The hist() statements produce the separate histograms with titles along the
$x-$axes. A direct comparison of these two graphs in Fig. 3.4 is difficult. We cannot
easily tell, for example, if the one-year CD4 values are generally larger or smaller
than those at baseline. It is not clear which of these two sets of values has a wider
range. This figure would be adequate if we were only interested in the number of
values below the 200 thresholds after one year.

We need to look at these two groups in a manner allowing a quick comparison. The
plot(x, y) command plots a scatterplot of $x - y$ values. We can plot the baseline
and one-year values and then we can see a correlation between the two values of
each subject.

That is, the **R** command

```
plot(cd4$baseline, cd4$oneyear, xlab = "Baseline", ylab = "At 1 year")
```

produces the plot appearing in Fig. 3.5.

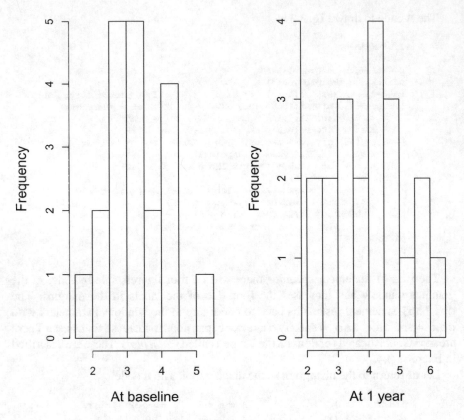

Figure 3.4 Histograms of CD4 counts, values in 100's

This figure demonstrates baseline and one-year values are positively correlated within individuals but still do not allow a direct before-and-after comparison.

In order to compare the values, we need other graphical methods. These appear in Fig. 3.6. The membership variable `group` is discrete and a plot of this along the *x*−axis results in two vertical stripes in the left-most plot in Fig. 3.6.

It is sometimes better to add a small amount of random noise to scatter these values just enough to see the underlying distribution. These *jittered* values are plotted in the center of the three plots. A number of observations will often occlude others in a plot such as this, even with a modest sample size. The `jitter(group)` command takes the group values and adds a small amount of random noise.

The program producing Fig. 3.6 is given in Output 3.2. In Fig. 3.6, we can see the one-year values are more variable than the baseline values. This comparison is easier to make with the jittered grouping values.

The *spaghetti plot* links every individual's paired values. From the spaghetti plot, we can see if subjects with high baseline values are associated with high one-year values. A few individuals' values decrease, but clearly there is an overall trend of increasing values among the scattered lines.

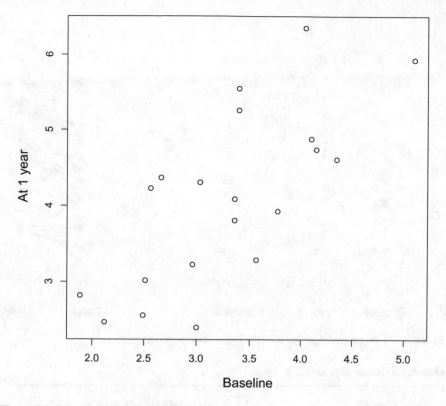

Figure 3.5 Basic scatterplot of CD4 counts

3.3 Displays for Bivariate Data

Let's have a look at the well-known scatterplot. Consider the data given in Table 1.1 for the values of apartment rents and house prices for each state. The values are contained in a data.frame called housing in **R** so we have

```
> housing

     Apartment House
AK         949 237.8
AL         631 121.5
AR         606 105.7

       .    .    .


WI         704 173.3
WV         528  95.9
WY         636 188.2
```

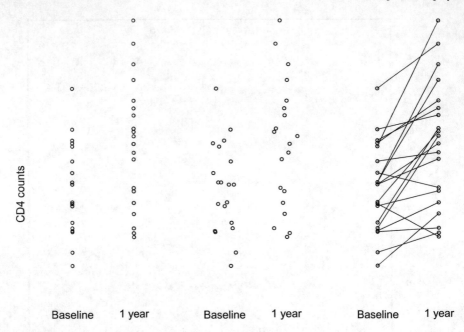

Figure 3.6 CD4 counts by group, with jittering, and as spaghetti

Output 3.2 **R** code to produce Fig. 3.6

```
library(boot)                           # contains the cd4 dataset
n <- length(cd4$baseline)               # sample size
join <- c(cd4$baseline,cd4$oneyear)     # concatenate all CD4 values
group <- rep(c(0, 1), each = n)         # assign group membership
par(mfrow = c(1, 3))                    # three side by side plots on one page
plot(group, join,                       # 1st plot with simple X axis
   ylab = "CD4 counts", xlab = "", axes = FALSE,
   ylim = c(0, max(join)), xlim = c(-.25,1.25))
text(c(0,1), c(1,1), labels = c("Baseline", "1 year"))

plot(jitter(group), join,               # 2nd plot with jittered X-axis
   ylab = "", xlab = "", axes = FALSE,
   ylim = c(0, max(join)), xlim = c(-.25, 1.25))
text(c(0,1), c(1,1), labels = c("Baseline", "1 year"))

plot(group, join,                       # 3rd plot: spaghetti
   ylab = "", xlab = "", axes = FALSE,
   ylim = c(0, max(join)), xlim = c(-.25, 1.25))
text(c(0,1), c(1,1), labels = c("Baseline", "1 year"))
for (i in 1:n)                          # draw individual connecting lines
   lines(c(0,1), c(cd4$baseline[i], cd4$oneyear[i]))
```

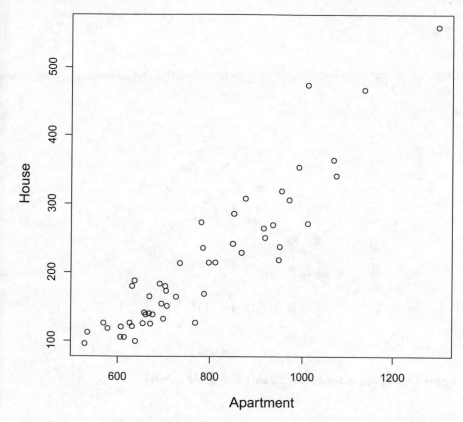

Figure 3.7 Basic scatterplot of housing data

A simple command

```
> plot(housing)
```

produces the scatterplot in a familiar format, given in Fig. 3.7.

The figure contains labels for the two axes because they are defined as column names in the `data.frame`. This figure conveys the basic information: The prices of houses are correlated with apartment rents and the values are skewed toward the high ends of both. Let's try to improve upon this basic figure.

Any serious discussion of statistical graphics would be amiss if it failed to mention the series of books by E Tufte. Tufte (2001) recommends eliminating the *chart junk* or non-essential graphical items in order to draw our attention to the patterns in the data.

Specifically, in Fig. 3.7, the box containing the figure is purely decorative. Further, the numbers and tick marks along the two axes convey only a small amount of information about the range of values.

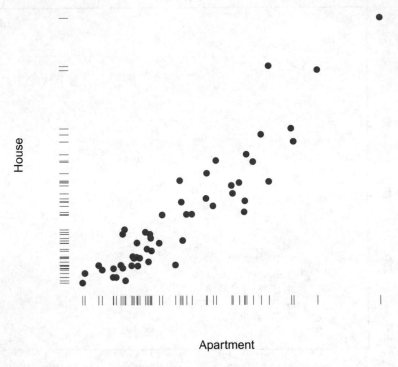

Figure 3.8 Plot with minimal chart junk and a high data to ink ratio

Tufte (2001) would urge us to maximize the *data to ink ratio*. The point of drawing a scatterplot is to examine the bivariate relationship between the variables of interest, in this case housing prices and apartment rents. A greater amount of "ink" should be dedicated to presenting the data instead of framing the picture with decorative axes. This brings us to the plot in Fig. 3.8 with no numbers in the axes, bold symbols emphasizing the data, and "rug fringes" displaying the two marginal distributions.

Figure 3.8 was produced using

```
require(graphics)                           # library for rug program
attach(housing)
boundA <- range(Apartment) * c(.95, 1)      # find bounds for plot area
boundH <- range(House) * c(.8, 1)

plot(housing, xlim = boundA, ylim = boundH, # Plot data with bounds
    axes = FALSE,                           # Omit the usual axes
    cex = 1.5, pch = 16,                    # Plot large solid circles
    col = "red")                            # Select color of points
rug(Apartment, side = 1, col = ''blue'')    # Add rug fringes
rug(House, side = 2, col = ''blue'')
```

where `rug` adds "fringes" corresponding to a univariate scatterplot of the marginal distributions. Tufte (2001) refers to the style of Fig. 3.8 as a *dot-dash-plot*. One problem with the graph in Fig. 3.8 is our eyes can get distracted and wander away from the figure because it lacks a bounding box to frame the figure and focus our attention.

3.3.1 Plot Options, Colors, and Characters

Let us describe some of the many options available when using the `plot` function in **R**.

The bounds of the original `plot()` statement, above, are modified to move the rug fringes a little away from the bivariate data points. This is done using the `xlim=` and `ylim=` options. This last example illustrates the use of the `cex=` option to magnify or shrink the size of the plotted characters. The `axes=FALSE` suppresses the usual axes and their numerical values.

The `plot` statement in this last example uses the `pch=` option to choose the plotting character. The most commonly used `pch=` options are

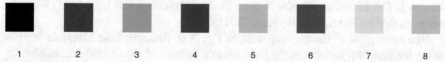

Colors may also be used using the `col=` option. The colors can be addressed by name or by number. Eight colors can be addressed by number:

A complete spectrum of colors is available. See the `help` file on `rainbow` and `palette`. There are also a large number of named colors including such inventive names as `seashell2`, `peachpuff3`, and `papayawhip`. See `color()` for the complete list.

The `rainbow(n)[i]` function divides the visible spectrum into n shades and `[i]` picks the i-th of these.

As an example of the `rainbow` function, the **R** code

```
plot( c(0,1), c(0,1), type="n", xlab=" ", ylab=" ", axes=
   FALSE)
n <- 125
for (i in 1:n)
   {
      lines(rep(i/(n+1), 2),  c(0,1), lwd=4,
        col=rainbow(n)[i])
   }
```

produces Fig. 3.9.

The sizes of plotted objects can be changed. The `cex=2` option, for example, will double the size of plotted characters. Similarly, `cex=.5` will shrink characters by half. The `cex.lab=` option is used to change the size of the font used on the axes.

Figure 3.9 An example of
the rainbow() function

3.3.2 *More Graphics for Bivariate Data*

In contrast to Fig. 3.8, let us consider a scatterplot with a lot of processing and detail
attached. The *bivariate boxplot* is described by Goldberg and Iglewicz (1992) and
programmed by Everitt and Hothorn (2011).

The scatterplot of the housing data in Fig. 3.10 illustrates the bivariate boxplot
using the program bvbox in the MVA library. Instead of the central box containing
50% of the univariate data as in a univariate boxplot of Fig 3.3, the bivariate boxplot
includes a pair of estimated ellipses, the inner one containing approximately 50%
of the data and the outer one containing about 95%. For ease of interpretation, we
have added text to the figure allowing us to identify the three outliers: California,
Hawaii, and Washington DC.

The **R** code to produce Fig 3.10 is

```
library(MVA)                              # library for bvbox
extreme <- c( "DC", "HI", "CA")           # Three extreme states
exst <- match(extreme, rownames(housing)) # identify index in data

bvbox(housing, xlab = "Apartment", ylab = "House",
   pch = 19, cex = 1.25, col = "red")
text(housing$Apartment[exst], housing$House[exst],
   labels = extreme, cex = .8,             # label names, small font
   pos = c(2,2,3))                         # position labels: L,L, top
```

See Exercise 3.6 on modifying the graphical options in the bvplot routine.

The match() statement is discussed in Sect. 2.1.2 and is used to identify the
subscript (index or observation number) associated with each of the named three

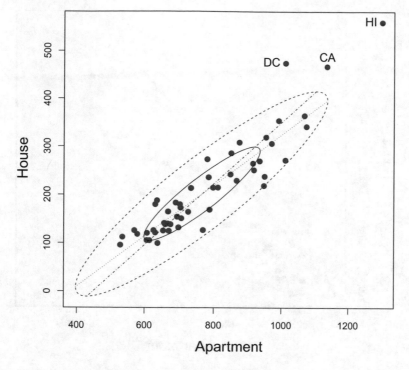

Figure 3.10 Bivariate boxplot of housing data

extreme states. In this example, `match()` is used to identify the index of each of the three names of extreme values among the `rownames` of the `data.frame`.

The two lines inside the ellipses of Fig. 3.10 are estimates of the regression line. The darker line is the usual least squares line using all of the observations. The lighter line is a more robust estimate reducing the influence of any extreme outlying data values. See Chap. 9 for a full discussion of linear regression. See also Exercise 14.1 for an examination of the most extreme values in these data and whether these can be considered as outliers.

Let us end this section on two-dimensional plots with a discussion of the *convex hull*. The convex hull is a lot like wrapping an irregularly shaped object with the smallest amount of gift paper: The most extreme points in any direction will define the ultimate shape of the package. Mathematically, the convex hull is the smallest convex polygon containing all of the data. In **R**, the `chull` function returns the indices of the data points most extreme in each direction:

```
> chull(housing)

[1] 34 10 44 26 50 29  8 12
```

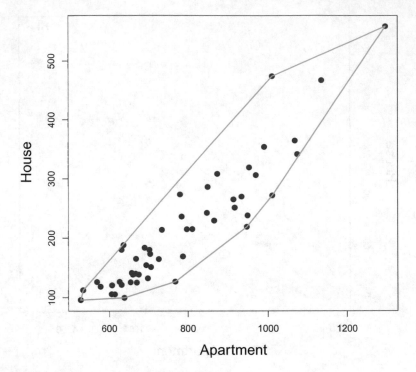

Figure 3.11 Convex hull of the housing data

We can redraw the housing data from Fig. 3.7 and identify those points on the convex hull. The program

```
ch <- chull(housing)          # find the indices of the convex hull
ch <- c(ch,ch[1])             # loop back to the beginning
plot(housing, pch = 19, col = 2,
    cex = 1.25)               # plot the original data
lines(housing$Apartment[ch], housing$House[ch],
    type = "l", col = 3, lwd = 2) # bold, green lines
```

draws Fig. 3.11.

The `lines` command adds lines to the figure with the `type="l"` option. The lines also need to return back to the beginning, so the list of indices `ch` from the convex hull program `chull` must repeat the first observation at the end of this list in order to complete the polygon. In this example, the `lwd=` option in `lines` controls the width of the lines.

The convex hull in Fig. 3.11 identifies the extremes in the data. Some might argue not all of these observations should be considered outliers. If there are outliers, the convex hull will pick some of these out. If there are several outliers, as identified in Fig. 3.10, then they might hide behind the largest of these. California is an outlier but

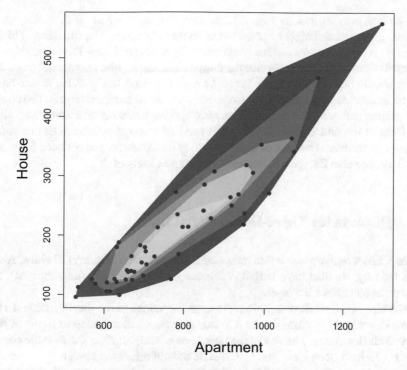

Figure 3.12 Five peeling convex hulls and color-fill for the housing data

is dwarfed by the larger outlier of Hawaii. Such a problem is called *masking*, where one extreme outlier obscures others in the data.

Suppose we omitted the observations on the convex hull and looked at what remains. This would remove the most extreme values to reveal those less extreme. We might then draw the convex hull of those remaining observations. It is also useful to repeat this process several times. The net effect is much like peeling an onion, successively removing the outermost layers, one at a time. This repeated process will give a better idea about the underlying shape of the data.

The program lines

```
library(aplpack)
nlev <- 5                  # Number of levels
colors <- heat.colors(9)[3:(nlev+2)]
plothulls(housing, n.hull = nlev, col.hull = colors,
    xlab = "Apartment", ylab = "House",
    lty.hull = 1:nlev, density = NA, col = 0, main = " ")
points(housing, pch = 16, cex = 1, col = "blue")
```

draw and then peel away five successive convex hulls to produce Fig. 3.12. Each successive layer is plotted in a different color by `plothulls`.

The best way to look at Fig. 3.12 is as a five-layer wedding cake. Layers on the inside are stacked higher and on top of those further out. The smaller and higher cake layers represent areas with a greater density of observations. The baker might be accused of being sloppy, but notice the convex hull has no bias about what these data layers should look like. Compare Fig. 3.12 with Fig. 3.10. In Fig. 3.10, we see layers are perfect and parallel ellipses, regardless of what the data might suggest. The convex hull peeling in Fig. 3.12 is the nonparametric approach making no assumptions about the form of the underlying data. We can see these nested convex hulls are almost ellipses, so the best summary of these data may lie somewhere in between Figs. 3.10 and 3.12. See also Exercise 3.7 on drawing convex hulls of data.

3.4   Displays for Three-Dimensional Data

Table 3.1 lists January maximum temperature data in each of many US cities. Along with the city, we also have latitude (degrees north), longitude (degrees east), and altitude in feet above sea level.

The size of the circle or bubble represents the values of the third variable. In this example, we plot US cities on the XY-axis as a conventional map in terms of their latitude and longitude. The size of the bubble represents altitude. Cities at the corners of Fig 3.13 have been identified by the state to help orient the reader.

The bubble sizes show cities on the east and west coasts are all at sea level. Midwest cities are situated at slightly higher altitudes. The highest altitude cities are in the Rocky Mountains in the west. The program producing this figure is given in Output 3.3.

Longitude is measured as the distance from Greenwich, England, and needs to be reversed in order to have this map display east and west in their familiar right/left orientation. Puerto Rico and the three states Alaska, Hawaii, and Massachusetts are identified to help the reader.

The with() and text() commands are used to add symbols and labels to this plot. The symbols command sets the size of the circles proportional to the altitude. Options in the symbols command include inches= to scale the sizes of the circles, fg= to set the color, and lwd= to create thick or thin lines.

Another useful display for three dimensions is based on *kriging*. Kriging is named after Daniel Krige[1] who was examining the grades of gold taken from several small exploratory mine shafts. He developed kriging, a smooth mathematical function summarizing the underlying concentration of gold. He used this method for interpolating between the data values observed in the mines. We can perform the same process to model the altitude data examined in Fig. 3.13.

Figure 3.14 should look familiar to us as a weather map. Small local deviations are smoothed out, and a simplified version of reality is presented. The map clearly identifies sea-level cities on the coasts and the high-altitude cities in the Rocky

---

[1] Daniel Gerhardus Krige, (1919–2013). South African mining engineer.

Table 3.1 Maximum January temperature (T, in degrees Fahrenheit), latitude, longitude, and altitude in feet above sea level, for some of the largest U.S. cities

T	Lat	Long	Alt	Name	T	Lat	Long	Alt	Name
61	30	88	5	Mobile AL	59	32	86	160	Montgomery AL
30	58	134	50	Juneau AK	64	33	112	1,090	Phoenix AZ
51	34	92	286	Little Rock AR	65	34	118	340	Los Angeles CA
55	37	122	65	San Francisco	42	39	104	5,280	Denver CO
37	41	72	40	New Haven CT	41	39	75	135	Wilmington DE
44	38	77	25	Washington DC	67	30	81	20	Jacksonville FL
74	24	81	5	Key West FL	76	25	80	10	Miami FL
52	33	84	1,050	Atlanta GA	79	21	157	21	Honolulu HI
36	43	116	2,704	Boise ID	33	41	87	595	Chicago IL
37	39	86	710	Indianapolis IN	29	41	93	805	Des Moines IA
27	42	90	620	Dubuque IA	42	37	97	1,290	Wichita KS
44	38	85	450	Louisville KY	64	29	90	5	New Orleans LA
32	43	70	25	Portland ME	44	39	76	20	Baltimore MD
37	42	71	21	Boston MA	33	42	83	585	Detroit MI
23	46	84	650	Sault Ste Marie	22	44	93	815	Minneapolis MN
40	38	90	455	St Louis MO	29	46	112	4,155	Helena MT
32	41	95	1,040	Omaha NE	32	43	71	290	Concord NH
43	39	74	10	Atlantic City NJ	46	35	106	4,945	Albuquerque NM
31	42	73	20	Albany NY	40	40	73	55	New York NY
51	35	80	720	Charlotte NC	52	35	78	365	Raleigh NC
20	46	100	1,674	Bismark ND	41	39	84	550	Cincinnati OH
35	41	81	660	Cleveland OH	46	35	97	1,195	Oklahoma City

(continued)

Table 3.1 (continued)

T	Lat	Long	Alt	Name	T	Lat	Long	Alt	Name
44	45	122	77	Portland OR	39	40	76	365	Harrisburg PA
40	39	75	100	Philadelphia PA	61	32	79	9	Charleston SC
34	44	103	3,230	Rapid City SD	49	36	86	450	Nashville TN
50	35	101	3,685	Amarillo TX	61	29	94	5	Galveston TX
37	40	111	4,390	Salt Lake City	25	44	73	110	Burlington VT
50	36	76	10	Norfolk VA	44	47	122	10	Seattle WA
31	47	117	1,890	Spokane WA	26	43	89	860	Madison WI
28	43	87	635	Milwaukee WI	37	41	104	6,100	Cheyenne WY
81	18	66	35	San Juan PR					

Source Mosteller and Tukey (1977, pp. 73–4), with corrections.

Output 3.3 Program to create the bubbleplot in Fig. 3.13

```
JanTemp <- read.table(file="JanTemp.txt", header=TRUE)
require(MASS)
attach(JanTemp)
longe <- 180 - long                              # Reverse East and West

plot(longe,lat, pch = 16,   cex = .7,            # Plot dots at cities
    xlab="Longitude, east", ylab = "Latitude", col = "red")
with(JanTemp,symbols(longe,lat,circles = alt, # Altitude sized circles
    inches = .3,  add = TRUE,  lwd = 3,  fg = "green"))
    landmarks <- c( "AK", "HI", "MA", "PR")      # Four landmark states
    lmi <- match(landmarks, state) # identify landmark's indexes in data
    text(longe[lmi],lat[lmi],labels = landmarks,  # Identify landmarks
      pos=c(1,1,4,3), col = "blue")
```

Mountains. In this case, the altitude values have been approximated and smoothed. The program to generate this figure appears in Output 3.4.

The surf.ls(4,...) program approximates the altitude values as a fourth-degree polynomial in both latitude and longitude. You can try other values: lower polynomial degrees are smoother but may be unrealistic, while large values result in rough plots. The actual fitting uses least squares regression to estimate the altitude values. Least squares and other regression methods are described in Chap. 9.

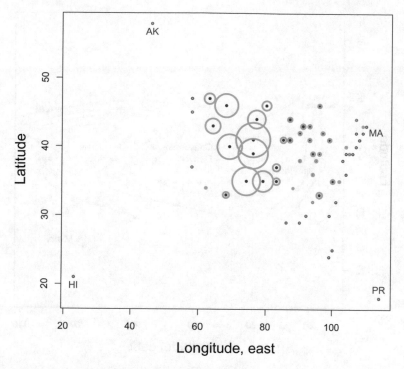

Figure 3.13 Bubble plot of altitudes of US cities

Output 3.4 Program to produce the krig plot in Fig. 3.14

```
library(MASS)
library(spatial)
attach(JanTemp)
longe <- 180 - long                 # Longitude, east
alt.kr <- surf.ls(4, longe, lat, alt) # Kriging surface
altsur <- trmat(alt.kr, 55, 110,
       28, 50, 50)          # Set limits of plot, excluding outliers
eqscplot(altsur, xlab = "Longitude, east", cex.lab = 1.5,
    ylab = "Latitude",type = "n")    # plot in equal scale   coordinates
contour(altsur, levels = c(0, 1000, 2000, 4000),
    add = TRUE, col = "blue") # specify contour colors and levels
points(longe, lat, pch = 16, col = "red") # add original cities
ex <- c("Miami", "Seattle", "SanFrancisco",
    "Denver", "Cheyenne")            # List of special cities
exi <- match(ex, name)               # index for these cities
text(longe[exi], lat[exi], labels = ex, # label special cities
    pos = c(4, 3, 4, 4, 4), cex = 1)
```

The eqscplot() program creates a plotting area in which the *x*- and *y*-axis are presented on the same scale. You may have noticed the scatterplot US map in Fig. 3.13 (plotted using the plot function) appears narrow and tall. The use of

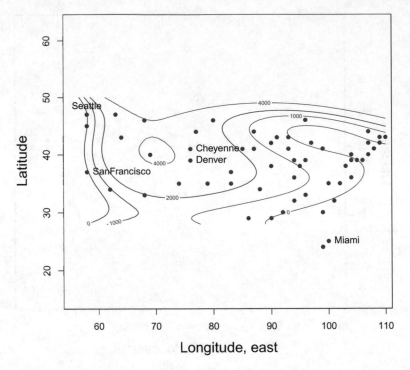

Figure 3.14 Kriging plot of altitudes of US cities

`eqscplot` function in this present program sets up and labels the axes, but does no actual plotting because of the `type="n"` option. The remainder of this program plots all of the cities, except the extremes: Juneau, San Juan, and Honolulu. Finally, the program identifies specified individual cities with printed labels using the `text` statement.

3.5 Displays for Higher Dimensional Data

How can we generalize the display of multivariate data with several dimensions? This area is ripe for creative development. Here are a few helpful methods available in **R**.

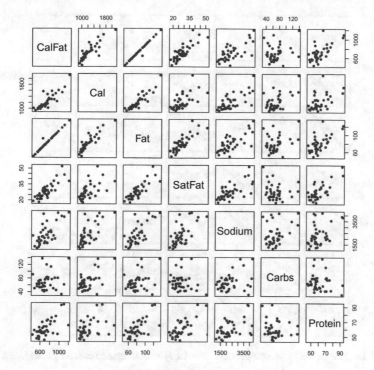

Figure 3.15 Basic matrix scatterplot of hamburger data

3.5.1 Pairs, Bagplot, Coplot, and Corrplot

One straightforward approach is to consider these two at a time and draw all possible bivariate scatterplots. Then we can do it all again, this time, with the axes reversed. An example appears in Fig. 3.15.

The pairs() command in **R** produces a matrix of scatterplots. As an example, the matrix scatterplot of the burger data in Table 1.6 is presented in Fig. 3.15. The names of the variables (calories, fat, sodium, and carbohydrates) run down the diagonal. Every possible pair of these variables is plotted twice with the axes reversed above and below the diagonal.

In this figure, we see carbohydrates and sodium each exhibit a few extreme outliers. Fat and calories from fat are linearly related, but one value seems to be calculated incorrectly. Calories are closely related to fat. Carbohydrates and sodium appear unrelated. This figure was produced using

```
pairs(burger, pch = 16, col = "red")
```

We can improve on this basic pairs() plot and use some additional options, adding color, different plotting characters, and a smoothed regression line called

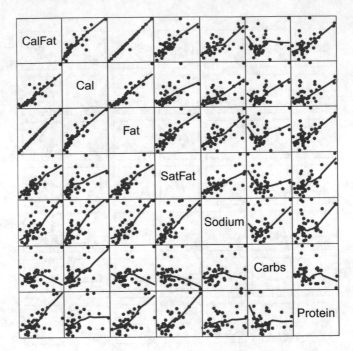

Figure 3.16 Scatterplot of hamburger data with loess smoothing and cleaner presentation

loess. The loess line is a compromise between smoothness and small deviations away from the observed data.

The program to produce Fig. 3.16 is given by

```
pairs(burger, lwd = 3, pch = 16, cex = 1.25, col = "red",
      gap = 0, xaxt = "n", yaxt = "n",
      panel = panel.smooth, col.smooth = "blue")
```

The loess lines help us see non-linear relationships between carbohydrates and each of the other variables in the upper half of this figure. A number of other options produce a cleaner presentation: `gap=0` removes the spacing between the panels, `xaxt = "n"`, `yaxt = "n"` removes the numbers in the axes, and contrasting colors separate the data from the fitted model.

The *bagplot.pairs* routine combines several features we have covered: the bivariate boxplot, the convex hull, and the pairs scatterplot. The bagplot contains a scatterplot of bivariate data. The outer polygon of each bagplot is a convex hull, excluding extreme outliers. The inner polygon (the "bag") of the bagplot contains the central 50% of the data. Data points between the two convex hulls are connected with lines to the central, bivariate median. Figure 3.17 was produced using

```
library(aplpack)
bagplot.pairs(burger[ , 4 : 7], gap = 0, col.baghull = "green")
```

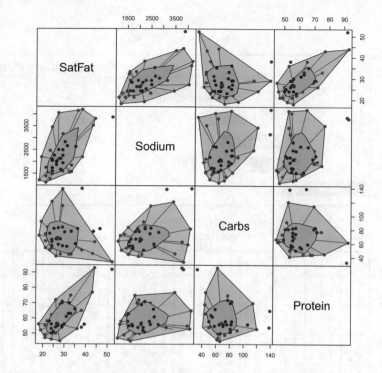

Figure 3.17 Bagplot pairs of hamburger data

The pairwise approach to examining multivariate data reduces the problem back to two dimensions and looks at it as a series of pairs of scatterplots. This simplification overlooks the multivariate character of the data. After all, if there are complex relationships, we need a way to display these simultaneously.

One improvement on the pairwise scatterplot matrix is to look at a series of scatterplots, each representing a view of a slice of a third variable. Chambers (1992) calls this a conditioning plot or *coplot*. In the hamburger data, for example, Fig. 3.15 shows calories and sodium do not have a strong relationship. There is also an outlier with very high values of both sodium and calories. Suppose we want to examine the relationship between calories and sodium across different values of the variable measuring fat content.

The coplot function in the **R** code

```
library(graphics)
coplot(Cal ~ Sodium | Fat,  data=burger,
    rows=1, pch=16, cex=1.75, col="red",
    bar.bg = c(num = "blue", fac = gray(0.95) ))
```

produces Fig. 3.18.

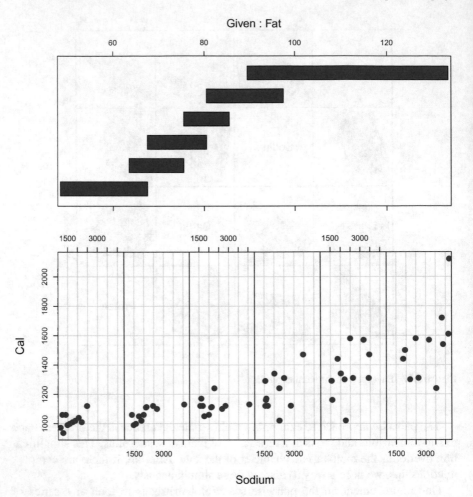

Figure 3.18 Burger coplot of calories and sodium, stratified by fat

The program code Cal ~ Sodium | Fat specifies calories and sodium will be plotted against each other for stratified values of fat. In particular, the top of Fig. 3.18 shows how the coplot program cuts the range of fat values into a series of six overlapping intervals. For each of these intervals of the fat variable, there is a scatterplot of calories plotted against sodium at the bottom half of this figure.

As we look at the scatterplots on the bottom half, from left to right, we see a changing relationship between calories and sodium. For the lowest values of fat, both calories and sodium are small. Larger values of fat are associated with larger values of both calories and sodium. The large outlier between sodium and calories only appears within the highest range of fat. At no value of fat does there appear to be a strong relationship between calories and sodium.

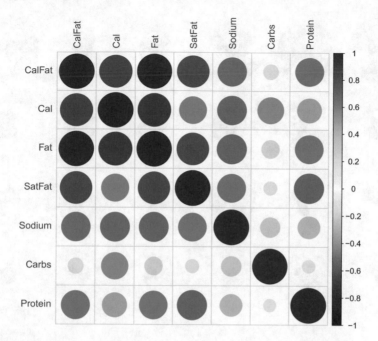

Figure 3.19 The `corrplot` of the hamburger data

If we need to address scalability, the methods in this subsection will lose their usefulness if there are too many observations to be contained in a small scatterplot. The small boxes will fill with observations making visual inference difficult. In this case, we might reduce the data to a correlation matrix, using a single number to describe the relationship between a pair of variables.

The correlation is a matrix of values needing its own graphical display. The `corrplot()` takes the correlation matrix of the burger data and the code

```
corrplot(cor(burger))
```

produces the plot in Fig. 3.19.

The `corrplot` program has many possible options and we just accepted the defaults in this example. In Fig. 3.19, the individual correlations are displayed both by color and size. Correlations close to zero are both smaller and paler in color.

3.5.2 Glyphs: Stars, Radar, and Faces

The *star plot* summarizes each data item as a circle with different-sized wedges. An example of the hamburger data appears in Fig. 3.20. Every star is an individual (row) and every wedge on the star represents a different variable (column) in the data.

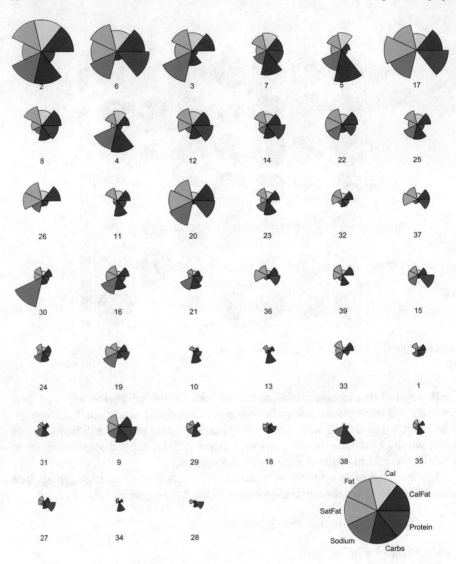

Figure 3.20 Star plot of burgers, ordered by calories, with key

The radius of each wedge in the star indicates the size of the scaled values for each individual, relative to all other measurements for each variable. These variables are listed in different colors and directions. The key for this is given in the lower-right corner of the figure. The radius of each wedge is scaled and can be used to compare the relative magnitude of each variable value across all individuals.

To aid in organization, all burgers have been ordered by their calorie values, in reading order, from largest at the top, to smallest. We can sort in decreasing order by sorting on the *negative* values, in the code given below. The numbers in the figure refer to the listing order of `row.names` in the `data.frame`. Figure 3.20 was produced using the **R** commands

```
library(graphics)                        # for the stars program
palette(rainbow(7))                      # set colors
burs <- burger[ order(-burger$Cal), ]# order by Cal, decreasing
stars( burs, len=1, cex=0.5, key.loc=c(12.5, 2),
    labels=row.names(burs), draw.segments=TRUE)
```

which labels each object and provides a useful guide to the directions of the stars in the lower-right corner. The help for this command `help(stars)` explains a large number of options available for this graphical display.

In Fig. 3.20, we can see the burgers in the top two rows are simultaneously extreme in most dimensions. The first few burgers are different from the others and extreme in most of the seven dimensions. Outside of the top two rows, the stars for the burgers are not very different from each other and only a few are extreme in more than one dimension.

Stars are an example of a *glyph*. A glyph is a general class of graphics in which the shape of the plotted character is indicative of the multivariate characteristics of the observation. In addition to stars, a simple glyph appears in Fig. 3.13 in which the size of the plotted circle is related to the altitude of the respective city.

The stars can be placed on top of each other, creating what is called a *radar* or *spider plot*. An example of this appears in Fig. 3.21 for the six burgers with the highest calories.

The program to produce this figure is given in Output 3.5. The program begins by identifying the highest caloric burgers. The `radarchart` program is in the `fmsb` library and requires each column of values to begin with the values of the maximum and minimum values. This program has many options to modify the presentation. The `legend` statement adds a useful key to the plot.

An advantage of the radar plot over the star plot is it facilitates a comparison of one burger to another. A downside of this radar plot is the figure becomes very cluttered if we include more than six items.

Let us examine the most extreme example of a glyph. Chernoff (1973) used cartoon faces as a glyph to demonstrate multivariate information. Each variable can represent some aspect of the face: head size and color, degree of smile or frown, amount and shape of the hair, the spacing and size of eyes, and so on.

An example of *Chernoff's faces* appears in Fig. 3.22 for the nine highest calorie burgers in Table 1.6. The first three or so of these faces are over-sized and outlandish, corresponding to the extreme, high data values. We can see a gradual trend of lower values in the last row of faces in this figure. These correspond to smaller head sizes, less hair, smaller eyes, and mouths. The faces for the omitted burgers are similar to those of the last row in this figure. The `faces` program to draw these is available in the `aplpack` package.

Radar plot for high calorie hamburgers

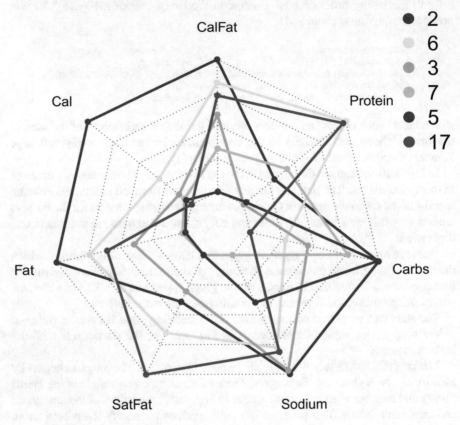

Figure 3.21 Radar (spider) plot of highest calorie burgers

3.5.3 Parallel Coordinates

Consider multivariate data categorized into a small number of groups. We have several graphical methods to describe group membership as well as distinguishing characteristics for each group. This is the data examined by RA Fisher[2] which motivated the initial study of discriminant analysis. (See Sect. 10.5.) In this well-known example of multivariate data, three species of iris flowers are measured in terms of their

- petal length;
- petal width;
- sepal length;
- sepal width.

---

[2] Ronald Aylmer Fisher (1890–1962). British geneticist and statistician.

Output 3.5 Program to produce the radar plot, Fig. 3.21

```
burger <- read.table(file = "burger.txt", header = TRUE,
                     row.names = 1)
nbur <- 6                    #  number of burgers to plot
hical <- order(burger[ , 2], decreasing = TRUE)[1 : nbur]
short_bur <- burger[hical, ] #  data for the highest caloric burgers
ncols <- dim(burger)[2]      #  number of columns
brr <- NULL                  #  build table of column ranges
for (j in 1 : ncols) brr <- cbind(brr, range(short_bur[, j])[2 : 1])
brr                          #  rows of column maximums and minimums

       [,1] [,2] [,3] [,4] [,5] [,6] [,7]
 [1,] 1197 2120  133   52 4200  139   93
 [2,]  639 1540   90   29 2490   33   53

colnames(brr) <- colnames(burger)    #  row and column names
row.names(brr) <- c("max", "min")    #       for range values
rad_burger <- rbind(brr, short_bur)  #  add ranges to data
rad_burger                           #  list data: max, min, then raw data

      CalFat  Cal Fat SatFat Sodium Carbs Protein
max    1197 2120 133     52   4200   139     93
min     639 1540  90     29   2490    33     53
2      1197 2120 133     38   4200   139     65
6      1098 1720 122     44   3819    62     93
3       963 1610 107     36   4150    81     53
7       820 1580  91     29   2490   114     70
5       639 1570  90     29   3170   138     54
17     1044 1540 116     52   3880    33     92

line_color <- rainbow(nbur)[1 : nbur]  #  define colors
library(fmsb)                          #  library with the program
radarchart(rad_burger, plty = 1, plwd = 3,pcol = line_color,
          title = "Radar plot for high calorie hamburgers")
legend(x=1.05,   y=1.4, legend = hical, bty = "n",
         pch=20 , col = line_color, cex = 1.5, pt.cex = 2.5)
```

The data is available in the MASS library in **R**. The *parallel coordinate* display (sometimes called the *parallel axes* display) plots the separate coordinate axes parallel to each other, rather than as at right angles to each other, as we often think of in terms of axes.

To product this display, begin by re-scaling each of these separate measurements so they are all on the same scale, usually between 0 and 1. The multidimensional values for each item are connected with lines so we can follow these across the different dimensions. In this example, we can also plot each of these series of lines in a different color for each of the iris species. The plot in Fig. 3.23 displays these data, with each species in a different color. Every jagged line traces the four values for one flower across each of the four dimensions.

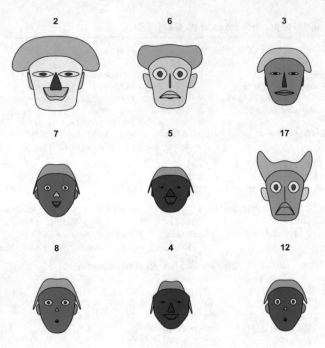

Figure 3.22 Chernoff faces display for the nine highest caloric hamburgers

The **R** program to produce this figure is

```
library(MASS)
ir <- rbind(iris3[ , , 1], iris3[ , , 2], iris3[ , , 3])
parcoord(log(ir)[ , c(3, 4, 1, 2)],   # Order the axes
    col = c(rep("red", 50), rep("green", 50), rep("blue", 50)))
```

In **R**, the data is listed as a three-dimensional data frame, where the third subscript indicates each of the three separate species. The rbind statement creates a
data.frame called ir where the three species are listed one after the other as
rows.

The parcoord program draws the parallel axes plot given in Fig. 3.23. The data
values are scaled on each of the four axes after taking logs of all data. The ordering
of the four axes in this plot is specified. You can try other orderings to obtain a more
pleasing result. In this case, we chose the ordering here so the three species separate
well in the plot. The different colors for each of the species are specified using the
col= option.

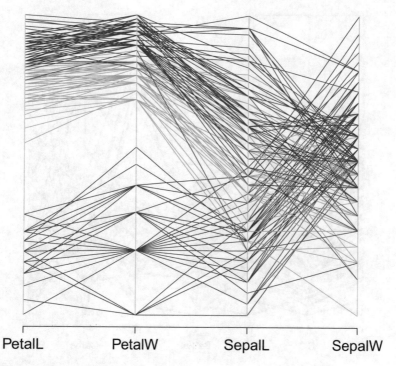

Figure 3.23 Parallel coordinate plot for the iris data

Specifically, the three colors, `col=` values, and species in this figure are as follows:

Color	Species
Red	*Setosa*
Green	*Versicolor*
Blue	*Virginica*

We can see the *Setosa* (in red) has the lowest values of petal length and width. *Setosa* generally also has relatively large values of sepal width. *Virginica* (in blue) and *Versicolor* (in green) have an ordering with larger values of *Virginica* in most cases across all four of the measured variables.

The parallel coordinate plot is also useful when there are no identified categories of individuals. Figure 3.24 plots the hamburger data. There are no categories of burgers but we can create these by identifying the nine with the highest calorie values. In this figure, we can see those with the highest calories and also generally highest for each of the other nutritional values as well.

The parallel coordinate plot is not very different from the star plot or the radar plot. If we could imagine pinching the bottom of Fig. 3.24 into a point and rotating

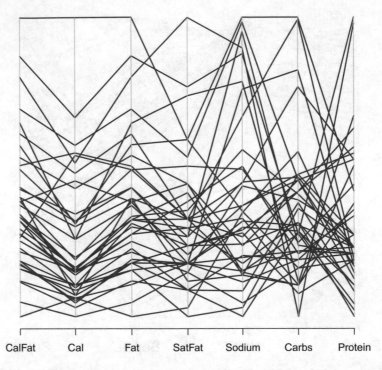

CalFat   Cal   Fat   SatFat   Sodium   Carbs   Protein

Figure 3.24 Parallel coordinate plot for the hamburger data. The highest calorie burgers are identified in *red*

the top into a circle, we would have the star plot in Fig. 3.20 or the radar plot of Fig. 3.21.

3.6 Additional Reading

The field of statistical graphics is open to new developments. There is so much more left to do. The good news is the field is so accessible because it does not require an extensive mastery of mathematical and computational expertise before one can make an innovative and lasting contribution. Perhaps the biggest disappointment is in the twenty-first century we are still limited to two-dimensional paper in a printed book as did publishers since Guttenberg,[3] over 500 years ago. Some software packages allow us to slowly rotate a three-dimensional object. This may allow our spatial perception

---

[3] Johannes Gutenberg (1398–1468). German, invented movable type. This led to the wide availability of books, which, in turn, was instrumental in the Renaissance and the following scientific development.

to find patterns and is usually aided by the inclusion of factor methods, described in Chap. 8.

Innovation in the field of statistical graphics has come at a steady pace with several notable pioneers. Tukey[4] was ahead of his time. When we look at Tukey (1977), we take many of his ideas for granted because they are now a part of our everyday language. At a time when working at a computer meant waiting for a 110 baud teletype machine to clunk and chug along, Tukey developed a boxplot, the innovative histogram printed in only three lines. He coauthored Chambers *et al* (1983) and inspired Cleveland (1993).

The books by Tufte are artistic and passionate contributions to the field. You don't have to have a rigorous background in mathematical statistics to appreciate what is being conveyed. Perhaps a rigorous background in statistics trains us to think in certain rigid ways and this can be a distraction.

Wilkinson (1999)[5] describes a new language codifying and unifying the whole of statistical graphics. This is a new direction taking us away from specific examples into a discussion of what is possible, sometimes combining two or more methods of display. An applied version of this in **R** has been the development of the `ggplot2` function. An introduction to `ggplot2`, and graphics in **R** more generally, is provided in Chang (2013).

The lattice plot builds on the earlier trellis plot. The `lattice` package is a large suite of useful graphics available in **R** and more fully described in Sarkar (2008). One example is the violin plot, as part of Exercise 3.4.

Ideally, we should explore data in an interactive environment allowing us to use sliders alongside plots to visualize the effects of different amounts of smoothing. For three-dimensional data, there is no substitute for rotations in a dynamic setting. Some of these tools are available in the `aplpack` library but cannot be adequately appreciated until they are experienced first hand.

3.7 Exercises

3.1 Describe the *pie chart*. What type of data is this best suited for? What are its limitations?

3.2 How does the sample correlation change when we remove successive layers of convex hulls from our two-dimensional data? Add `cor(x,y)` inside the loop of the program generating the convex hull peeling in Fig. 3.25. What do you think are the reasons for this change as we deleted those extreme observations?

---

[4] John Wilder Tukey (1915–2000). American statistician and mathematician.

[5] Leland Wilkinson (1944-2021) American statistician and computer scientist. His book cited here played an important role in the development of the `ggplot` package in **R**.

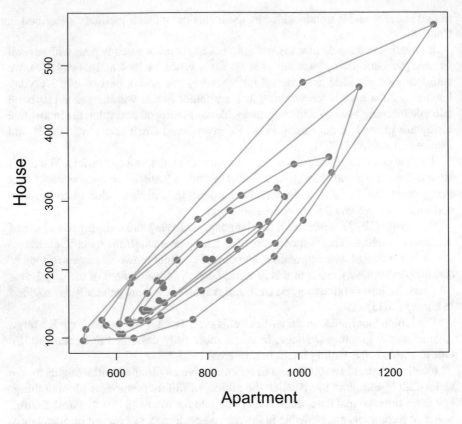

Figure 3.25   Five peeling convex hulls of the housing data

3.3 Look at the relationship between fat and sodium content for each of the 40
burgers in Fig. 3.15. Sodium values seem to rise quickly for higher levels of fat.
Does this look like a linear relationship?

    a. Plot fat and sodium using a bivariate boxplot and also as a single convex
hull. Do these methods assist or mislead us?

    b. In this same data set, calories and fat seem to exhibit an hourglass shape
with greater variability at both the high and low ends. Examine the bivariate
boxplot and convex hull of this pair of variables. Are these methods useful
in this situation?

3.4 In the `lattice` package, there is a data set called `singer` which gives the
heights of singers in the New York Choral Society, a serious amateur vocal
group. Heights are given separately by each of the different voice parts, high to
low (soprano, alto, tenor, bass). Each of these is further divided into tiers (1 and
2) for higher and lower voices within each part.

     a. In **R**, explore graphical methods such as jittering and boxplots to show the characteristics and distributions of heights by voice group. The general trend is taller people have deeper singing voices, but also comment on the shape of the distributions within each vocal group. The documentation for `singer` provides other useful displays of these data.

     b. The *violin plot* is an improvement over the boxplot. Read about violin plots in the help file under the name `panel.violin` and examine these data. Explain the various features of these graphical displays and use them to describe additional features of these data.

3.5 a. Consider a set of randomly generated faces:

```
faces(matrix(rnorm(192),16,12),main="Random Faces")
```

     What is the tendency for us to identify patterns and similar-looking individuals in such a sample? Is this a good feature or a shortcoming of the method?

     b. Similarly, generate randomly distributed data and plot these using `pairs()` with `panel.smooth`. Again, what is the tendency for us to see patterns when there is no reason for these to exist?

3.6 The `bvbox` in the `MVA` library produces the bivariate boxplot appearing in Fig. 3.10. Modify this code to create a new program with more options for the graphical output. Copy the program code into a text editor and add options to change the colors, line types, and line widths of the ellipses and the regression lines. See Fig. 6.1 for an example of how the output might look.

3.7 Write a program in **R** to draw and peel away successive convex hulls in bivariate data. As an example, five convex hulls of the housing data is displayed in Fig. 3.25. Hint: Recall a negative subscript in a list will omit the item.

3.8 The `anorexia` data set in the `MASS` library lists the pre- and post-treatment weights of 72 young women with anorexia. There were three different treatments: control or no treatment, behavioral coaching, or family intervention. Find a suitable way to display these data using colors to identify the three different interventions.

Chapter 4
Some Linear Algebra

M ANY OPERATIONS performed on multivariate data are facilitated using vector and matrix notation. In this chapter, we introduce the basic operations and properties of these and then show how to perform them in **R**.

4.1 Apples and Oranges

A single numerical value is called a *scalar*, as in the price of an apple. With multivariate data, we like to talk about several different values at the same time. We can combine these as a *2-tuple* (apple, banana) or a *3-tuple* (apple, banana, orange) and so on up to the more general *n*-tuple. This collection of information would be referred to as the *vector* of fruit prices. The order of the items in the list matters, of course.

Mathematically, a vector is expressed as a vertical list:

$$\textbf{fruit price} = \begin{pmatrix} \text{Apple price} \\ \text{Banana price} \\ \text{Orange price} \end{pmatrix}$$

Sometimes, it is convenient to express this as a horizontal, rather than a vertical list. To do this, we have the *transpose* operation giving

$$\textbf{fruit price}' = (\text{Apple price}, \ \text{Banana price}, \ \text{Orange price}),$$

where the prime (') exponent indicates the transpose.

Notice how we also use a **bold font** to indicate a vector, to distinguish it from a scalar which appears in a normal font.

Vectors are added component-wise. So for example, if each fruit has its own tax

© Springer Nature Switzerland AG 2022
D. Zelterman, *Applied Multivariate Statistics with R*, Statistics for Biology and Health,
https://doi.org/10.1007/978-3-031-13005-2_4

$$\textbf{fruit tax} = \begin{pmatrix} \text{Apple tax} \\ \text{Banana tax} \\ \text{Orange tax} \end{pmatrix}$$

then

$$\textbf{fruit price} + \textbf{fruit tax} = \begin{pmatrix} \text{Apple price} + \text{Apple tax} \\ \text{Banana price} + \text{Banana tax} \\ \text{Orange price} + \text{Orange tax} \end{pmatrix}$$

Suppose we have a shopping list with the quantities of each fruit:

$$\textbf{fruit quantity} = \begin{pmatrix} \text{\# of Apples} \\ \text{\# of Bananas} \\ \text{\# of Oranges} \end{pmatrix}$$

The scalar-valued *inner product* of two vectors is defined by

$$\begin{aligned} \textbf{fruit quantity}' \ \textbf{fruit price} = {}& \text{\# of Apples} \times \text{Apple price} \\ &+ \text{\# of Bananas} \times \text{Banana price} \\ &+ \text{\# of Oranges} \times \text{Orange price} \end{aligned}$$

which we would interpret as our total price of the fruit.

Notice the inner product is a linear operator with the property

$$\begin{aligned} \textbf{fruit quantity}\,'(\,\textbf{fruit price} + \textbf{fruit tax}) = {}& \textbf{fruit quantity}' \ \textbf{fruit price} \\ &+ \textbf{fruit quantity}' \ \textbf{fruit tax} \end{aligned}$$

so the price we pay for our groceries, including the taxes, can be calculated in either manner.

We can combine all this information about fruit in a matrix:

$$\textbf{FRUIT} = \begin{pmatrix} \text{Apple price} & \text{Apple tax} & \text{Apple quantity} \\ \text{Banana price} & \text{Banana tax} & \text{Banana quantity} \\ \text{Orange price} & \text{Orange tax} & \text{Orange quantity} \end{pmatrix}$$

where we interpret the columns as prices, taxes, and quantities, respectively, and the rows correspond to the different fruit.

The notation for a matrix always appears in a **CAPITAL BOLD** font.

The transpose of the **FRUIT** matrix reverses the roles of columns and rows so

$$\textbf{FRUIT}' = \begin{pmatrix} \text{Apple price} & \text{Banana price} & \text{Orange price} \\ \text{Apple tax} & \text{Banana tax} & \text{Orange tax} \\ \text{Apple quantity} & \text{Banana quantity} & \text{Orange quantity} \end{pmatrix} .$$

Again we use the prime ($'$) to perform a transpose.

When it comes to multivariate data, it is very handy to talk about the data arranged in columns and rows such as in this example. Data arranged in tables such as in the examples of Chap. 1 will list observed items as rows and attributes or variables measured on each as columns. In matrix notation, we can easily describe arithmetic operations performed in parallel, on the whole data set in a more compact manner.

4.2 Vectors

Let's begin with the basic arithmetic operations for vectors and (in the following section) matrices. In Sect. 4.5, we move on to more advanced matrix properties.

A *scalar* is a single numerical value and a *vector* is a *n-tuple* or collection of numerical values listed in a prescribed order.

We use **bold**, lower-case letters to denote vectors. The notation for a vector x is

$$x = \begin{pmatrix} x_1 \\ x_2 \\ \vdots \\ x_n \end{pmatrix}$$

and the *transpose* is $x' = (x_1, x_2, \ldots, x_n)$. Two vectors are equal if they have an equal number of components and are equal in each of these components.

A vector x can be multiplied by a scalar constant c

$$cx = \begin{pmatrix} cx_1 \\ cx_2 \\ \vdots \\ cx_n \end{pmatrix}.$$

The sum of two vectors x and $y' = (y_1, y_2, \ldots, y_n)$ is

$$x + y = y + x = \begin{pmatrix} x_1 + y_1 \\ x_2 + y_2 \\ \vdots \\ x_n + y_n \end{pmatrix}.$$

As with scalar arithmetic, vector addition is commutative so

$$x + y = y + x.$$

Vector addition is only defined when the vectors have the same length. The *zero vector* $0' = (0, 0, \ldots, 0)$ with all zero components is the additive identity. That is,

$$x + 0 = 0 + x = x .$$

The number of components in the zero vector is usually not specified, but is assumed, so the arithmetic operation is defined whenever it appears.

Vector subtraction is similarly defined:

$$x - y = \begin{pmatrix} x_1 - y_1 \\ x_2 - y_2 \\ \vdots \\ x_n - y_n \end{pmatrix}$$

and $x - 0 = x$.

The scalar-valued *inner product* is defined by

$$x'y = \sum_{i=1}^{n} x_i y_i . \tag{4.1}$$

Again, this operation is only defined for vectors of the same length.

The inner product is symmetric in its arguments so

$$x'y = y'x$$

and is a linear operator so that

$$x'(y + z) = x'y + x'z . \tag{4.2}$$

As an example of the operations defined up to this point, suppose

$$x = \begin{pmatrix} 1 \\ 5 \\ 2 \end{pmatrix} \text{ and } y = \begin{pmatrix} 3 \\ -1 \\ 6 \end{pmatrix} .$$

Then we have

$$x' = (1, 5, 2),$$

$$3x = \begin{pmatrix} 3 \\ 15 \\ 6 \end{pmatrix} ,$$

$$x + y = \begin{pmatrix} 4 \\ 4 \\ 8 \end{pmatrix} ,$$

and

$$x'y = (1 \times 3) + (5 \times -1) + (2 \times 6) = 10.$$

Two vectors with an inner product equal to zero are said to be *orthogonal*. The zero vector $\mathbf{0}$ of is orthogonal to all other vectors.

A pair of vectors x_1 and x_2 are said to be *linearly dependent* if there exists a scalar c with $x_1 = cx_2$.

More generally, a set of vectors $x_1, x_2, \ldots, x_n$ are linearly dependent if there exist scalars $c_1, c_2, \ldots, c_n$ not all zero, with

$$c_1 x_1 + c_2 x_2 + \cdots + c_n x_n = \mathbf{0}. \tag{4.3}$$

The implication of linear dependence in least one vector can be expressed as a linear combination of the others. Conversely, vectors are said to be *mutually independent* if (4.3) does not hold. That is, if vectors $x_1, x_2, \ldots, x_n$ are mutually independent and if (4.3) holds then we must have $c_1 = c_2 = \cdots = c_n = 0$. Mutually orthogonal vectors are linearly independent, but linearly independent vectors need not be orthogonal. See Exercise 4.5.

The *Euclidean*[1] *length* (or more simply, the *length*) of a vector) is the square root of the inner product with itself:

$$||x|| = (x'x)^{1/2} = \sqrt{x_1^2 + x_2^2 + \cdots + x_n^2}. \tag{4.4}$$

In a two-dimensional plane, the Euclidean length is how we interpret distance. As an example, if we travel to a point one unit east and two units north away from where we began, then the distance (as the crow flies) is $\sqrt{5}$, just as we would determine using the result of Pythagoras.

4.3 Basic Matrix Arithmetic

A matrix generalizes a vector to an array of values. We use bold **CAPITAL** letters to denote matrices. An n by m matrix X has n rows and m columns and has elements indexed by two subscripts:

$$X = \begin{pmatrix} x_{11} & x_{12} & \ldots & x_{1m} \\ x_{21} & x_{22} & \ldots & x_{2m} \\ \vdots & \vdots & \ddots & \vdots \\ x_{n1} & x_{n2} & \ldots & x_{nm} \end{pmatrix}.$$

---

[1] Euclid, mathematician in ancient Greece, lived around 300 BCE.

The transpose X' of a matrix X takes its values and turns it on its upper-left and lower-right diagonal. The transpose of an $n \times m$ matrix has dimensions $m \times n$. The transpose has the effect of reversing the subscripts, so

$$X' = \begin{pmatrix} x_{11} & x_{21} & \ldots & x_{n1} \\ x_{12} & x_{22} & \ldots & x_{n2} \\ \vdots & \vdots & \ddots & \vdots \\ x_{1m} & x_{2m} & \ldots & x_{nm} \end{pmatrix}.$$

A matrix is said to be *symmetric* if it is equal to its transpose, *i.e.,* $X' = X$. Only square matrices can be symmetric.

A matrix X can be multiplied by a scalar c:

$$cX = \begin{pmatrix} cx_{11} & cx_{12} & \ldots & cx_{1m} \\ cx_{21} & cx_{22} & \ldots & cx_{2m} \\ \vdots & \vdots & \ddots & \vdots \\ cx_{n1} & cx_{n2} & \ldots & cx_{nm} \end{pmatrix}$$

and two matrices with the same dimensions can be added:

$$X + Y = \begin{pmatrix} x_{11} + y_{11} & x_{12} + y_{12} & \ldots & x_{1m} + y_{1m} \\ x_{21} + y_{21} & x_{22} + y_{22} & \ldots & x_{2m} + y_{2m} \\ \vdots & \vdots & \ddots & \vdots \\ x_{n1} + y_{n1} & x_{n2} + y_{n2} & \ldots & x_{nm} + y_{nm} \end{pmatrix}.$$

We can also define matrix multiplication. As with the inner product for vectors, the dimensions must be correct for matrix multiplication to be defined. If X is n by m and Y is m by p then

$$\underset{(n \times p)}{Z} = \underset{(n \times m)}{X} \quad \underset{(m \times p)}{Y}$$

is defined.

Notice the "middle" dimensions of X and Y need to be equal. That is, we can multiply the matrices X and Y if the number of columns of X is equal to the number of rows in Y. The elements of the resulting matrix product Z has dimensions n by p. The (ij)-th element of Z is equal to the inner product of the i-th row of X and the j-th column of Y.

As an example of these matrix operations suppose

$$X = \begin{pmatrix} 5 & -1 & 3 \\ 2 & 4 & 1 \\ 3 & 1 & 2 \\ -2 & 5 & 2 \end{pmatrix}$$

and

$$Y = \begin{pmatrix} 2 & 3 \\ 4 & 1 \\ 3 & 5 \end{pmatrix}.$$

Then

$$3X = \begin{pmatrix} 15 & -3 & 9 \\ 6 & 12 & 3 \\ 9 & 3 & 6 \\ -6 & 15 & 6 \end{pmatrix},$$

$$Y' = \begin{pmatrix} 2 & 4 & 3 \\ 3 & 1 & 5 \end{pmatrix},$$

and

$$XY = \begin{pmatrix} (5 \times 2) + (-1 \times 4) + (3 \times 3) & (5 \times 3) + (-1 \times 1) + (3 \times 5) \\ (2 \times 2) + (4 \times 4) + (1 \times 3) & (2 \times 3) + (4 \times 1) + (1 \times 5) \\ (3 \times 2) + (1 \times 4) + (2 \times 3) & (3 \times 3) + (1 \times 1) + (2 \times 5) \\ (-2 \times 2) + (5 \times 4) + (2 \times 3) & (-2 \times 3) + (5 \times 1) + (2 \times 5) \end{pmatrix}$$

$$= \begin{pmatrix} 15 & 29 \\ 23 & 15 \\ 16 & 20 \\ 22 & 9 \end{pmatrix}.$$

In this example, we see matrix multiplication is not *commutative*. That is, XY is not necessarily equal to YX nor is YX necessarily defined. See also Exercise 4.4.

A square *diagonal matrix* has zero entries off the main diagonal:

$$\mathbf{Diag}(a_1, a_2, \ldots, a_n) = \begin{pmatrix} a_1 & 0 & \cdots & 0 \\ 0 & a_2 & \cdots & 0 \\ \vdots & \vdots & \ddots & \vdots \\ 0 & 0 & \cdots & a_n \end{pmatrix}.$$

The *identity matrix* I

$$I = \begin{pmatrix} 1 & 0 & \cdots & 0 \\ 0 & 1 & \cdots & 0 \\ \vdots & \vdots & \ddots & \vdots \\ 0 & 0 & \cdots & 1 \end{pmatrix}$$

is a square, symmetric matrix with 1's running down the diagonal and all other entries equal to zero.

The identity matrix has the property it has no effect when multiplied by another matrix:

$$IX = X$$

just as multiplying by 1 in scalar arithmetic.

The dimensions of the identity matrix I are usually inferred from context. In this last equation, the dimensions of I have to be the same as the first dimension of X in order for this matrix multiplication to be defined. To make this point in a different way, if we assume the $(n \times m)$ matrix X is not square then we can also write somewhat ambiguously

$$\underset{(n \times n)}{I} \quad \underset{(n \times m)}{X} = \underset{(n \times m)}{X} \quad \underset{(m \times m)}{I} = \underset{(n \times m)}{X}$$

where the two appearances of I represent different-sized matrices within the same mathematical expression. For this reason, we will sometimes include the dimensions of matrices in equations when this removes the confusion.

4.4 Matrix Operations in R

The basic mathematical operations for vectors and matrices described in Sects. 4.2 and 4.3 can easily be implemented in **R**. The advanced matrix functions covered in Sect. 4.5 will be introduced using **R** to facilitate the discussion. The advanced operations involving determinants, inverses, and eigenvalues, for examples, are best described in terms of their computational procedures. The use of these procedures will be more fully appreciated in subsequent chapters.

We add two vectors $x + y$ using the same notation in **R**: namely x+y. The inner product of a vector with its self $x'x$ is computed by omitting the second argument: crossprod(x).[2] All of these operations are only defined when x and y have the same length. The following dialog illustrates these operations:

```
> x <- seq(2,8,2)
> x

[1] 2 4 6 8

> y <- 4:1
> y

[1] 4 3 2 1
```

---

[2] There should be no confusion here with the a totally different operation familiar to physicists and engineers called the *vector cross product* only valid for vectors in three dimensions of two vectors $x'y$ is defined at (4.1) and computed using crossprod(x,y).

```
> x+y

[1] 6 7 8 9

> crossprod(x,y)

      [,1]
[1,]   40

> crossprod(x)

      [,1]
[1,]  120
```

Notice the `crossprod` function returns a 1×1 matrix, not a scalar.
The * operation for vectors performs a component-wise product of vectors:

```
> x * y

[1]  8 12 12  8
```

and not the vector cross product.

The *outer product* xx' is an $n \times n$ matrix. This is computed using the %o% operator as in x %o% x. The vector outer product operation is illustrated in the following dialog:

```
> x

[1] 2 4 6 8

> x %o% x

      [,1] [,2] [,3] [,4]
[1,]    4    8   12   16
[2,]    8   16   24   32
[3,]   12   24   36   48
[4,]   16   32   48   64
```

Notice how **R** prints the matrix values, bordered by a useful index notation. The heading for each row and column reminds us of the subscripts we would use to address each row or column. So, for example, we have

```
> (x %o% x)[, 3]

[1] 12 24 36 48
```

```
> (x %o% x)[2 ,]
```

```
[1]   8 16 24 32
```

showing how we access the third column and second row of the matrix outer product, respectively. Both of these are treated as vectors.

We can easily build special types of matrices using `diag` to form a diagonal matrix and `matrix` to build a matrix with specified values.

So, for example,

```
> diag(1, 4, 4)

     [,1] [,2] [,3] [,4]
[1,]    1    0    0    0
[2,]    0    1    0    0
[3,]    0    0    1    0
[4,]    0    0    0    1
```

is a 4×4 identity matrix and

```
> matrix(1, 4, 4)

     [,1] [,2] [,3] [,4]
[1,]    1    1    1    1
[2,]    1    1    1    1
[3,]    1    1    1    1
[4,]    1    1    1    1
```

is a 4×4 matrix of all 1's.

We can also construct a 4×4 matrix with the counts $1, \ldots, 16$:

```
> matrix(1 : 16, 4, 4)

     [,1] [,2] [,3] [,4]
[1,]    1    5    9   13
[2,]    2    6   10   14
[3,]    3    7   11   15
[4,]    4    8   12   16
```

running down columns.

If we wanted the counts to run across the rows, we can transpose this matrix with the t function

```
> t(matrix(1 : 16, 4, 4))

     [,1] [,2] [,3] [,4]
[1,]    1    2    3    4
[2,]    5    6    7    8
[3,]    9   10   11   12
[4,]   13   14   15   16
```

The `diag` function can be used to both build diagonal matrices as well as extract the diagonal elements of an existing matrix:

```
> diag( t(matrix(1 : 16, 4, 4)))

[1]  1  6 11 16
```

We can add two matrices with A + B and multiply element-by-element A * B. These operations are valid only when A and B have the same dimensions.

```
> A

     [,1] [,2] [,3] [,4]
[1,]    1    2    3    4
[2,]    2    4    6    8
[3,]    3    6    9   12

> B

     [,1] [,2] [,3] [,4]
[1,]    2    4    6    8
[2,]    4    8   12   16
[3,]    6   12   18   24

> A + B

     [,1] [,2] [,3] [,4]
[1,]    3    6    9   12
[2,]    6   12   18   24
[3,]    9   18   27   36

> A * B

     [,1] [,2] [,3] [,4]
[1,]    2    8   18   32
[2,]    8   32   72  128
[3,]   18   72  162  288
```

The multiplication of two matrices is accomplished by writing A %*% B. This operation is illustrated as follows:

```
> A

     [,1] [,2] [,3] [,4]
[1,]    1    2    3    4
[2,]    2    4    6    8
[3,]    3    6    9   12
```

```
> t(B)

     [,1] [,2] [,3]
[1,]    2    4    6
[2,]    4    8   12
[3,]    6   12   18
[4,]    8   16   24

> A %*% t(B)

     [,1] [,2] [,3]
[1,]   60  120  180
[2,]  120  240  360
[3,]  180  360  540
```

Recall the product of a 3×4 matrix and a 4×3 matrix is a 3×3 matrix. We can also solve linear equations in **R**. Consider the system of linear equations

$$a_{11}x_1 + a_{12}x_2 + \cdots + a_{1,n}x_n = b_1$$
$$a_{21}x_1 + a_{22}x_2 + \cdots + a_{2,n}x_n = b_2$$
$$\vdots \qquad\qquad \vdots \qquad\qquad \vdots\ \vdots$$
$$a_{n1}x_1 + a_{n2}x_2 + \cdots + a_{n,n}x_n = b_n.$$

These equations can be written in the more compact, matrix notation

$$Ax = b$$

for known matrix $A = \{a_{ij}\}$ and vector $b = \{b_i\}$. We want to solve these equations for vector $x = \{x_i\}$ satisfying relationships. The solution in **R** is obtained by solve(A,b).

As a numerical example, suppose $b = \{9, 7, 5, 3\}$ and A is a 4×4 matrix of random values generated uniformly between 0 and 1.

```
> (b <- c(9, 7 5, 3)

[1] 9 7 5 3

> (A <- matrix(runif(16),c(4,4)))

          [,1]      [,2]      [,3]      [,4]
[1,] 0.6692485 0.5644291 0.4361838 0.7869338
[2,] 0.9458449 0.4710188 0.8120588 0.5741354
[3,] 0.3366968 0.1971159 0.3774943 0.3954844
[4,] 0.1841985 0.9128133 0.3773530 0.2363638

> solve(A,b)

[1] -1.9162283 -0.5453288  2.7192532 11.9503542
```

Algebraically, we can write $x = A^{-1}b$ where A^{-1} is the inverse of A. The inverse A^{-1} can be obtained in **R** using `solve(A)`:

```
> solve(A)

          [,1]         [,2]        [,3]        [,4]
[1,]   1.4205610   2.15995584  -5.478218  -0.8099599
[2,]   0.5768595   0.04273936  -1.881024   1.1229594
[3,]  -2.8628620   0.01850019   5.301603   0.6158308
[4,]   1.2357195  -1.87784541   3.069534  -0.4579570
```

The matrix inverse operation is explained in Sect. 4.5.2.

In the next section, we look at more advanced matrix operations. These are best introduced along with the corresponding **R** code.

4.5 Advanced Matrix Operations

The methods described in this section make the leap to beyond what a human could reasonably accomplish with pencil and paper alone. These concepts are important and are needed for subsequent chapters. To ease the discussion, we include the **R** code accomplishing these tasks in order to show the reader these methods can be implemented with a minimum amount of effort for any specific set of numerical values. The reader wishing to learn more about these advanced properties of matrices is referred to the classic textbook by Lang (2010).[3] Golob and Van Loan (1983) is another excellent reference for learning more about the computational aspects of matrix operations

4.5.1 Determinants

The *trace* of a square matrix is the sum of its diagonal elements. The *determinant* is another numerical value associated with a square matrix.

As an example, consider the 2×2 matrix

$$A = \begin{pmatrix} a & b \\ c & d \end{pmatrix}.$$

The trace of A is $a + d$ and the determinant is

$$\mathrm{Det}(A) = ad - bc. \tag{4.5}$$

---

[3] Serge Lang (1927–2005) French-born, American mathematician.

For another example, the trace of the 3×3 matrix

$$B = \begin{pmatrix} a & b & c \\ d & e & f \\ g & h & i \end{pmatrix}$$

is $a + e + i$ and the determinant is

$$\text{Det}(B) = a(ei - fh) + b(fg - id) + c(dh - eg). \tag{4.6}$$

As we can see from these two examples, the determinant is a polynomial in the matrix elements. These expressions quickly grow in complexity with the size of the matrix so, in general, it is best to find determinants numerically in **R** as in this example:

```
> (x <- matrix(rnorm(25), 5, 5))

            [,1]        [,2]        [,3]        [,4]        [,5]
[1,]  0.8773400  -0.5657782   1.7634118   1.8728550  0.9928573
[2,]  0.1017325  -0.3619644   0.8324341   1.4387591  0.2699057
[3,]  0.8026365  -0.6943805  -0.8926545   1.2955549  1.7452754
[4,]  0.9237657   1.2665737  -0.3078966  -0.2517838  1.0968427
[5,]  1.8795828  -0.5785956  -0.3837322   1.2007208  0.7950999

> det(x)

[1] -7.170792
```

In this example, we use **R** to generate a 5×5 matrix (denoted as x) whose elements are sampled from a standard normal distribution. The det(x) function returns the determinant of this matrix.

Some special cases of determinants are worth mentioning. The determinant of a diagonal matrix is the product of its diagonal entries. So we have

$$\text{Det}(\mathbf{Diag}(x_1, x_2, \ldots, x_n)) = \text{Det} \begin{pmatrix} x_1 & 0 & \cdots & 0 \\ 0 & x_2 & \cdots & 0 \\ \vdots & \vdots & \ddots & \vdots \\ 0 & 0 & \cdots & x_n \end{pmatrix} = x_1 x_2 \cdots x_n.$$

Similarly, the determinant of the identity matrix I is equal to 1 regardless of its size. The determinant of a matrix is equal to the determinant of its transpose, so

$$\text{Det}(A) = \text{Det}(A').$$

The determinant of a scalar c multiple of an $n \times n$ matrix A satisfies

$$\text{Det}(cA) = c^n \, \text{Det}(A) \, .$$

The determinant of a product of square matrices is the product of the individual determinants:

$$\text{Det}(AB) = \text{Det}(A) \, \text{Det}(B) \, .$$

The *rank* of a matrix is the maximum number of linearly independent rows and columns when these are considered as vectors. A square matrix whose rank is equal to the number of rows (or columns) is said to be of *full rank* or *nonsingular*. A square matrix with less than full rank has a determinant of zero and is said to be *singular*.

4.5.2 Matrix Inversion

The *inverse* of a square matrix A (when it exists) is denoted by A^{-1} and has the property the product

$$A^{-1}A = A A^{-1} = I$$

is equal to the identity matrix.

Let us draw comparisons between inverses of matrices and the parallel in scalar operations. The inverse of a matrix is analogous to what the reciprocal is to a scalar. The scalar 1 is its own reciprocal, just as the identity matrix I is its own inverse. Corresponding to the scalar value zero, which does not have a reciprocal, a matrix with a zero determinant does not have an inverse. Conversely, any square matrix with a non-zero determinant will have an inverse.

In the 2×2 matrix

$$A = \begin{pmatrix} a & b \\ c & d \end{pmatrix}$$

the inverse is given by

$$A^{-1} = \frac{1}{ad - bc} \begin{pmatrix} d & -b \\ -c & a \end{pmatrix} \tag{4.7}$$

provided the determinant $ad - bc$ is non-zero.

The inverse of the 3×3 matrix

$$B = \begin{pmatrix} a & b & c \\ d & e & f \\ g & h & i \end{pmatrix}$$

is given by

$$B^{-1} = \frac{1}{\text{Det}(B)} \begin{pmatrix} A & B & C \\ D & E & F \\ G & H & I \end{pmatrix}$$

where $\mathrm{Det}(B)$ is the determinant given at (4.6). This inverse exists only when the

$$A = ei - fh \qquad B = ch - bi \qquad C = bf - ce$$
$$D = fg - di \qquad E = ai - cg \qquad F = cd - af$$
$$G = dh - eg \qquad H = bg - ah \qquad I = ae - bd$$

determinant is non-zero.

As with a matrix determinant, we see the mathematical complexity of finding the inverse increases greatly with the size of the matrix. Fortunately for us, matrix inverses can be calculated numerically in **R** with little effort on our part. The following example illustrates this, continuing with the same matrix x generated earlier in this section to illustrate the determinant.

Here is the x matrix again:

```
> x

             [,1]        [,2]        [,3]        [,4]       [,5]
[1,]  0.8773400  -0.5657782   1.7634118   1.8728550  0.9928573
[2,]  0.1017325  -0.3619644   0.8324341   1.4387591  0.2699057
[3,]  0.8026365  -0.6943805  -0.8926545   1.2955549  1.7452754
[4,]  0.9237657   1.2665737  -0.3078966  -0.2517838  1.0968427
[5,]  1.8795828  -0.5785956  -0.3837322   1.2007208  0.7950999
```

We use the solve() function to find the inverse:

```
> solve(x)

             [,1]        [,2]        [,3]         [,4]        [,5]
[1,]   0.1588468  -0.3984637  -0.33113613   0.04831542   0.59711329
[2,]  -0.5552320   1.1185653  -0.28424175   0.69540112  -0.02176659
[3,]   0.6985182  -0.5875821  -0.19048830  -0.04702547  -0.18979125
[4,]  -0.6586654   1.4906931  -0.04002048   0.18067946   0.15505461
[5,]   0.5522533  -0.7788176   0.54445190   0.09628027  -0.49543987
```

Just to check, we can multiply the matrix x by its inverse:

```
> x %*% solve(x)

             [,1]         [,2]         [,3]          [,4]          [,5]
[1,]   1.000000e+00  -6.661338e-16  1.110223e-16   4.163336e-17  -1.110223e-16
[2,]   1.665335e-16   1.000000e+00  5.551115e-17   2.775558e-17   0.000000e+00
[3,]   0.000000e+00  -2.220446e-16  1.000000e+00   1.387779e-16  -1.110223e-16
[4,]   1.110223e-16  -2.220446e-16  0.000000e+00   1.000000e+00  -1.110223e-16
[5,]  -5.551115e-17   1.110223e-16  1.110223e-16  -1.387779e-17   1.000000e+00
```

The resulting product is very nearly an identity matrix: There are 1's running down the diagonal and the off-diagonal entries are either zero or quantities within rounding error of zero (about $\pm 10^{-16}$). This is another reminder that performing numerical computations will usually result in very small numerical errors which (hopefully) do not greatly distort the final answers. The study of numerical algorithms and the corresponding rounding errors are examined in the mathematical field of *numerical analysis*.

A useful relationship between matrix determinants and inverses is

$$\text{Det}\left(A^{-1}\right) = 1/\text{Det}(A).$$

The inverse of a matrix is not always needed when it is part of a more complex mathematical expression. As an example of avoiding the use of the matrix inverse, suppose we want to compute the quadratic form $b'A^{-1}b$ in **R**. (We will need to calculate similar expressions when we evaluate the multivariate normal density function, given at (7.2)). We can obtain this in **R** as

```
b %*%  solve(A,b)
```

without having to separately find the inverse matrix A^{-1}.

There are closely related matrix operations including inverses when these exist, and other similar properties when they don't. These generalized inverses of matrices are described in Sect. 4.5.5.

4.5.3   *Eigenvalues and Eigenvectors*

Let us introduce another advanced topic in matrix algebra. Every square matrix has an associated set of *eigenvalues* and *eigenvectors*. If A is a square matrix, then consider the linear equation

$$Ax = \lambda x \tag{4.8}$$

for some eigenvector x and a scalar eigenvalue λ.

Intuitively, (4.8) says the effect of multiplying the vector x by A is the same as multiplying it by a scalar. Multiplication of a vector by a scalar results in changing its length by either stretching $(\lambda > 1)$, shrinking $(0 < \lambda < 1)$, or reversing direction by changing its signs $(\lambda < 0)$. A vector x satisfying (4.8) is called an eigenvector of A and the value λ corresponding to x is called the eigenvalue. If one solution exists to (4.8) then there are an infinite number of these solutions. If (x, λ) is a solution to (4.8), then, for example, $(2x, \lambda/2)$ is also a solution. See Exercise 4.10 for more details. One useful way to avoid this ambiguity in **R** is to find a set of eigenvectors x all of unit length and are mutually orthogonal. Vector length is defined at (4.4).

The identity matrix I leaves vectors unchanged

$$Ix = x$$

so the eigenvalues λ's of the identity matrix are all equal to 1, and every vector x is an eigenvector of the identity matrix.

Here are some useful properties of eigenvalues in relation to other topics already discussed. The eigenvalues $\lambda_1, \lambda_2, \ldots, \lambda_n$ of an $n \times n$ matrix A are related to the trace

$$\text{Trace}(A) = \lambda_1 + \lambda_2 + \cdots + \lambda_n \tag{4.9}$$

and the determinant

$$\text{Det}(A) = \lambda_1 \lambda_2 \cdots \lambda_n . \tag{4.10}$$

The *characteristic polynomial*

$$p(\lambda) = \text{Det}(A - \lambda I) \tag{4.11}$$

is a polynomial in λ and the roots of the equation $p(\lambda) = 0$ determine the eigenvalues. In practice, **R** uses a different algorithm to find eigenvalues.

An $n \times n$ matrix will have n eigenvalues. Just as a polynomial may have multiple roots, some of the eigenvalues may be repeated, corresponding to multiple roots[4] of $p(\lambda) = 0$. A polynomial may have complex roots, and the eigenvalues may be *complex numbers*. Complex numbers are expressible as $\alpha + \beta i$ where $i^2 = -1$. Complex roots will appear as *complex conjugates*. That is, if $\alpha + \beta i$ is a complex root of a polynomial with real-valued coefficients, then $\alpha - \beta i$ will also be a root of this polynomial.

Eigenvalues and eigenvectors can be obtained in **R** using

```
evs <- eigen (A)
```

for a symmetric matrix A. Then evs$val is the vector of eigenvalues and evs$vec are the corresponding eigenvectors.

For very large matrices, we might only require the eigenvalues. In which case, to save computing time, use

```
eigen(A, only.values =TRUE)$values
```

and only the eigenvalues are computed.

In **R** we can calculate the eigenvalues of the 5×5 matrix x examined previously,

```
> eigen(x)$values

[1]  3.502643+0.0000i -1.124313+1.140676i -1.124313 -1.140676i
[4] -1.589936+0.0000i  0.501957+0.0000i
```

---

[4] A quadratic equation, for example, always has two roots and we say $x^2 = 0$ has a root at $x = 0$ of multiplicity two.

In this numerical example, we see two of the five eigenvalues are complex conjugates. We also have

```
> prod(eigen(x)$values)

[1] -7.170792+0i

> det(x)

[1] -7.170792
```

illustrating the equality of the determinant and the product of the eigenvalues as stated in (4.10).

A square matrix A is said to be *positive definite* if for every non-zero vector x we have

$$x'Ax > 0$$

and nonnegative definite if $x'Ax \geq 0$.

See Exercise 4.11 for some properties of positive definite matrices and how to identify these. A useful property of positive definite matrices is all of their eigenvalues are real and nonnegative.

4.5.4 Diagonalizable Matrices

A square matrix A is said to be *diagonalizable* if it is expressible as

$$A = XDX^{-1} \tag{4.12}$$

for a diagonal matrix D.

The numerical identification of the components of a diagonalizable matrix is very simple in **R** using the `eigen` function. The diagonal matrix D in (4.12) is the diagonal matrix of the eigenvalues of A. The eigenvectors provided by `eigen` are expressed as a matrix whose columns are mutually orthogonal vectors. That is, the X in (4.12) is the matrix of eigenvectors.

Let us verify all of these statements in **R**. We begin by constructing a positive definite matrix called `apa`:

```
> (a <- matrix(rnorm(15), 5, 3))   # 5x3 matrix with random entries

             [,1]         [,2]        [,3]
[1,]   0.4968134  -0.97565489  -0.6246059
[2,]   1.4922367  -0.10939041  -1.3471900
[3,]   1.5666928   1.82600963  -0.5806661
[4,]   1.3176006  -0.22123894  -1.2764140
[5,]  -0.6809085  -0.07426517  -1.8700602
```

```
> (apa <- t(a) %*% a)                    #  pos definite a'a matrix

          [,1]       [,2]       [,3]
[1,]   8.210201 -4.913078 -2.044630
[2,]  -4.913078  3.886116  1.608089
[3,]  -2.044630  1.608089  0.733343
```

We find the eigenvalues and eigenvectors:

```
> (ax <- eigen(apa))    # eigenvalues and eigenvector as a matrix

$values
[1] 12.01145060   0.76052212   0.05768692

$vectors
            [,1]          [,2]            [,3]
[1,]   0.8137227 -0.5811763  -0.009462608
[2,]  -0.5363584 -0.7444990  -0.397543559
[3,]  -0.2239980 -0.3285656   0.917534510
```

We can check the matrix of eigenvectors is orthogonal:

```
> ax$vectors %*% t(ax$vectors)

             [,1]            [,2]            [,3]
[1,]   1.000000e+00 -1.439820e-16 -1.908196e-17
[2,]  -1.439820e-16  1.000000e+00 -1.665335e-16
[3,]  -1.908196e-17 -1.665335e-16  1.000000e+00
```

which is very close to being an identity matrix, except for rounding errors in entries off the main diagonal.

Finally, we can verify the diagonalization process of (4.12)

```
> ax$vectors %*% diag(ax$values) %*% t(ax$vectors)

          [,1]       [,2]       [,3]
[1,]   8.210201 -4.913078 -2.044630
[2,]  -4.913078  3.886116  1.608089
[3,]  -2.044630  1.608089  0.733343
```

returning the original matrix apa given above.

Properties of diagonalizable matrices are examined in Exercise 4.13.

4.5.5   Generalized Inverses

We may want to talk about matrices that are not invertible. The *generalized inverse* (or sometimes referred to as the *Moore–Penrose inverse*) corresponds to the matrix inverse when it exists and has a similar property when it doesn't. The generalized inverse A^- of A has the property

$$AA^-A = A.\qquad(4.13)$$

The generalized inverse is not unique. We show how to construct one in Exercise 4.12.

In **R** we can obtain a generalized inverse using the function `ginv` in the MASS library. Here is an example of its use. We begin by including the MASS package:

```
> library(MASS)

Attaching package: 'MASS'

> (z <- matrix(rnorm(15), 3, 5))

          [,1]       [,2]       [,3]        [,4]      [,5]
[1,] -1.019293 -1.1105161 -0.8835698 -1.56692865 0.3841926
[2,] -1.706265  0.5660277 -1.8179978  0.29282216 0.6521679
[3,]  0.556425 -0.5469372 -0.9581269  0.02266884 0.7840144

> (q <- t(z) %*% z)

           [,1]       [,2]       [,3]       [,4]       [,5]
[1,]  4.2599060 -0.1381812  3.4694761  1.1101408 -1.0681307
[2,] -0.1381812  1.8527737  0.4762167  1.8934466 -0.4863137
[3,]  3.4694761  0.4762167  5.0038186  0.8304212 -2.2762859
[4,]  1.1101408  1.8934466  0.8304212  2.5415241 -0.3932605
[5,] -1.0681307 -0.4863137 -2.2762859 -0.3932605  1.1876054
```

The matrix Z is a 3×5 matrix of standard normal variates and

$$Q = Z'Z\qquad(4.14)$$

is a 5×5 symmetric, positive nonnegative definite matrix.

The eigenvalues of Q should all be real and positive:

```
> eigen(q)$values

[1]  9.269311e+00  3.794984e+00  1.781333e+00 -1.290715e-16 -3.613510e-16
```

These eigenvalues are all real but the two smallest are within rounding error of zero reflecting the fact the 5×5 matrix Q is of rank 3. See Exercise 4.8 for more details.

The generalized inverse of Q is

```
> ginv(q)
```

```
             [,1]          [,2]          [,3]          [,4]          [,5]
[1,]    1.7573935   0.58990933    0.35307232   -0.18596570   -1.3996771
[2,]    0.5899093   0.33810377    0.06772675   -0.16774283   -0.5864543
[3,]    0.3530723   0.06772675    0.30962523   -0.09430042   -0.1568524
[4,]   -0.1859657  -0.16774283   -0.09430042    0.13993652    0.2003483
[5,]   -1.3996771  -0.58645427   -0.15685241    0.20034835    1.2424363
```

and we can check this solution satisfies (4.13) using

```
> q %*% ginv(q) %*% q   -q
```

```
             [,1]           [,2]           [,3]           [,4]           [,5]
[1,]  -2.220446e-16  -2.220446e-16  -1.942890e-16   4.440892e-16   2.498002e-16
[2,]   2.220446e-16   2.220446e-16  -1.526557e-16   2.220446e-16  -1.665335e-16
[3,]  -1.387779e-16  -5.551115e-17  -8.881784e-16   4.440892e-16  -1.110223e-16
[4,]   2.220446e-16  -6.661338e-16   2.220446e-16   4.440892e-16   4.024558e-16
[5,]   1.110223e-16  -5.551115e-17   2.220446e-16   8.326673e-17   0.000000e+00
```

because this difference between

$$Q'Q(Q'Q)^- Q'Q$$

and Q is within rounding error (about 10^{-16}) of zero in all 25 elements of this 5×5 matrix.

4.5.6 Matrix Square Root

To end this section on advanced matrix operations, we note there is also a *matrix square root*. By analogy to the scalar operation with the same name, for a square matrix Z, is there a square matrix X with the property $X^2 = Z$? The answer is not every matrix Z will have a square root, and when there is a square root, it may not be unique. When the square root exists, we write $X = Z^{1/2}$ using a familiar notation. See Exercise 4.14 to show the square root may not be unique.

The matrix square root of a diagonal matrix with nonnegative entries $\{d_1, d_2, \ldots d_n\}$ is just the diagonal matrix with the square roots of the entries. That is, if

$$D = \mathbf{Diag}(d_1, d_2, \ldots, d_n)$$

then

$$D^{1/2} = \mathbf{Diag}(d_1^{1/2}, d_2^{1/2}, \ldots, d_n^{1/2}). \tag{4.15}$$

Just as there is no (real-valued) square root of a negative number, the square root only exists for nonnegative definite matrices. A nonnegative definite matrix will have no negative eigenvalues, so this provides an easy check for us in **R**.

An easy way to find the square root of a matrix is to express it as in the diagonalizable form given at (4.12) and use Exercise 4.12. The following **R** program includes a check for a nonnegative definite matrix:

```
msqrt <- function(a)    # matrix square root of positive definite matrix
    {
    a.eig <- eigen(a)
    if ( min(a.eig$values) < 0) # check for positive definite
        warning("Matrix not positive definite")

    a.eig$vectors %*% diag(sqrt(a.eig$values)) %*% t(a.eig$vectors)
    }
```

Let us provide a numerical example of this program and its use.

```
> (x <- matrix(rnorm(35), 7, 5)) # 7x5 matrix of normals

           [,1]        [,2]        [,3]        [,4]        [,5]
[1,]   0.3798194   0.2114649   1.2076177   1.0124777  -1.49971761
[2,]   1.5125906  -0.9378462   0.4264717   1.3007917  -0.20352177
[3,]  -0.2841299  -1.1639801  -2.0819616  -1.8749218  -0.52516122
[4,]  -1.2978443  -1.0741596   1.7710925  -1.8331337  -0.54667111
[5,]   0.3154816  -0.7757654   2.4617252  -1.5434827  -0.63295035
[6,]  -1.0363971   1.0355279   0.9133007  -0.6332664   0.41377237
[7,]  -0.1596910  -0.9360372   1.5617765  -0.8657940   0.08946316
```

is a 7×5 of standard normals.

From this, we create a 5×5 symmetric, positive definite matrix:

```
> (z <- t(x) %*% x)        # pos definite, symmetric 5x5 matrix

           [,1]        [,2]       [,3]        [,4]        [,5]
[1,]   5.3964714  -0.7819263  -1.022616   5.5716021  -0.6615621
[2,]  -0.7819263   5.9832371  -2.049524   4.4976418   1.9079767
[3,]  -1.0226159  -2.0495241  18.444907  -3.2958671  -2.8132511
[4,]   5.5716021   4.4976418  -3.295867  13.1258459   0.8410505
[5,]  -0.6615621   1.9079767  -2.813251   0.8410505   3.4450550
```

We can see the symmetry and check the matrix is positive definite:

```
> eigen(z)$values        # check positive definite

[1] 22.2951500 14.0726580   7.0743534   2.2363879   0.7169668
```

because all of the eigenvalues are positive.

We can find the matrix square root $Z^{1/2}$ using the `msqrt` program given above:

```
> (sqrtz <- msqrt(z))        # find matrix square root

            [,1]        [,2]        [,3]         [,4]         [,5]
[1,]   1.9849903  -0.4102019  -0.1244228   1.11419094  -0.17640021
[2,]  -0.4102019   2.1943311  -0.2449349   0.87546138   0.41648139
[3,]  -0.1244228  -0.2449349   4.2449391  -0.38357917  -0.45032400
[4,]   1.1141909   0.8754614  -0.3835792   3.31074757   0.09904232
[5,]  -0.1764002   0.4164814  -0.4503240   0.09904232   1.74008050
```

Finally, we can check the the difference between $(Z^{1/2})^2$ and Z:

```
> sqrtz %*% sqrtz - z     # check properties of matrix sqrt

            [,1]         [,2]         [,3]         [,4]          [,5]
[1,]  -2.664535e-15  1.443290e-15 -1.332268e-15 -1.154632e-14   2.109424e-15
[2,]   1.665335e-15 -8.881784e-15 -1.332268e-15 -1.776357e-15  -1.776357e-15
[3,]  -1.110223e-15 -8.881784e-16 -3.552714e-14  5.329071e-15   7.549517e-15
[4,]  -1.065814e-14 -1.776357e-15  3.552714e-15 -3.907985e-14   1.998401e-15
[5,]   1.998401e-15 -1.332268e-15  7.549517e-15  1.776357e-15  -4.884981e-15
```

This difference is within the rounding error of a matrix of all zeroes, confirming the properties of the matrix square root in **R**.

4.6   Exercises

4.1 Let $x' = (2, 1, -5)$ and $y' = (2, 1, 1)$.

    a. Find $x + y$.
    b. Show x and y are orthogonal.
    c. Find a non-zero vector z orthogonal to both x and y.
    d. Show any vector orthogonal to both x and y must be a scalar multiple of z.

4.2 For vectors x, y, and z with the same dimensions and scalar c, verify

    a. $x'y = y'x$.
    b. $||cx|| = |c|\,||x||$ where $|c|$ is the absolute value of c.
    c. $||x|| = 0$ if and only if x is the zero vector.
    d. Verify (4.2).

4.3 Let X denote an $n \times n$ square matrix and y is an n-tuple vector of all 1's. Interpret $y'X$ and Xy.

4.4 Suppose X, Y, and Z are matrices with the appropriate dimensions so multiplication is defined.

    a. Prove $(XY)Z = X(YZ)$.
    b. Prove $(XY)' = Y'X'$. Also $(XYZ)' = Z'Y'X'$.
    c. Suppose X and Y are square matrices with the same dimensions. Show XY is not necessarily equal to YX.

4.5 a. Find a pair of linearly independent vectors but are not orthogonal.

b. Suppose the vectors $x_1, x_2, \ldots, x_k$ are mutually orthogonal. Show they are also linearly independent. *Hint:* If they are linearly dependent and orthogonal then they must all have zero length.

4.6 Consider the matrix

$$A = \begin{pmatrix} 2 & 1 \\ 1 & 1 \end{pmatrix}.$$

a. Find the trace, determinant, and inverse of this matrix.

b. Multiply this matrix by its inverse and verify your solution is correct.

c. Use (4.9) and (4.10) to find the eigenvalues for this matrix.

4.7 Let $X = \{x_{ij}\}$ denote a matrix with n rows and p columns.

a. Show $X'X$ is a symmetric matrix.

b. Verify the ith diagonal element of $X'X$ is

$$\sum_{k=1}^{n} x_{ki}^2$$

and the (i, j) off-diagonal elements of $X'X$ are

$$\sum_{k=1}^{n} x_{ki} x_{kj}$$

for $i \neq j = 1, 2, \ldots, p$.

c. Suppose $A = \{a_{ij}\}$ is a $p \times p$ symmetric matrix. Then verify $B = XAX'$ is symmetric with diagonal elements

$$b_{ii} = \sum_{s=1}^{p} \sum_{t=1}^{p} a_{st} x_{is} x_{it}$$

and off-diagonal elements

$$b_{ij} = b_{ji} = \sum_{s=1}^{p} \sum_{t=1}^{p} a_{st} x_{is} x_{jt} .$$

4.8 Show the rank of a $n \times m$ matrix cannot be larger than the smaller of n and m. As a consequence, show the 5×5 matrix Q constructed at (4.14) cannot have rank greater than 3.

4.9 A *linear space* S is a set of vectors with the properties:

(i) The zero vector $\mathbf{0}$ is an element of S.

(ii) If x and y are in S then $x + y$ is also in S.

a. Show for any vector x, the set

$$S(x) = \{cx \;\; \text{for every scalar} \;\; c\}$$

of every scalar multiple of x is a linear space. We say $S(x)$ is the space *spanned* by the vector x.

b. More generally, consider the set of every linear combination of the vectors $x_1, x_2, \ldots, x_n$:

$$S(x_1, x_2, \ldots, x_n) = \{c_1 x_1 + c_2 x_2 + \cdots + c_n x_n \;\; \text{for all scalars} \;\; c_i\}.$$

Show this is a linear space. Such a set is called the *linear space spanned by the vectors* $x_1, x_2, \ldots, x_n$ or more simply, the *span* of $x_1, x_2, \ldots, x_n$.

4.10 Show the set of all solutions in x of (4.8) form a linear space. Specifically show the following:

a. The zero vector $x = (0, 0, \ldots, 0)$ satisfies (4.8).
b. If the eigenvectors x_1 and x_2 are both solutions to (4.8) with respect to an eigenvalue λ then the sum $x_1 + x_2$ of these eigenvectors will also solve (4.8).

4.11 Let Z denote an arbitrary $n \times m$ matrix.

a. Show $Z'Z$ is symmetric.
b. Show $Z'Z$ is nonnegative definite. *Hint:* If $y = Zx$ then $y'y = x'Z'Zx$.
c. Show every eigenvalue of $Z'Z$ must be nonnegative. *Hint:* If λ is an eigenvalue with eigenvector x then $Z'Zx = \lambda x$. If we multiply on the left by x' then we also have

$$x'Z'Zx = \lambda x'x.$$

4.12 Let Z denote an arbitrary $n \times m$ matrix. The previous exercise showed eigenvalues of $Z'Z$ are all real and nonnegative. Let us denote these by

$$\lambda_1 \geq \lambda_2 \geq \cdots \geq \lambda_r \geq \lambda_{r+1} = \lambda_{r+2} = \cdots = \lambda_m = 0$$

with corresponding eigenvectors $x_1, x_2, \ldots, x_m$. Refer to (4.13) and show the matrix

$$\sum_{i=1}^{r} (1/\lambda_i) \, x_i x_i'$$

is a generalized inverse of $Z'Z$.

4.13 Suppose the matrix A is expressible as in (4.12). Find A^{10}.

4.14 In this exercise, we explore the properties of the matrix square root.

a. Verify (4.15).

b. Consider the 2×2 identity matrix

$$I = \begin{pmatrix} 1 & 0 \\ 0 & 1 \end{pmatrix}.$$

Show the matrix square root of I is not unique.

Specifically, consider any numbers r and s, at least one of which is non-zero. Then define

$$t = \sqrt{r^2 + s^2}$$

and define

$$J = 1/t \begin{pmatrix} \pm s & \pm r \\ \pm r & \mp s \end{pmatrix}.$$

Show $J^2 = I$.

Chapter 5
The Univariate Normal Distribution

THE NORMAL DISTRIBUTION is central to much of statistics. In this chapter and the two following, we develop the normal model from the univariate, bivariate, and then, finally, the more general distribution with an arbitrary number of dimensions.

Historically, the normal distribution was developed as an approximation to the binomial distribution by de Moivre[1] in 1738 but the more common attribution is to Gauss[2] in 1809. As a result, the normal distribution is often referred to as the *Gaussian distribution* or frequently as the *bell curve* because of the familiar shape of its density function.

5.1 The Normal Density and Distribution Functions

The density function of the *standard normal distribution* is

$$\phi(x) = (2\pi)^{-1/2} \exp(-x^2/2) . \tag{5.1}$$

The distribution is called the standard normal because a random variable X sampled from this distribution will have zero mean and unit variance. This function is available in **R** as dnorm().

Of course we are not restricted to the use of standard normal variates. If X is a standard (zero mean, unit standard deviation) normal then the linear transformation

$$Z = \mu + \sigma X$$

is also normally distributed with mean μ and variance σ^2.

---

[1] Abraham de Moivre (1667–1754). French mathematician and probabilist.
[2] Carl Friedrich Gauss (1777–1855). German mathematician and physicist.

© Springer Nature Switzerland AG 2022
D. Zelterman, *Applied Multivariate Statistics with R*, Statistics for Biology and Health,
https://doi.org/10.1007/978-3-031-13005-2_5

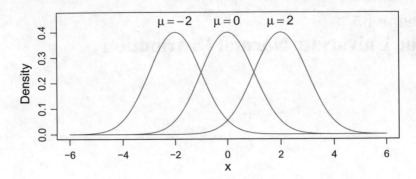

Figure 5.1 The normal distribution density function (5.2) for specified mean values, all with a standard deviation $\sigma = 1$

This more general and useful form of the distribution of $Z = \mu + \sigma X$ defined for $\sigma > 0$ has density function

$$\phi(z \mid \mu, \sigma) = \sigma^{-1}(2\pi)^{-1/2} \exp\{-(z - \mu)^2/2\sigma^2\}. \tag{5.2}$$

In Fig. 5.1, we see the familiar bell curve is shifted left and right by varying the value of the mean μ. When the value of the standard deviation σ is varied, Fig. 5.2 demonstrates the curve can also have a sharp peak (when σ is small) or be broad and flat (when σ is large).

The cumulative distribution or area under the normal curve is much more important than the bell curve itself. That is, we usually want to describe the probability of an interval under the bell curve, but almost never need the value of the bell curve itself.

Specifically, let

$$\Phi(x) = \int_{-\infty}^{x} \phi(t)\,dt \tag{5.3}$$

denote the cumulative probability up to the value x.

The tail areas are symmetric so

$$\Phi(-x) = 1 - \Phi(x)$$

for every value of x.

This integral, for the standard normal ($\mu = 0$ and $\sigma = 1$), is evaluated by pnorm() in **R**. The shape of Φ may be unfamiliar to many readers, so we present some examples in Fig. 5.3. In each of the curves of Φ in Fig. 5.3, we see that all these begin close to zero on the left and increase monotonically up to one on the right. The curves shift from left to right as the mean increases. Smaller standard deviations cause the curve to rise more quickly. The shape of the normal density in Figs. 5.1 and 5.2 should be familiar to the reader, but the shape in Fig. 5.3 is rarely displayed.

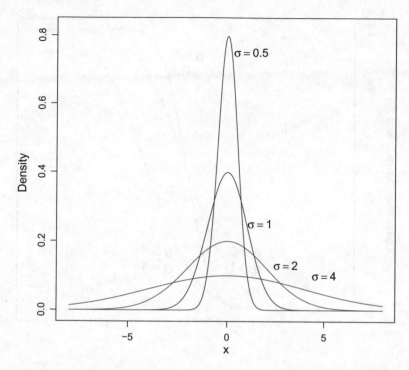

Figure 5.2 The normal distribution density function (5.2) with mean 0 and different values of the standard deviation as given

In **R** we can generate random samples from a standard normal distribution using the `rnorm()` function. This function was also illustrated in Sects. 2.5 and 4.5. The argument to `rnorm()` specifies how many random values are generated:

```
> rnorm(4)

[1]   1.1624076 -1.9219944   0.4634357 -2.5063903

> rnorm(5)

[1] -2.5397705   0.5856622 -1.3165089   3.3851341   1.5616724
```

Notice the random values generated are different with every invocation of `rnorm`. Your values will differ from these as well.

We calculate values of the standard normal density function ϕ given at (5.1) using `dnorm()` which may take a vector argument. Similarly, the cumulative normal Φ at (5.3) with $\mu = 0$ and $\sigma = 1$ is found using `pnorm()`.

We can illustrate these functions in **R** by plotting the values using

```
> x <- (-50:50)/12
> plot(x, dnorm(x), type = "l")
```

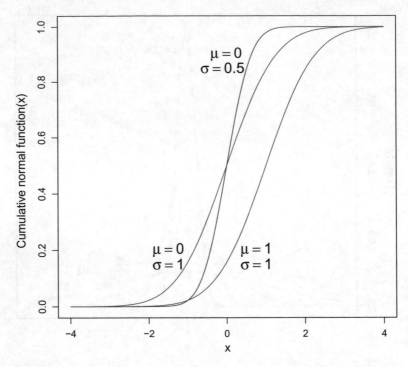

Figure 5.3 The cumulative normal distribution function (5.3) for means μ and standard deviations σ as given

to plot the standard normal density function in Fig. 5.1 and then

```
> plot(x, pnorm(x), type = "l")
```

to illustrate the cumulative distribution function with mean zero and standard deviation one, as in Fig. 5.3.

There is also the function qnorm() to calculate the *quantile function* from the normal distribution. The quantile is the inverse of Φ. That is, for any probability p $(0 < p < 1)$, the normal quantile $x = x(p)$ is value solving the equation

$$\Phi(x) = p. \tag{5.4}$$

You may be familiar with the use of this function for finding the critical value of a statistical test. Specifically, a standard normal distribution has 95% of its area between the familiar values -1.96 and $+1.96$. We can obtain these values in **R** using the qnorm function:

```
> qnorm(.05/2)

[1] -1.959964
```

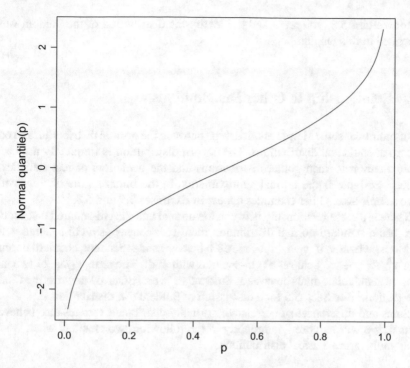

Figure 5.4 The quantile function $\Phi^{-1}(p)$ of the standard normal distribution

```
> qnorm(1 - .05/2)

[1] 1.959964
```

We use the argument of .05/2 because we want half of the .05 probability in each of the two tails of the normal curve. A plot of the qnorm() function is given in Fig. 5.4. As p approaches either 0 or 1, then this curve tends to $-\infty$ or $+\infty$, respectively.

To illustrate another use of this function in **R**, we generate a set of probabilities uniformly distributed between (but not including) 0 and 1 and then find the corresponding normal quantiles:

```
> x <- runif(6)
> x

[1] 0.6828715 0.4100933 0.5086939 0.7548347 0.8098490
[6] 0.7866481

> qnorm(x)

[1]  0.47574359 -0.22730502  0.02179419  0.68978305
[5]  0.87733996  0.79484489
```

In Exercise 5.8, you are asked to identify the distribution of the random values generated in this fashion.

5.2   Relationship to Other Distributions

Let us point out some simple relationships between the normal distribution and other important statistical distributions. The normal distribution is frequently used as an approximation to many other distributions and the behaviors of test statistics. A popular example is the normal approximation to the binomial distribution with a large sample size. Other examples appear in Exercises 2.9 and 5.8.

There is a close relationship between the normal and the chi-squared distribution. If x has a standard normal distribution then x^2 behaves as a chi-squared with 1 df. More generally, if $x_1, x_2, \ldots, x_k$, each behave as independent, standard normals, then $x_1^2 + \cdots + x_k^2$ behaves as chi-squared with k df. The ratio x_1/x_2 of two independent standard normals behaves as Student's t with 1df, also known as the *Cauchy distribution*.[3] See Sect. 5.5 for a discussion of Student's t distribution.

Sums and differences of correlated, normally distributed variates also behave as normal. We will explore this property in the following two chapters when we talk about multivariate normal distributions.

5.3   Transformations to Normality

If you are reading this section, then it is likely you are already suspicious your data is not exactly normally distributed. In this section, we will provide statistical tests to see if your data is "close enough" to being normal and some things you can do about it if it isn't. Of course, there are times when it is not worth testing for normality or even pretending the data are normally distributed, because the non-normal shape is obvious. In this case, other techniques are available to us such as robust, nonparametric methods not relying on the assumption of normally distributed data. As an example, if the data values are binary valued, then the normal distribution is not appropriate and no amount of transformation will make these data look normal.

As a case study for this section, let us examine the median apartment rents for each of the 50 US states and DC given in Table 1.1.

The best way to start is to draw a histogram. In **R** we draw a histogram using the `hist(x)`. This command is discussed in Sect. 3.1. The histogram of the rent values appears in the upper left corner of Fig. 5.5. The data values have a longer right tail than the left (right skewed), and we are going to show how to repair this. There is also some evidence of a gap in the middle of the distribution, perhaps indicating the

---

[3] Augustin-Louis Cauchy 1789–1857. French mathematician.

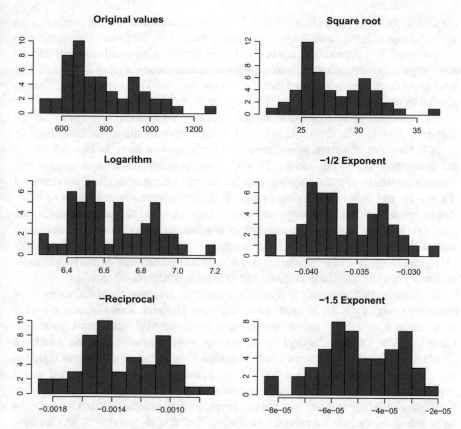

Figure 5.5 Histograms of the median apartment rents in Table 1.1. The data has been transformed using the power transformation (5.5)

data is sampled from two different populations. This bimodal feature is much harder to fix than the asymmetry, which we will discuss next.

It is possible and often useful to transform skewed data values in order to make them more symmetric. Clearly, a linear transformation will not change the basic shape of the histogram. A non-linear transformation is needed. The *power transformations* attributed to Box and Cox (1964) can be summarized as

$$\text{Power}(x) = \begin{cases} -x^{\lambda} & \text{for } \lambda < 0 \\ \log(x) & \text{for } \lambda = 0 \\ x^{\lambda} & \text{for } \lambda > 0 \end{cases} \qquad (5.5)$$

for positive valued data (x) and any specified value of λ. This function is called `bct` and is available in the `TeachingDemos` library.

The further λ is from 1, the greater the effect of the transformation. Values of $\lambda < 1$ in this transformation will have the effect of pulling in a long right tail and spreading out values in a short left tail. This is what is needed for the rent data and we will explore these next. A negative sign is needed in the power transformation for values of $\lambda < 0$ because reciprocals of large numbers are small numbers and we need to preserve the order of the data, not reverse it. Values of $\lambda > 1$ in (5.5) will tend to push out the right tail of the distribution and this is the opposite of what is needed to make the distribution of the rent data more symmetric.

Histograms of transformed median rent values are given in Fig. 5.5. These include values of $\lambda = 1, 1/2, 0, -1/2, -1,$ and -1.5. Choosing the appropriate value of λ calls for more of a sense of esthetics than mathematical rigor. In Fig. 5.5 we see the square root ($\lambda = 1/2$) and log ($\lambda = 0$) transformations result in more symmetric improvements over the original data but are not strong enough. The reciprocal ($\lambda = -1$) and $\lambda = -1.5$ appear to overdo the transformation and begin to introduce a longer left tail. The reciprocal square root ($\lambda = -1/2$) seems to be a nice compromise, producing a more symmetric distribution, although there is not much we can do about the bimodal character of the data. Ideally, a separate statistical analysis could be applied to help identify characteristics and membership in two or more different populations. These methods are described in Chaps. 10 and 11.

Next we examine methods to check for normality. A simple graphical method for checking normality is the quantile-quantile plot or *QQ plot*. This plot compares the quantiles of the observed values with those of the theoretical distribution, hence the name QQ. The QQ plot displays the sorted, observed values against the values we would expect to observe had they been sampled from a theoretical normal distribution. If the observed data was sampled from a normal distribution, then we would expect these values to form a nearly straight line.

What are the expected values from an ordered normal sample? To find these, begin by recalling the cumulative normal distribution function Φ given at (5.3). Consider then, a sorted sample $x_1 \leq x_2 \leq \cdots \leq x_n$ from a standard normal distribution with mean $\mu = 0$ and standard deviation $\sigma = 1$.

We would expect these ordered, standardized values to obey

$$\Phi(x_1) = 1/(n+1), \quad \Phi(x_2) = 2/(n+1), \quad \cdots \quad , \Phi(x_n) = n/(n+1). \quad (5.6)$$

In other words, the theoretical, expected sample values should be spread out evenly with all n observations having equal cumulative probabilities between each. See Exercise 5.2 for more details.

We can take the set of equations in (5.6) and invert Φ using the normal quantile function to obtain the expected normal quantiles. These values are close approximations to where the ordered values should be expected to occur in the sample. Specifically, the expected quantiles for the QQ plot are

$$\widehat{x_1} = \Phi^{-1}(1/(n+1)), \quad \widehat{x_2} = \Phi^{-1}(2/(n+1)), \quad \ldots \quad \widehat{x_n} = \Phi^{-1}(n/(n+1)). \quad (5.7)$$

The quantile function $\Phi^{-1}()$ is plotted in Fig. 5.4 and can be calculated using the `qnorm()` function in **R**.

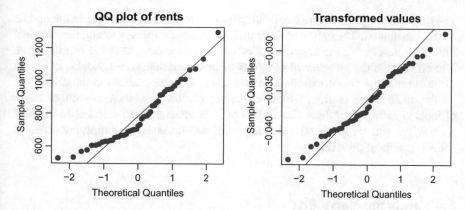

Figure 5.6 QQ plot of the original apartment rent values on left and power transformed with $\lambda = -1/2$ on the right

The QQ plot consists of a scatterplot of the paired values $(\widehat{x}_i, x_i)$. Ideally, this should appear as a straight line if the x_i were a "perfect" sample with all observations appearing exactly where we would expect them to be. In the QQ plot we should expect to see the greatest deviations from the straight line at its ends, partly because the sampled values at the extremes will have greater variability than those observations nearer to the center of the distribution.

An example of a QQ plot for the rent data appears in Fig. 5.6. The plot on the left is for the raw data. The graph on the right is of the transformed data raised to the power $\lambda = -1/2$. This was the power we decided was best in the histogram plots of Fig. 5.5.

In **R** we draw a QQ plot for data in y with the code

```
qqplot(y)
qqline(y)
```

The qqplot() command produces the data plot, and the qqlines() command adds the diagonal line as a useful visual reference. The line is drawn between the first and third quartiles of the observed data. The quartiles divide the observed data into four equal sized groups so 1/4 of the data values are below the first quartile and 1/4 are above the third quartile. The qqplot() statement accepts the options pch=, cex=, and col= to control the plot character, its size, and its color.

The QQ plot of the original rent values on the left half of Fig. 5.6 shows that the lower (left) tail is short relative to where the normal distribution would expect it. The sample in the first quartile is higher than the line anticipates, and the lower tail is not as spread out as it should be if the data more closely followed a normal distribution. The upper (right) tail looks about correct for the original data values.

The QQ plot for the $\lambda = -1/2$ transformed data on the right half of Fig. 5.6 follows the line more closely but both the upper and lower tails of this transformed distribution are slightly shorter than what the normal distribution would anticipate.

The center of this plot shows a small bump indicative of the bimodal gap in the middle of the distribution. The center of the transformed values appears to hug the diagonal line more closely, but the upper tail does not have as good a fit as the original data. The extremes of the sample will generally be more variable, so we should not expect the tails to follow the normal model as closely as the observations in the center.

To conclude this section, the power transformation gives us a continuous range of tools to reshape our data. The choice of λ is more art than science. In the next section, we will try to quantify the degree of non-normality by applying different statistical tests to the data.

5.4   Tests for Normality

There are many ways in which the data can appear non-normal. Similarly, there are a wide range of tests of normality we can apply. Each of these looks for a different deviation from the normal model. Using the words of hypothesis testing, the null hypothesis of the data has been sampled from a normal population, but there are many possible deviations from this model to consider as alternative hypotheses. Similarly, we need to know what attributes of the normal distribution are being examined in each test. The **R** libraries `fBasics` and `nortest` provide a number of useful tests of normality. In this section, we will review a few of these.

Begin with a random sample $x = (x_1, \ldots, x_n)$ with sample mean $\bar{x}$. The simplest and most intuitive test available examines the observed and expected histograms. Suppose we cut up the real line into a small number of non-overlapping intervals. Then we count the number of observations falling into each of these categories, just as we would when constructing a histogram. The theoretical normal distribution also provides the number of counts expected in each of these intervals. Finally, the observed and expected counts can be combined in a Pearson[4] chi-squared statistic.

If obs_i and exp_i are the observed and expected counts in the i-th interval then

$$\sum_i (\mathrm{obs}_i - \mathrm{exp}_i)^2/\mathrm{exp}_i$$

is the Pearson chi-squared statistic.

The `pchiTest` test in the `fBasics` library does the calculations for this test, including the p-value obtained from the corresponding chi-squared reference distribution. (This test is also available as `pearson.test` in the `nortest` library.) The default number of categories chosen by this method is the largest integer in $2n^{4/5}$ so the number of interval categories[5] increases almost in proportion to the sample size. There are options in the test allowing you to vary the number of categories.

---

[4] Karl Pearson (1857–1936). British historian, lawyer, and mathematician.

[5] There is mathematical theory to suggesting $n^{4/5}$ is about the correct number of categories needed when drawing a histogram. See Tapia and Thompson (1978, p 53) for details on this.

The cutpoints of the intervals are chosen so each interval has the same expected number of counts. See Exercise 5.8 for an example of how this is done.

Here is an example of the use of the Pearson test. Consider the original apartment rents we examined in Sect. 5.3 as a candidate for transformation:

```
> library(fBasics)
> pchiTest(housing$Apartment,
+          description="Original apartment values")

Title:
  Pearson Chi-Square Normality Test

Test Results:
  PARAMETER:
    Number of Classes: 10
  STATISTIC:
    P: 12.7255
  P VALUE:
    Adjusted: 0.07909
    Not adjusted: 0.1754

Description:
  Original apartment values
```

In this case, 10 interval categories are examined and two different methods for calculating the reference p-values. The adjusted p-values (adjusted for small sample sizes) provide a small amount of evidence to reject the null hypothesis of an underlying normal population. Ideally, the next step would be to examine the frequencies in each of the ten categories to see where the lack of fit occurs. See Exercises 5.8 and 5.9 for more detail on this test of the normal distribution for the transformed apartment rent data.

Let us examine a different test of the normal distribution based on higher moments of the sampled data. The *Jarque–Bera test* examines the third and fourth moments of the sampled data. The *skewness* of the sample is defined by the third moment about the sample mean:

$$\widehat{\gamma_3} = \text{skewness} = n^{-1} \sum (x_i - \overline{x})^3 / \text{var}(\boldsymbol{x})^{3/2} .$$

Skewness measures asymmetry of the sampling distribution. The skewness should have a value near zero for normally distributed data. Values far from zero indicate that the data was sampled from an asymmetric distribution. Positive skewness means the right, upper tail of the data is longer than the left tail.

The *kurtosis*

$$\widehat{\gamma_4} = \text{Kurtosis} = n^{-1} \sum (x_i - \overline{x})^4 / \text{var}(\boldsymbol{x})^2 - 3$$

is the fourth moment of the data, centered about its mean.

There is a "3" in the definition of kurtosis because in the normal distribution, the fourth central moment is $3\sigma^4$. Positive or negative values of the kurtosis indicate the tails of the sampling distribution are longer (heavier) or shorter (lighter), respectively, than a normal distribution. A large positive kurtosis may also indicate the presence of outliers in the data. Similarly, a negative kurtosis may be the result of the truncation of extremes in the data. Skewness and kurtosis may be computed in **R** on data using functions of the same name in the fBasics library.

The Jarque–Bera statistic

$$JB = n/6 \left(\text{skewness}^2 - \text{kurtosis}^2/4 \right)$$

provides a test of the normal distribution by combining both the skewness and kurtosis for a data sample. (Jarque and Bera 1987)

This statistic behaves as chi-squared with 2df under the null hypothesis of normally distributed data. Statistically, large values of JB are indicative of a poor fit for the normal distribution. In **R**, the jbTest() function calculates the value of the JB statistic and provides the corresponding p-value of the reference chi-squared statistic. This function is part of the fBasics library.

As an example of the use of this test, let us look at the apartment rents. The following examines the original, untransformed values and gives the **R** output:

```
> library(fBasics)
> jbTest(housing$Apartment,
+        title="Original apartment rents")

Title:
 Original apartment rents

Test Results:
  PARAMETER:
    Sample Size: 51
  STATISTIC:
    LM: 5.499
    ALM: 6.3
  P VALUE:
    LM p-value: 0.043
    ALM p-value: 0.053
    Asymptotic: 0.064
```

The jbTest() calculates both a finite sample (LM) and asymptotic (ALM) version of the JB statistic as well as their corresponding p-values. In this example, the three p-values are close in value to indicate a consensus of methods and small enough for us to question the adequacy of the fit of the normal distribution.

Let us run this test again on the transformed apartment rents using the transformation we found in Sect. 5.3. The **R** code and output in part are as follows:

```
> jbTest(-housing$Apartment^(-1/2),
+        title="Transformed apartment rents")

    .    .    .

    P VALUE:
      LM p-value: 0.29
      ALM p-value: 0.331
      Asymptotic: 0.429
```

The three p-values given here provide good evidence of data sampled from a normal population. This is quantitative evidence of the benefit of transforming these data values. See also Exercise 5.9.

The *Kolmogorov–Smirnov test*[6,7] is a nonparametric examination of the cumulative distribution function. This test compares the maximum difference between the cumulative distribution function of the data with the theoretical normal distribution. Intuitively, this statistic measures how far the cumulative, ordered data values are from where we would expect them to appear. This is similar to the visual inspection we apply when we perform the QQ-plot as in Fig. 5.6 except it only measures the largest vertical difference between the ordered data and the fitted straight line.

In **R**, this test expects the data values to be standardized with respect to the mean and standard deviation. Here is an example, again examining the apartment rents:

```
> z <- housing$Apartment
> z <- ( z -mean(z)) / sd(z)
> ksnormTest(z)

Title:
 One-sample Kolmogorov-Smirnov test

Test Results:
  STATISTIC:
    D: 0.1597
  P VALUE:
    Alternative Two-Sided: 0.1484
    Alternative       Less: 0.5633
    Alternative    Greater: 0.07421
```

The test method provides three p-values for alternative hypotheses, and the largest difference of the two distribution functions are either one- or two-sided. Unless we have strong *a priori* concerns, the two-sided alternative hypothesis is the preferred approach. In this example, none of these three p-values indicates a large deviation from the normal distribution.

The *Shapiro–Wilk* test statistic is

---

[6] Andrey Nikolaevich Kolmogorov (1903–1987). Soviet mathematician and probabilist.

[7] Nikolai Vasil'evich Smirnov (1900–1966). Soviet probabilist.

$$W = \left(\sum a_i x_{(i)} \right)^2 \Big/ \text{std dev}(x)$$

where a_i are constants depending only on the sample size (Shapiro and Wilk 1965).[8,9]

The $x_{(i)}$ are the ordered data values $x_{(1)} \le x_{(2)} \le \cdots \le x_{(n)}$. As with the Kolmogorov–Smirnov test, this statistic also measures how far the ordered data values are from where we would expect them to appear. Informally, the Shapiro–Wilk test examines how far the observed data deviate from the QQ plot and the Kolmogorov–Smirnov test examined the maximum difference in the QQ plot, measured on a vertical scale.

The `shapiro.test()` in **R** provides a formal p-value for the W statistic. Here is an example of its use:

```
> shapiro.test(housing$Apartment)

        Shapiro-Wilk normality test

data:   housing$Apartment
W = 0.9346, p-value = 0.007472

> shapiro.test(-housing$Apartment^(-1/2))

        Shapiro-Wilk normality test

data:   -housing$Apartment^(-1/2)
W = 0.9737, p-value = 0.3136
```

The first of these two tests shows a large discrepancy between the original apartment rent data and a normal distribution. The second use of the `shapiro.test` demonstrates how much better the transformed values follow the normal distribution.

As we have shown in the past two sections, there are tests for normality and transformations to make our data look more normal. We point out this exercise in transforming and testing is not the final goal. Usually, our interest is in inference made on the data using some statistical method depending on a normal distribution for its validity. The motivation for testing normality, then, is our inference requires it, but normality is not an end unto itself.

But if this is indeed the case, then we should not be asking if our data are normally distributed. The real question is whether our data are close enough to the normal distribution in order to obtain valid statistical inference. Instead, we need to question the sensitivity of the statistical method to the assumptions of normality. Simulation methods in **R** are ideal for addressing such issues. Simulation methods are discussed in Sects. 2.2 and 2.6.

---

[8] Samuel Sanford Shapiro (1930–till date) American statistician and engineer.

[9] Martin Bradbury Wilk (1922–2013) Canadian statistician and former Chief Statistician of Canada.

5.5 Inference on Univariate Normal Means

In this section, we want to describe statistical inference on the population parameter μ. Given a random sample $x_1, x_2, \ldots, x_n$ from a univariate normal distribution with mean μ and variance σ^2.

The sample average $\overline{x}$ is

$$\overline{x} = n^{-1} \sum_i x_i$$

is used to estimate μ.

The standard error of $\overline{x}$ is $\sigma/\sqrt{n}$. This standard error would be ideal, except σ is rarely known in practice and needs to be estimated. The usual point estimate for σ^2 is

$$s^2 = (n - 1)^{-1} \sum (x_i - \overline{x})^2 . \tag{5.8}$$

In Sect. 5.6, we will describe inference on σ^2.

For a long while, researchers would substitute the value s for the unknown σ and treat $\overline{x}/(s/\sqrt{n})$ as normally distributed. Gosset[10] pointed out the appropriate distribution while working at the Guinness Brewery in Dublin. His work was considered a trade secret so he published it in 1908 under the pen name "Student," leading to the present name of "Student's t-distribution."

The distribution of $\overline{x}/(s/\sqrt{n})$ is Student's t with $n - 1$ df if the underlying observed values $x_1, x_2, \ldots, x_n$ are sampled from a standard normal distribution. Figure 5.7 plots the Student t-distribution for 1, 2, 5, and 10df and compares these to a standard normal distribution. The lower df distributions have much longer tails than the normal, and above 10df, these distributions are indistinguishable from the normal. The normal distribution corresponds to the t-distribution with infinitely many df.

We can now discuss inference on the mean μ of a normal population. There are three important forms of statistical inference we can draw: a confidence interval of μ, a hypothesis test whether μ is equal to a specified value, and equality of means sampled from two different populations. A good way to illustrate these is to have **R** generate a random sample of normally distributed data for us.

In **R** we can generate standard normal variates and find their sample average, estimated variance, and standard deviation as in the dialog:

```
> sample <- rnorm(6)
> sample

[1] -1.0763316  0.1058763 -2.3284413  1.1132752  0.4492566 -1.1717192

> mean(sample)

[1] -0.4846807
```

---

[10] William Sealy Gosset (1876–1937). British mathematician.

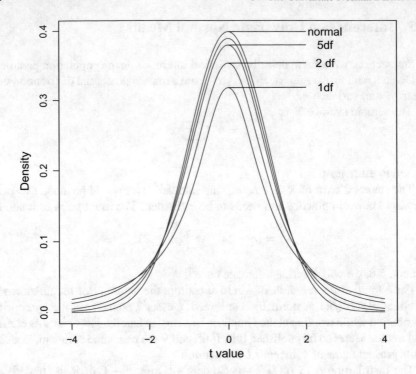

Figure 5.7 Density of normal and Student's t with 1,2,5, and 10df

```
> var(sample)

[1] 1.599197

> sd(sample)

[1] 1.264594
```

The one sample t.test program for this sampled data

```
> t.test(sample)

        One Sample t-test

data:  sample
t = -0.9388, df = 5, p-value = 0.3909
alternative hypothesis: true mean is not equal to 0
95 percent confidence interval:
 -1.811790  0.842429
sample estimates:
 mean of x
-0.4846807
```

calculates a 95% confidence interval for the normal population mean μ and tests the hypothesis whether μ is equal to zero. In this present sample, there is no evidence against this hypothesis. Your values will be different every time you run this example.

To test other hypotheses about μ you can specify a known value for the null hypothesis, as in this example

```
> t.test(sample, mu=2)

          One Sample t-test

data:  sample
t = -4.8128, df = 5, p-value = 0.004829
alternative hypothesis: true mean is not equal to 2
95 percent confidence interval:
 -1.811790  0.842429
sample estimates:
 mean of x
-0.4846807
```

in which the small p-value .0048 shows that there is little evidence μ is equal to 2.

The third important form of inference concerns the comparison of means from two different populations. So for example,

```
> sample2 <- rnorm(5) + 1.5
[1] -0.5277086  2.5294779  3.0055344  2.9060771  3.2043778
```

generates a sample with a population mean of 1.5.

The corresponding two-sample t-test of equality of population means

```
> t.test(sample, sample2)

          Welch Two Sample t-test
s      data:  sample and sample2
t = -3.1238, df = 7.735, p-value = 0.01476
alternative hypothesis: true difference in means is not equal to 0
95 percent confidence interval:
 -4.7194790 -0.6969859
sample estimates:
 mean of x  mean of y
-0.4846807  2.2235518
```

produces a relatively small p-value (.014) providing evidence the two population means are not equal. The 95% confidence interval is of the *difference* of the two population means. The Welch[11] t-test is a modification of the usual t-test accommodating unequal population variances by introducing fractional df.

Let us use the t.test function to simulate the behavior of the univariate confidence interval. Specifically, Output 5.1 generates 50 different normal random samples and finds a (univariate) 95% confidence interval of the mean of each sample. In

---

[11] Bernard Lewis Welch (1911–1989). English statistician.

Output 5.1 Program to produce Fig. 5.8 of simulated univariate confidence intervals for a normal mean

```
reps <- 50                  # number of intervals to generate
sim.mean <- 2               # true population mean
cover <- 0                  # count of coverage of true value
ints <- NULL                # start a list of intervals
for (i in 1 : reps)         # generate the confidence intervals
  {
    int <- t.test(rnorm(25, mean = sim.mean, sd = 5))$conf.int[1 : 2]
    ints <- rbind(ints, int)
    if(int[1] <= sim.mean &&
       int[2] >= sim.mean) cover <- cover + 1
  }
ints                        # print these intervals
cover <- cover / reps
cover                       # percent coverage of true values

pdf(file = "simCI.pdf")     # capture graphics in file
op <- par(mfrow = c(1, 2))# side-by side plots

plot(0,0, xlim = c(min(ints[ , 1]) - .5, max(ints[ , 2]) + .5),
    ylim = c(0, reps), type = "n", ylab = "Simulation number",
    xlab = "Confidence interval") # create an empty frame
for (i in 1 : reps)             # plot the intervals
  {
    lines(ints[i, ], c(i, i), col = rainbow(6)[4], lwd = 3.5)
    points(ints[i, ], c(i, i), col = "red", pch = 16, cex = .5)
  }
lines(rep(sim.mean, 2), c( -5, reps + 5), lty = 3, col = "blue")

lengths <- ints[ , 2] - ints[ , 1]
hist(lengths, xlab = "Lengths of intervals",
   main = " ", breaks = 10, col = rainbow(7)[5])

dev.off()                   # return to R graphics window
par(op)                     # reset plotting option
```

Fig. 5.8, we plot each of the confidence intervals and provide a histogram of their lengths.

In each of the 50 samples, the observed mean and standard deviations will vary, producing intervals of different lengths and centered at different places. The location of the true population mean is indicated with a dotted line, but of course, this value would not be known to us in practice. The confidence intervals include the true value in 98% of these fifty samples, which is close to the claimed coverage rate of 95%. Fig. 5.8 also includes a histogram of the lengths of these intervals.

The use of Fig. 5.8 is to help interpret confidence intervals, in general. This is an awkward concept to explain and can only be interpreted in the context of many repeated samples from the same population. The data is random, and so the endpoints of the confidence interval are as well. We will never know the true population mean, but with repeated sampling from the population, these random intervals are

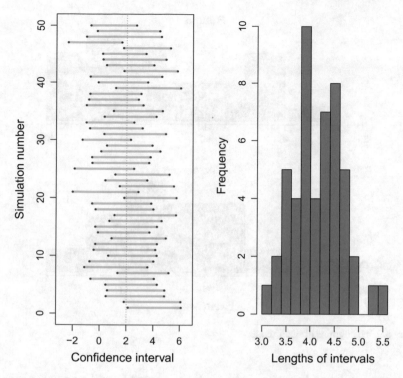

Figure 5.8 Simulated confidence intervals of a normal mean. The program in Output 5.1 produces this figure

Table 5.1 Mathematics examination scores, by gender

Women	Men
94 90 96 73 71 75 52	77 57 79 65 68 65 55
86 93 86 50 30 46 36	72 66 29 69 85 82 43
82 55 75 47 80 92 56	60 64 82 91 51 60 76
43 77 63 76 67 99 93	43 82 87 32 71 77 77
75 90 92 88 76 61 77	79 97 56
49 67 81 89 88 42 51	
58 98 46 96 90 46 50	
67 83 85	

Source Sullivan (2008).

constructed in such a way they should cover the true value 95% of the time. Unfortunately, we usually only observe one sample from the population so the single observed confidence interval will either cover the true value or not. We cannot correctly talk about a probability associated with this single interval. The confidence interval is only associated with repeated sampling from the population.

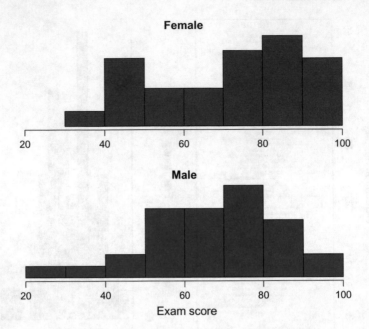

Figure 5.9 Histograms of math scores

Let us complete this section with a real-data example. Sullivan (2008) gives the data in Table 5.1 of the mathematics scores of a group of men and women. These were students in an elementary algebra course, enrolled at a community college over two semesters.

A good place to begin is to look at the separate histograms, given in Table 5.9. Even though we see in this figure the male students have a wider range, the women students have a larger standard deviation of values: 19.0 for women and 16.5 for men. One explanation for this discrepancy is more women students had values at the extremes of their range but few males scored near their endpoints.

Another good first step is to check for normality using the QQ plot described in Sect. 5.4. The QQ plots in Fig. 5.10 confirm the deviations from normality, apparent in Fig 5.9. Specifically, the female observations have shorter tails than would be expected under a theoretical normal sample. This does not look too deviant to question the assumption of normally distributed data. The values of the male students look closer to a normal sample. No outliers are apparent in either male or female data.

These tests do not indicate problems with the normal distribution assumptions, so we can proceed and test the hypothesis of equality of population means:

```
> t.test(score[sex == female], score[sex == male])

        Welch Two Sample t-test
```

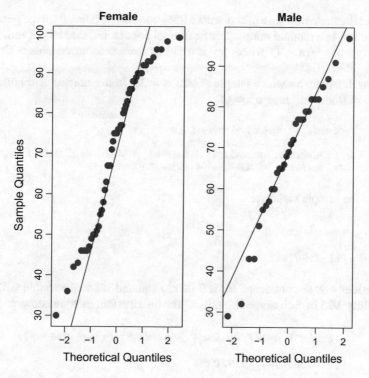

Figure 5.10 QQ plots of math scores

```
data:  score[sex == female] and score[sex == male]
t = 1.0226, df = 70.327, p-value = 0.31
alternative hypothesis: true difference in means is not equal to 0
95 percent confidence interval:
 -3.845393 11.939686
sample estimates:
mean of x mean of y
 71.69231  67.64516
```

The female students have a larger average score than the males. The p-value of .31 gives us no evidence the population means are different from each other.

We next examine statistical inference on the normal variance parameter.

5.6 Inference on Variances

As we did in Sect. 5.5, let us begin by assuming we have a random sample $x_1, x_2, \ldots, x_n$ from a normal distribution with mean μ and variance σ^2. The variance is estimated by s^2 given at (5.8) and this is calculated using the var() function in **R**.

Let us illustrate how we can construct a 95% confidence interval for the population variance σ^2. In a random sample from a normal population, the sample variance s^2 behaves as $\sigma^2 \chi^2/(n-1)$ where χ^2 is a chi-squared random variable with $n-1$ df.

Let us illustrate this with a sample of size $n = 10$ from a normal distribution with mean $\mu = 0$ and variance $\sigma^2 = 6$:

```
> (sample <- sqrt(6) * rnorm(10))

[1]   5.8661171   0.3683464   0.8060940   0.1836058  -1.6013981   2.2258245
[7]   0.6948691  -0.2916154  -4.9956032  -1.8808992
```

and find the sample variance:

```
> var(sample)

[1] 7.957982
```

Consider a 95% confidence for a 9 df chi-squared random variable with equal probability .025 in each of the two tails of the distribution. In **R** we compute this as

```
> (chis95 <- c( qchisq(.975, 9), qchisq(.025, 9)))

[1] 19.022768  2.700389
```

so the 95% confidence interval for σ^2 from our sample is then

```
> 9 * var(sample) / chis95

[1]   3.765059 26.522781
```

We can also construct a *one-sided confidence interval* for σ^2 with all of the uncertainty at one end:

```
> (chis05 <- qchisq(.95, 9))

[1] 16.91898
```

so the one-sided 95% confidence interval for σ^2 is all values greater than

```
> 9 * var(sample) / chis05

[1] 4.233225
```

so all of the uncertainty is expressed at the lower estimate for σ^2.

Exercise 2.5 describes several tests available in **R** for testing the equality of variances in different populations. These include the bartlett.test() test. Other tests of equality of variances available in **R** are var.test(), flinger.test(), ansari.test(), and mood.test(). Use the help() file to read about these tests.

5.7 Maximum Likelihood Estimation, Part I

In this section, we want to introduce a very general process of parameter estimation and show how we can do this in **R**. We start with a simple example: estimating the mean and standard deviation from a normal sample. The reason for this apparent backward motion is to become familiar with a new method when the answer is already well known to us. Then we can use the new method and advance to more difficult problems where the solution is not obvious.

Let's begin by generating a random sample from the normal distribution with a specified mean and standard deviation:

```
> z <- rnorm(25, mean = 5, sd = 10)
> z[1 : 5]

[1]   3.861693   9.953657 14.686397 17.601439 -8.863527

> mean(z)

[1] 3.949079

> sd(z)

[1] 10.33858
```

This example generates 25 random values from a normal population with mean 5 and standard deviation 10 using the rnorm function. This function is previously described in Sect. 5.1, but notice how we are now using the mean= and sd= options. The mean() and sd() functions return the average and standard deviation of the sample. These are not the population values, of course, but are within sampling error of the true values. (It would take an extremely large sample to obtain the population parameters.)

Now suppose we didn't know how to estimate the mean and standard deviation and **R** did not include these functions to make it so easy for us. To estimate these parameters, we will need to introduce two important principles: (1) the likelihood of the data and (2) estimate the parameters using those values to maximize this likelihood function.

The *likelihood* of a normal observation is the density function $\phi(z \mid \mu, \sigma)$ given at (5.2). The likelihood function is evaluated using the dnorm() function in **R**. Different likelihood functions will be used for different statistical distributions and models, but we will stay with this example for now.

The observations z_i are independent in this example so the *joint likelihood* is the product of the individual likelihood functions:

$$\phi(z \mid \mu, \sigma) = \prod_i \phi(z_i \mid \mu, \sigma) \qquad (5.9)$$

The principle of *maximum likelihood* directs us to find the values of μ and σ maximizing this quantity. On one level this may seem counterintuitive because Figs. 5.1 and 5.2 seem to suggest the parameters μ and σ are fixed and only z varies in ϕ. We now need to think about the likelihood function differently and consider the observed data z as fixed. That is, we are fixing the data values in ϕ and letting the parameters vary.

Intuitively, the likelihood tells us how likely the observed data was to be observed. Maximum likelihood estimates are those parameter values making the observed data as likely to occur as possible. In words, the observations are all we have in order to estimate parameters. Maximizing the likelihood is a method to make the observed data look as good as possible. Such parameter estimates are called *maximum likelihood estimates* and are frequently abbreviated *mle's*.

Next we need to find values of μ and σ to maximize $\phi(z \mid \mu, \sigma)$. Notice the data in z remains the same, while the parameters μ and σ are meant to vary. We can evaluate the likelihood for z at any given parameter values using the dnorm() function in **R**. This is best performed as a function. (We discuss writing functions in **R** in Sect. 2.5).

The function

```
lik <- function(parm) prod( dnorm(z, mean = parm[1], sd = parm[2]))
```

of a single, vector-valued argument evaluates the normal likelihood given at (5.9). The data in z is external and is understood by the function.

The vector argument to the lik function is a 2-tuple consisting of the mean and the standard deviation. We can evaluate it at the known, true parameter values

```
> lik(c(5,10))
```

```
[1] 2.468186e-41
```

and see the value of the likelihood near its maximum is an extremely small number.

The reason the likelihood is so small (about 2×10^{-41}) is each term $\phi(z_i)$ in (5.9) is smaller than 1, and some of these terms can be quite small. Multiplying these together results in a very small number. A problem with working with the likelihood, then, is in sufficiently large sample sizes, the likelihood can be an extremely small number and **R** might round this number down to zero.

A useful way to avoid such extreme numbers is to take the *logarithm* of the likelihood function. The resulting log-likelihood

$$\Lambda(\mu, \sigma) = \log\{\phi(z \mid \mu, \sigma)\} = \log\left\{\prod_i \phi(z_i \mid \mu, \sigma)\right\} = \sum_i \log\{\phi(z_i \mid \mu, \sigma)\}$$

$$(5.10)$$

is much easier to work with because it consists of *sums* of terms, rather than a *product* of terms. (Throughout this book, we always take logarithms to the base $e = 2.718\ldots$)

The corresponding log-likelihood in (5.10) is calculated by the **R** function

```
llik <- function(parm) sum( dnorm(z, mean = parm[1],
        sd = parm[2], log = TRUE ))
```

using the `log = TRUE` option in `dnorm`.

We then evaluate this function

```
llik(c(5, 10))

[1] -93.5025
```

and obtain a more useful number. The log-likelihood is a negative number because it represents the log of a fraction.

Is it acceptable to use the log of a function we are maximizing rather than the original function itself? Taking logs is a reasonable approach because the maximum of the function will also occur at the same place its logarithm is maximized. There are several reasons for using the logarithm as we will see. In statistical practice, when we talk about the likelihood function, we almost always mean the *log* of the likelihood so we often forget to use the word *log* in writing and speaking. See Exercise 5.3 for more on this example.

Next, let's have a look at this log-likelihood function. Fig. 5.11 illustrates the log-likelihood function $\Lambda(\mu, \sigma)$ in (5.10). This figure is plotted using the code given in Output 5.2. This code uses the `persp` function which plots three-dimensional objects with options for different perspectives and shading.

The perspective plot of the log-likelihood $\Lambda(\mu, \sigma)$ is given in Fig. 5.11. This figure shows us the log-likelihood Λ is a function of the parameters θ and σ. There is a clear single maximum in these two parameters, and then the log-likelihood falls off as we move away from its maximum. In Exercise 5.3 we find the exact mathematical expressions for the location of this maximum.

How do we use **R** to find the estimates of the mean and standard deviation parameters to maximize the log-likelihood? The `nlm` program is a very handy program, and we will make repeated use of it. Given a function of several variables and a reasonable set of starting values for the parameters, `nlm` will numerically locate the maximum as well as approximate the first and second derivatives at this minimum. (The `nlm` function was introduced in Sect. 2.7.)

The `nlm` program was written to find the *minimum*, but we are interested in finding a *maximum*. We work around this by defining the *negative log-likelihood*:

```
nll <- function(par)        # negative, normal log-likelihood
```

Output 5.2 Code to produce Fig. 5.11

```
trange <- seq(from = 0, to = 10, length = 25) # range of theta
srange <- seq(from = 6, to = 14, length = 25) # range of sigma
drawll <- function(th,sig)                       # the log-likelihood
    {
      sum(dnorm(z, mean = th, sd = sig, log = TRUE))
    }
# evaluate the log-likelihood at every pair of parameter values
zvals <- matrix(0, length(trange), length(srange))
for (i in 1 : length(trange))
    { for (j in 1 : length(srange))
      { zvals[i, j] <- drawll(trange[i], srange[j])
    } }

persp( x = trange, y = srange, z = zvals, cex.lab = 1.2,
       zlim=c(min(zvals), max(zvals) + .5),
       xlab = "mean", ylab = "std deviation",
       zlab = "Log likelihood", col = rainbow(6)[3],
       axes = TRUE, box = TRUE, theta = -30, shade = .3)
```

Figure 5.11 The
log-likelihood
function (5.10)

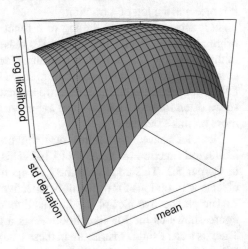

```
-sum(dnorm(z, mean = par[1], sd = par[2], log = TRUE))
```

which will be minimized.

As with the `llik` function, this function calculates the negative log-likelihood function. It is defined by a vector of arguments representing the two parameters to be estimated. The first, `parm[1]` is the mean, and the standard deviation is `parm[2]`.

The `nlm` program is invoked with the name of the function followed by a set of reasonable starting values:

```
nlm(nll, c(10, 15))   # call nlm with neg log-lik and initial values
```

The output from this program contains the minimum of the negative log-likelihood, estimates of where this occurs, estimated gradient, the number of iterations it took, and finally, an error message:

```
$minimum
[1] 90.06128

$estimate
[1] 7.127638 8.877439

$gradient
[1] 1.870154e-06 5.884479e-06

$code
[1] 1

$iterations
[1] 11

Warning messages:
1: In dnorm(x, mean, sd, log) : NaNs produced
```

Let's explain this output in reverse order, beginning with the error message. The nlm program looks for a function minimum and tries many different parameter values in order to get there. The program does not know the standard deviation must be a positive number and may have tried something invalid in its search. This produced several error messages along the way.

The $gradient is a numerical estimate of the first derivatives in each of the two directions of μ and σ. These values are both very close to zero. This is a good indication the extreme of the function has been achieved. Intuitively, we are at the top of the mountain when the landscape is flat in every direction.

The $estimate is the set of parameter values maximizing the log-likelihood (and minimize the negative log-likelihood). The first of this pair is exactly the same as the sample mean (7.127638) except possibly differing in the last digit.

The sample standard deviation (9.060493) and the maximum likelihood estimate of σ (8.877439) are noticeably different, however. The difference is explained in Exercise 5.3. Briefly, the usual estimate of the sample variance s^2 given at (5.8) divides the summation by $n - 1$ but the maximum likelihood estimate of σ^2 divides by n. That is, the maximum likelihood estimator of σ^2 is

$$\text{maximum likelihood estimator}(\sigma^2) = n^{-1} \sum (z_i - \overline{z})^2 \qquad (5.11)$$

and not the more familiar $n - 1$ denominator given by s^2 at (5.8). In other words, these two estimates of σ should differ by a factor of $\{n/(n - 1)\}^{1/2}$.

In Sect. 2.7, we showed how to capture the output from nlm. This ability allows us to use portions of the output in subsequent steps of **R**. For example, we may want to use the values of the parameter estimates in later steps.

In such simple examples as the estimation of the mean and standard deviation, the mathematics and computer output confirm each other. We will continue the discussion of maximum likelihood estimation in Sect. 6.5. We will end this section with a numerical method and will bring us to more complicated examples where the mathematics can become burdensome and the answer may not be known in advance.

In this next example, suppose we have data from a normal distribution and want to estimate the *ratio* of the mean to the standard deviation. That is, the (positive valued) normal mean is denoted by $\mu > 0$ and the standard deviation obeys the relationship

$$\sigma = \alpha\mu$$

for some parameter $\alpha > 0$ we also need to estimate. This example might arise in a setting where larger values of the mean are associated with less precise measurements such as where the *relative error* (α) remains the same.

In this example, we need to estimate the parameters α and μ. It is not obvious what the analytic form of the maximum likelihood estimates is without resorting to calculus. The point of this exercise, then, is to tackle a problem which would otherwise be difficult for us to solve without the help of **R**.

The negative, log-likelihood function for this model

```
prop <- function(par)                # negative log-likelihood
      -sum(dnorm(z, mean = par[1],
         sd = par[1] * par[2], log = TRUE ))
```

is a function of two parameters: par[1] is the mean μ and par[2] is the parameter α.

We can then generate some random data values for this problem and use nlm to fit the model:

```
(z <- rnorm(50, mean = 10, sd = 20)) # generate some data
nlm( prop, c( 5,5))                  # maximize with starting values
```

In this example, we generate 50 normal variates with known mean ($\mu = 10$) and standard deviation ($\sigma = 20$) so the true ratio α is equal to 2. The nlm function minimizes the negative log-likelihood, based on initial starting values of 5 for μ and 5 for α. Usually, our starting values for nlm are just good guesses in the neighborhood of the answer. You might try other starting values to see how well nlm works, and perhaps, whether it works at all. See Exercise 5.6 for more details.

A portion of the output from `nlm` includes the following:

```
$minimum
[1] 218.96

$estimate
[1] 9.090690 2.123380

$gradient
[1] -1.067062e-05 -4.542913e-05
```

The estimates are then $\widehat{\mu} = 9.09$ and $\widehat{\alpha} = 2.12$. Both of these estimates are reasonably close to the population values of 10 and 2, respectively. The two gradient values are close to zero indicating good convergence to an extreme minimum of the negative log-likelihood.

There are also error messages, omitted here, indicating attempts by `nlm` to fit the log-likelihood function where it is not defined, specifically where a trial value of the standard deviation $\sigma = \alpha\mu$ might be a negative number. Sometimes `nlm` gets caught in these invalid regions and never seems to get out. One way to avoid this situation is for us to start with reasonable initial values in the search for maximum likelihood estimates. Again, see Exercise 5.6 for guidance.

In conclusion, in this section we showed how we can write programs in **R** allowing us to fit mathematical models unlike those we might see in a textbook. This is an important skill for the data analyst because it opens a much wider range of models to consider as we explore data. In Sect. 6.5 we examine other properties of maximum likelihood estimation in **R** including hypothesis testing of parameter values and approximating the standard errors of the estimated parameters. In Sect. 7.4, we use maximum likelihood to fit different models and compare these in terms of a formal test of hypothesis. This test of hypothesis allows us to compare different models of the covariance matrix in a multivariate normal distribution.

5.8 Exercises

5.1 Consider some data such as the apartment rent values or the CD4 counts. Transform these values to more normal-looking distributions using the Box-Cox transformation (5.5) for different values of λ. Find the value of λ providing the best fit according to the Jarque–Bera test, the Kolmogorov–Smirnov test, or the Shapiro–Wilk test. Are these different λ's close in value? Explain why this may (or not) be the case.

5.2 a. If u is distributed as uniform between 0 and 1, what is the distribution of the normal quantile x satisfying the equation $\Phi(x) = u$?

b. In an ordered sample $u_1 \le u_2 \le \cdots \le u_n$ of n observations sampled from a uniform distribution on $(0,1)$, intuitively, where would we expect these values to appear? Use this result to motivate the use of (5.6).

5.3 a. Use the functional form of ϕ given at (5.2) and find a mathematical expression for the likelihood function (5.9).

   b. Find a mathematical expression for the log of the likelihood.

   c. Show the maximum likelihood estimate of σ^2 of the normal log-likelihood is achieved at (5.11). Notice how this expression for the estimate of σ^2 differs from the usual estimate s^2 of the sample variance given at (5.8). The estimator s^2 has the property of being *unbiased*. Explain how, with large samples, it should not matter which of these two estimators we use.

5.4 The Poisson[12] distribution is defined on non-negative integers. In the Poisson distribution, the mean is equal to its variance. If X has a Poisson distribution with mean $\lambda > 0$ then

$$\Pr[\, X = j \,] = e^{-\lambda} \lambda^j / j! \tag{5.12}$$

for $j = 0, 1, \ldots$.

   a. Use `rpois(25, lambda=10)` to generate a sample of 25 observations from a Poisson distribution with mean 10.

   Examine the QQ plot and test these data for normality. Repeat this exercise using larger and/or small Poisson means. Comment on what you see. Confirm when the mean λ is large, then the Poisson distribution is very similar to the normal.

   b. Program the Poisson likelihood (5.12). Use `nlm` to obtain the maximum likelihood estimate of the single parameter λ for a sample of Poisson observations.

   c. What is the functional form of the one parameter normal distribution when the mean and the variance are equal?

   d. Program the likelihood of the one parameter normal distribution you found in part c. Use `nlm` to obtain the maximum likelihood estimate of the single parameter from the sample of Poisson observations you used in part b. How does this estimate compare with the estimate you obtained in part b?

   e. Use calculus to show the sample mean is the maximum likelihood estimator of λ in a Poisson sample. Does this agree with the estimate you obtained in part b?

   f. Use calculus to find a closed-form expression for the maximum likelihood estimator of the one parameter normal distribution in part c. Does this agree with the estimate obtained in part d?

---

[12] Siméon Denis Poisson (1781–1840). French mathematician and physicist.

5.5   a. Show the standard normal density function $\phi(x)$ is symmetric about $x = 0$. That is, show $\phi(x) = \phi(-x)$.

    b. Show $\phi(x \mid \mu, \sigma)$ is maximized in x at $x = \mu$. That is, the normal mean is also the mode.

    c. What does the cumulative normal distribution function $\Phi(x \mid \mu, \sigma)$ look like when σ becomes very large? What does this say about the distribution of samples from this population?

    d. What does Φ look like when σ is very small? Similarly, what does this suggest about samples from this distribution?

5.6   Try other starting values for the `nlm` program in Sect. 5.7 fitting a standard deviation proportional to the mean. What range of values provide reasonable answers with a relatively small number of iterations? Does your finding depend on the size of the normal sample `z`? What happens if you start with invalid parameter values, such as negative estimates of the standard deviation?

5.7   Consider the housing data examined in Sect. 2.3. Suppose the average apartment cost is expressible as a linear function of housing costs. That is,

$$\text{Apartment rent} = \alpha + \beta \text{ Housing cost} + \text{error}$$

for parameters (α, β) where the errors are normally distributed with mean zero and variance σ^2.

    a. Does this seem to be a reasonable model for the data? Refer to Fig. 3.7, for example, to make your case. Interpret this model in terms of real estate values in different states.

    b. Write a function in **R** to calculate the negative log-likelihood in terms of the three parameters (α, β, σ) for this model. Use `nlm` to obtain the maximum likelihood estimates of these parameters.

5.8   Find the cut off points of the categories of the `phiTest` of normality. Specifically, begin with a dataset and estimate the mean $\hat{\mu}$ and standard deviation $\hat{\sigma}$. The cut points defined at (5.7) for a standard normal distribution determine the limits of k categories with equal probabilities.

5.9   a. Examine the transformed apartment rents with $\lambda = -.5$ to see if this provides a better normal fit for these data.

    b. Find the value of λ providing the best transformation according to the Pearson test. Does this transformation yield a more normal-looking QQ plot than the one in Fig. 5.6?

    c. Similarly, find the power transformation value of λ yielding the best fit according to the Jarque–Bera test. Compare this value of λ to the value you obtained in part b.

5.10 Write a program in **R** to fit a model for normally distributed data in which the variance σ^2 is proportional to the squared mean μ^2. That is, $\sigma^2 = \alpha\mu^2$ for some $\alpha > 0$ to be estimated. To avoid any problems `nlm()` might run into, put a check in your program to verify α is a positive number. One way around this possible error is to express α as e^{θ} for an arbitrary value of θ.

5.11 The `hills` dataset in the `MASS` library in **R** contains the record times of foot races held in Scottish hills. Obtain the data by in **R** as a `data.frame` using

```
> library(MASS)
> hills

                dist climb    time
Greenmantle      2.5   650  16.083
Carnethy         6.0  2500  48.350
    .    .   .
Cockleroi        4.5   850  28.100
Moffat Chase    20.0  5000 159.833
```

For each of 35 hills, the dataset provides the length of the race, the gain in altitude, and the time of the winning runner in 1984.

a. Use **R** to find means and standard deviations of the distances, altitudes, and times. Are these useful summaries of these data? Do these measurements capture the multivariate character of the observations?

b. Why might you expect the distribution of race times, altitudes, and distances to be skewed?

c. Plot the data in **R** and verify this is indeed the case. See if transformations of the data provide more symmetric distributions. Use the `pairs()` display or other graphical methods described in Chap. 3 to help you make your point.

d. There was debate about whether the time value for Knock Hill should be 18.65 or 78.65. Which of these values do you think is the correct one? What statistical evidence can you provide?

Chapter 6
Bivariate Normal Distribution

T HE BIVARIATE NORMAL DISTRIBUTION helps us make the important leap from the univariate normal to the more general multivariate normal distribution. To accomplish this, we need to make the transition from the scalar univariate notation of the previous chapter to the matrix notation of the following chapter.

Let us begin with an exploration of the swiss data given in the data sets library of **R**. These data are a collection of six demographic variables from 47 French-speaking cantons (provinces) of Switzerland in 1888. At the time, Switzerland was undergoing a *demographic transition* from a time of high fertility rates to the lower rates more commonly associated with developed nations. The help(swiss) for these data in **R** contains more details on the other variables in this data set as well as links for additional data for other parts of Switzerland. This data set will be examined again in Exercise 11.7.

Consider the paired observations made on young men drafted into the army. Figure 6.1 contains a scatterplot of the 47 provinces, plotting the percentage of men who claimed agriculture as their principal occupation and the percentage of men with academic examination scores at the highest level. Every canton is represented by one observation in this figure. (The options for changing graphical output in the bivariate boxplot routine bvbox are discussed in Exercise 3.6.)

One way to think about these observations is as a cloud scattered in the figure. At the center of the cloud, observations are more densely gathered, resulting in a thicker fog. At the edges of the scatter plot, observations are more widely dispersed and less frequent. The concept of density of observations will be continued in this chapter and is more formally expressed in the bivariate normal density function given at (6.1), below. Figures 3.10 and 3.25 also use graphical methods to estimate the density of similar sets of observations.

There are several features worth noting in Fig. 6.1. Chief among these is the high degree of association we see: Cantons with lower levels of agriculture are more likely to have higher examination scores. In regression methods (Chap. 9), we try to explain the means of one set of variables from the values of others. In this example,

© Springer Nature Switzerland AG 2022
D. Zelterman, *Applied Multivariate Statistics with R*, Statistics for Biology and Health,
https://doi.org/10.1007/978-3-031-13005-2_6

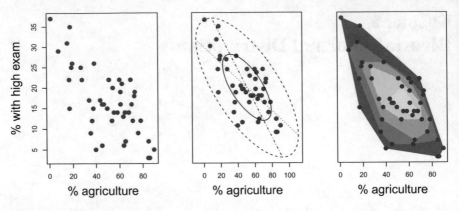

Figure 6.1 Scatterplot of percentage agriculture and high examination scores in 47 Swiss cantons. Data represented as raw scatterplot, bivariate boxplot, and as five-layer peeling convex hull

we cannot say one of these measurements directly causes the other. The examination scores and agriculture work appear to be negatively associated with each other. Both are probably the result of additional factors.

While there are attributes we can say about either agriculture or examination scores individually, the chief objective of multivariate analysis is to describe the *association* between these two measurements. In this chapter, we will use these data to motivate the bivariate normal distribution and show how we model the association between the paired observations of agriculture and examination scores.

6.1   The Bivariate Normal Density Function

Suppose X and Y have normal distributions with respective means (μ_X, μ_Y) and standard deviations (σ_X, σ_Y). Both of the standard deviations are positive valued. In addition to these four parameters, there is a *correlation coefficient* ρ of X and Y defined for $-1 < \rho < 1$.

The joint density function is given for all (x, y) by

$$\phi(x, y) = \frac{1}{2\pi \sigma_X \sigma_Y \sqrt{1 - \rho^2}}$$
$$\times \exp\left[-\frac{1}{2(1 - \rho^2)} \left\{ \frac{(x - \mu_X)^2}{\sigma_X^2} + \frac{(y - \mu_Y)^2}{\sigma_Y^2} - \frac{2\rho(x - \mu_X)(y - \mu_Y)}{\sigma_X \sigma_Y} \right\} \right]$$
$$(6.1)$$

This expression may be intimidating at first glance but a considerable simplification is possible. Notice every appearance of x is expressed as $(x - \mu_X)/\sigma_X$ which is the representation of a standard normal with mean zero and variance one. A similar expression holds for every appearance of y.

We can then write (6.1) in the much simpler form

$$K \exp \left\{ - \left(x^2 + y^2 - 2\rho xy\right) \Big/ 2(1 - \rho^2) \right\} \qquad (6.2)$$

where x and y represent *marginal* standard normal random variates.

When $\rho = 0$, both (6.1) and (6.2) can be expressed as the product of two normal density functions. A product of densities signifies independence so $\rho = 0$ is a special case. See Exercise 6.8 for details. In Exercise 6.3, we see uncorrelated normals are not necessarily independent. Uncorrelated bivariate normals must be independent.

A study of independence is antithetical to the purpose of multivariate data. We collect data on both x and y in which their relationship is one of the prime motivations of the study.

The value of $K = K(\rho)$ is chosen in (6.2) so the two-dimensional integral of this expression is equal to 1. In multivariate analysis, the word *marginal* refers to the variables taken individually. All values of ρ between -1 and $+1$ are possible. The limits are usually of little interest because $\rho = -1$ or $+1$ corresponds to settings where X and Y are exactly linear functions of each other.

Specifically, if $\rho = 1$, then Y is expressible as the linear combination

$$Y = \rho(X - \mu_X)\sigma_Y/\sigma_X + \mu_Y$$

with a positive slope σ_Y/σ_X. If $\rho = -1$, then this slope is negative.

If there is a perfect linear relationship between X and Y, then the bivariate data is expressible as a one-dimensional problem. As an example, knowing the temperature in Celsius does not tell us any more than knowing the value in Fahrenheit. The estimation of the slopes and intercepts of linear relationships and related linear regressions is discussed in Chap. 9.

In summary then, values of correlations near -1, 0, or $+1$ are all special cases to be treated differently. Most of our interest lies in situations where ρ is either between -1 and 0 or else between 0 and $+1$.

The marginal distribution is obtained by integrating out the other variable(s). The marginal distributions of X and Y are also normal with the same respective means and variances as given in the bivariate distribution (6.1). A simple approach to analyzing and modeling bivariate normal data, then, would be to consider each variable separately. This defeats the purpose of multivariate analysis in which we want to describe the relationship between X and Y.

In the discussion of the bivariate normal distribution, another parameter frequently discussed in describing the relationship between X and Y is the *covariance*. The covariance is defined as the expected value of

$$(X - \mu_x)\,(Y - \mu_y).$$

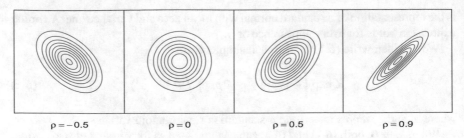

$$\rho = -0.5 \qquad\qquad \rho = 0 \qquad\qquad \rho = 0.5 \qquad\qquad \rho = 0.9$$

Figure 6.2 Contours of a bivariate normal density function with specified correlations

In terms of the parameters of the bivariate normal distribution, the covariance is equal to

$$\mathrm{Cov}(X, Y) = \rho\, \sigma_X \sigma_Y. \tag{6.3}$$

The covariance is represented by the symbol σ_{XY}^2. In Sect. 6.3, we discuss estimating the covariance.

It is often convenient to express the variances and covariance in a symmetric matrix, denoted by $\boldsymbol{\Sigma}$. The variances appear on the diagonal and the off-diagonal is the covariance:

$$\boldsymbol{\Sigma} = \begin{pmatrix} \sigma_X^2 & \sigma_{XY}^2 \\ \sigma_{XY}^2 & \sigma_Y^2 \end{pmatrix} = \begin{pmatrix} \sigma_X^2 & \rho\,\sigma_X \sigma_Y \\ \rho\,\sigma_X \sigma_Y & \sigma_Y^2 \end{pmatrix}. \tag{6.4}$$

There is also a matrix representation of (6.1). Let us define $\boldsymbol{\mu} = (\mu_1, \mu_2)$ to be the vector of means and use (6.4) to denote the matrix of variances and covariance. We can verify

$$\mathrm{Det}(\boldsymbol{\Sigma}) = \sigma_X^2 \sigma_Y^2 \left(1 - \rho^2\right)$$

from (4.5) and find $\boldsymbol{\Sigma}^{-1}$ at (4.7).

The density function of the bivariate normal distribution (6.1) can be written as

$$\phi(\boldsymbol{x} \mid \boldsymbol{\mu}, \boldsymbol{\Sigma}) = (2\pi)^{-1/2} \mathrm{Det}(\boldsymbol{\Sigma})^{-1/2} \exp\left\{-1/2(\boldsymbol{x} - \boldsymbol{\mu})' \boldsymbol{\Sigma}^{-1}(\boldsymbol{x} - \boldsymbol{\mu})\right\} \tag{6.5}$$

for $\boldsymbol{x} = \{x, y\}$, using matrix notation.

What does the bivariate normal density function look like? Figure 6.1 suggests ellipses stacked on top of each other. The appearance is similar to an oval wedding cake, as seen in Fig. 6.2. These images are all drawn with $\sigma_X = \sigma_Y$. If the marginal standard deviations were not equal, then these figures would be stretched vertically (for larger values σ_Y) or stretched horizontally (for larger σ_X).

The contours of constant density of $\phi(x, y)$ are ellipses. These are circular for a correlation of zero, indicating the shape is the same any way we rotate the figure. The ellipses will tilt either toward the right or the left depending on whether the correlation is positive or negative. It is clear the correlation in the Swiss data plotted in Fig. 6.1 corresponds to a negative correlation. Correlations close to either -1 or $+1$

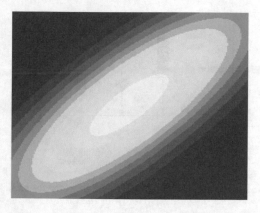 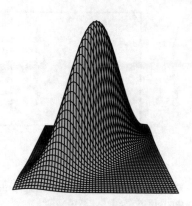

Figure 6.3 A bivariate normal density function with correlation .8, drawn using `image` and `persp`, both in the `graphics` package

result in thin ellipses corresponding to the almost perfect linear relationship between the two variables.

See Exercise 6.2 for details on how to draw the contour plots of Fig. 6.2. Two other graphical methods for depicting the bivariate normal density function are given in Fig. 6.3 using a heat image and a perspective plot.

In **R** there are a variety of computing options. The `fMultivar` library, for example, offers a variety of functions, specific to the bivariate normal distribution. In particular, the `dnorm2d` function in `fMultivar` calculates the bivariate normal density (6.1).

6.2   Properties of the Bivariate Normal Distribution

There are important features of the bivariate normal distribution described here: marginal and conditional distributions of the bivariate normal are also normally distributed, as are linear combinations. These features also hold in the more general multivariate normal distribution studied in the following chapter. The marginal distributions refer to X or Y considered alone. Conditional distributions refer to X at a given value of Y or vice versa.

The marginal distributions of the bivariate normal distribution are also normally distributed. This is generally a useful property because it suggests each variable in a multivariate data set can be examined individually. Of course, such an approach loses the multivariate character of the observations.

Another useful property of (6.1) is the conditional distributions are also normally distributed. Specifically, for any given value or range of X, the corresponding values of Y are also normally distributed. In practical terms of data analysis, this suggests we can examine the Y values as normals, separately for different ranges of X.

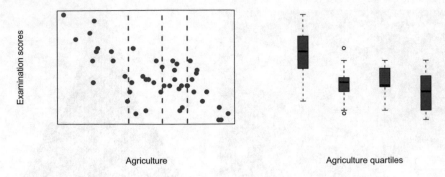

Figure 6.4 Scatterplot of Swiss agriculture and examination scores. Boxplots are given for each quartile of the agriculture values

As an example, Fig. 6.4 divides the agriculture rates into quartiles. (Each quartile contains one-quarter of the observations.) Within each quartile, we plot the corresponding set of examination scores giving a series of four boxplots. The model of the bivariate normal distribution suggests each of these four separate boxplots should depict a different normal distribution. This is a popular approach for examining bivariate data.

We should expect, for example, some ordering among the means across the data slices. We can exploit this property and use all of the observations to measure this trend, rather than look at the data through a number of small slices. In Chap. 9, we discuss linear regression which estimates the slope and intercept of this trend.

When we sample from the bivariate normal density function (6.1), the conditional distribution of Y for any given value of $X = x$ is also normally distributed with mean

$$\mu_Y + \rho(x - \mu_X)\sigma_Y/\sigma_X \tag{6.6}$$

and variance

$$(1 - \rho^2)\sigma_Y^2. \tag{6.7}$$

We can make several points on the basis of these last two equations. In (6.6), we see the conditional mean of Y is a linear function of a known value of X. This property is explored in Chap. 9 on linear regression. Notice the conditional variance of Y at (6.7) is always smaller than the marginal variance, σ_Y^2. This reduction in the variance demonstrated the benefit achieved by knowing the value of X. Further, the conditional variance in (6.7) is the same for every value of X. One assumption of linear regression is the constant variance, conditional on X, yet independent of the value of X.

Another important feature of the bivariate normal distribution is every linear combination of X and Y is also normally distributed. For any values of α and β, the random variable $\alpha X + \beta Y$ also has a (univariate) normal distribution. This is a useful property and will be more fully exploited in Chap. 8 when we seek to reduce the dimensionality of a multivariate problem by combining several variables together in this linear fashion.

We can use this property to transform a correlated bivariate normal pair into two independent normals. Specifically, suppose (X, Y) are a pair of random variables sampled from the density function (6.1) with some correlation ρ, not necessarily equal to zero.

Define

$$Z_1 = X \big/ \sqrt{2}\sigma_X + Y \big/ \sqrt{2}\sigma_Y \tag{6.8}$$

and

$$Z_2 = X \big/ \sqrt{2}\sigma_X - Y \big/ \sqrt{2}\sigma_Y. \tag{6.9}$$

Marginally, both Z_1 and Z_2 are distributed as standard normals. The joint distribution of (Z_1, Z_2) is also a bivariate normal with $\rho = 0$. Uncorrelated bivariate normal random variates are also independent. This construction of Z_1 and Z_2 illustrates we can begin with correlated normal variates and create an uncorrelated linear combination of these.

On the basis of a simple linear transformation of the data, we can create a pair of independent observations, remove the correlation, and eliminate the need to describe the multivariate character of the paired observations. The problem with this approach is Z_1 and Z_2 may not have simple interpretations. They represent linear combinations of measurements conceptually different from each other. This lack of simple interpretation results from two different combinations of the original measurements. In the Swiss data example, Z_1 and Z_2 represent sums and differences of agriculture rates X and examination scores Y. It is not intuitive how to interpret the sums and differences between these two measurements in the present example. However, in Chaps. 8 and 10, this feature will be exploited to identify groups of variables to be combined in order to reduce the dimensionality of the data.

In summary, the marginal and conditional distributions of the bivariate normal are also normally distributed. Linear combinations of normals are also normally distributed. These properties are also true of the more general multivariate normals distribution described in Chap. 7.

6.3 Inference on Bivariate Normal Parameters

We estimate the mean and standard deviation parameters of the bivariate normal distribution in the familiar manner used in the univariate distribution. So we have

$$\widehat{\mu}_X = \bar{x} = n^{-1} \sum_{i=1}^{n} x_i$$

and

$$\widehat{\sigma}_X^2 = s_X^2 = (n-1)^{-1} \sum_{i=1}^{n} (x_i - \bar{x})^2$$

with similar expressions for $\widehat{\mu}_Y$ and $\widehat{\sigma}_Y^2$.

The sample covariance σ_{XY} is estimated by

$$\widehat{\sigma}_{XY} = (n-1)^{-1} \sum_{i=1}^{n} (x_i - \bar{x})(y_i - \bar{y}).$$

The correlation ρ is estimated by the *Pearson correlation coefficient*

$$\widehat{\rho} = \sum_{i=1}^{n} (x_i - \bar{x})(y_i - \bar{y}) \Big/ \sqrt{\sum(x_i - \bar{x})^2 \sum(y_i - \bar{y})^2}. \qquad (6.10)$$

In **R**, we calculate these statistics using the functions mean, var, cov, and cor, respectively.

It is often convenient to express the collected estimators of variances and covariance in a symmetric matrix, denoted by S. The variances appear on the diagonal, and the off-diagonal is the covariance:

$$S = \begin{pmatrix} s_X^2 & \widehat{\rho}\, s_X\, s_Y \\ \widehat{\rho}\, s_X\, s_Y & s_Y^2 \end{pmatrix}.$$

This matrix is used to estimate the population variance matrix Σ introduced at (6.4).

Let's review with an example of the Swiss data. To find the means of the data in each column of this data.frame, we write

```
> colMeans(swiss[ , 2 : 3])

Agriculture Examination
   50.65957    16.48936
```

Note the data.frame variable labels are attached to the estimates.

Standard deviations of data.frame data are obtained using sapply(., sd) as in this example:

```
> sapply(swiss[ , 2 : 3], sd)

Agriculture Examination
  22.711218    7.977883
```

to estimate these univariate values.

The estimator S of variances and covariances

```
> var(swiss[ , 2 : 3])

              Agriculture Examination
Agriculture    515.7994    -124.39283
Examination   -124.3928      63.64662
```

is a symmetric matrix. The covariance, on the off-diagonal, is a negative number.

A separate estimate of the correlation coefficient ρ can be obtained using the `cor` function:

```
> cor(swiss[ , 2 : 3])

             Agriculture Examination
Agriculture    1.0000000   -0.6865422
Examination   -0.6865422    1.0000000
```

which is also expressed as a symmetric 2×2 matrix.

The correlation of a variable with itself is always equal to 1, so the correlation matrix will always have 1's running down the diagonal. The off-diagonal value $-.687$ confirms the negative correlation apparent in Fig. 6.1.

The `cor.test` function in **R** produces confidence intervals and tests the null hypothesis the population correlation coefficient is zero:

```
> cor.test(swiss[ , 2], swiss[ , 3])


        Pearson's product-moment correlation

data:  swiss[, 2] and swiss[, 3]
t = -6.3341, df = 45, p-value = 9.952e-08
alternative hypothesis: true correlation is not equal to 0
95 percent confidence interval:
 -0.8133545 -0.4974484
sample estimates:
      cor
-0.6865422
```

The t-test in this output refers to the *Pearson product-moment correlation* transformation

$$t = \widehat{\rho}\sqrt{(n-2)/(1-\widehat{\rho}^2)}.$$

This statistic should behave approximately as a t-statistic with $(n-2)$ df under the null hypothesis X and Y are independent and uncorrelated.

The *Fisher Z-transformation* of the correlation is

$$Z = 1/2 \ln\{(1+\widehat{\rho})/(1-\widehat{\rho})\}.$$

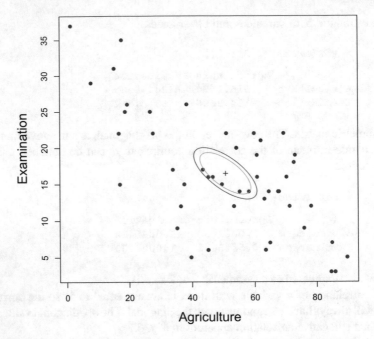

Figure 6.5 Joint 95 and 99% confidence ellipsoids for bivariate means of Swiss agriculture rates and education scores

With large sample sizes, Z should behave approximately as normal with mean zero and standard error $1/\sqrt{n-3}$ under the null hypothesis X and Y are uncorrelated. The functions `CIr`, `CIz`, `r2z`, and `z2r` in the `psychometric` library perform these transformations and create confidence intervals of the correlation coefficient.

There are nonparametric estimators of ρ, as well. See Exercise 6.1 for two nonparametric estimators useful when the data contains suspected outliers or may not have been sampled from a bivariate normal parent population.

Marginal confidence intervals for the mean parameter were described in Sect. 5.5. The joint confidence interval of the bivariate normal mean vector $\mu = (\mu_X, \mu_Y)$ is expressed as an ellipse.

The joint confidence contours are values of μ

$$(\overline{x} - \mu)' S^{-1} (\overline{x} - \mu) = \chi_2^2/n \qquad (6.11)$$

where χ^2 is the upper $1 - \alpha$ quantile of a chi-squared variate with 2 df.

An example of this appears in Fig. 6.5. This figure was drawn in **R** using the program code for the confidence ellipse of the bivariate means given in Output 6.1. The `bivCI` function returns m evenly spaced coordinates of the confidence ellipse of μ centered at the bivariate means. The ellipse is defined by (6.11) and much smaller than the range of the data. See Exercise 6.9 for more on this.

The `bivCI` function is defined and returns m points on a $1 - \alpha$ confidence ellipse. The code in this output plots the data. We next use `lines` to draw the 99 and 95% confidence ellipses. The last `lines` statement puts the "+" sign in the center of the figure.

Output 6.1 R code to draw Fig. 6.5

```
bivCI <- function(s, xbar, n, alpha, m)
#   returns m (x,y) coordinates of 1-alpha joint confidence ellipse
    of mean
{
    x <- sin(2 * pi * (0 : (m - 1)) / (m - 1)) # m points on a unit
      circle
    y <- cos(2 * pi * (0 : (m - 1)) / (m - 1))
    cv <-  qchisq(1 - alpha, 2)               # chi-squared critical value
    cv <- cv / n                              # value of quadratic form
    for (i in 1 : m)
    {
        pair <- c(x[i], y[i])        # ith (x,y) pair
        q <- pair %*% solve(s,pair)  # quadratic form
        x[i] <- x[i] * sqrt(cv / q) + xbar[1]
        y[i] <- y[i] * sqrt(cv / q) + xbar[2]
    }
    cbind(x, y)
}


plot(biv, col = "red", pch = 16, cex.lab = 1.5)
lines(bivCI(s = var(biv), xbar = colMeans(biv), n = dim(biv)[1],
       alpha = .01, m = 1000),
          type = "l", col = "blue")
lines(bivCI(s = var(biv), xbar = colMeans(biv), n = dim(biv)[1],
       alpha = .05, m = 1000),
          type = "l", col = "green", lwd = 1)
#  Add ``+'' sign
lines(colMeans(biv)[1], colMeans(biv)[2], pch = 3, cex = .8,
       type = "p",  lwd = 1)
```

6.4 Tests for Bivariate Normality

The test of bivariate, and more generally multivariate normality, has received considerable attention. Because there are so many ways in which the multivariate normal can fail, we can find a variety of tests for each of these. We begin by pointing out that verifying marginal normality for each of the two variables does not assure their joint distribution is bivariate normal. See Exercise 6.3 for an example of this behavior.

Rather than discussing tests specifically for the bivariate normal distribution, we will defer the discussion until Sect. 7.7 where we discuss tests for the more

general, multivariate normal distribution. Among the most frequently used tests in
R are mvnormtest in the mvShapiroTest library which performs a multivariate
Shapiro–Wilk test and mvnorm.etest in the energy library which performs the
energy test.

6.5 Maximum Likelihood Estimation, Part II

In this section, we will use the likelihood function to both estimate parameter values
and estimate standard errors of these estimates. We first introduced the concept of
maximum likelihood estimation in Sect. 5.7 and demonstrated how it can be used to
estimate parameters in models you may develop. These models may constrain the
parameters of the model, for example. The models can take a form unique to your
application. This section shows how maximum likelihood estimation also provides
estimates of the standard errors of the parameter estimates.

Refer back to Fig. 5.11. The peak of the likelihood function indicates the location
of the maximum likelihood estimates. We are only interested in the top so the derivative should be zero (or nearly so) in every direction. The $gradient estimate of
nlm is very close to zero indicating how flat the log-likelihood is at its maximum.

The *second derivative* tells us how curved the log-likelihood is at its maximum.
Informally, if the top of the peak is sharp, then there is little uncertainty about where
the maximum is located. Conversely, if the top of the peak is broad and flat, then the
estimate is less reliable.

The nlm procedure gives us an estimate of this curvature in the direction of each
parameter. The matrix of second derivatives is called the *Hessian*. The inverse of
the Hessian matrix is a useful approximation to the variances and covariances of the
estimated parameters. We will illustrate how to obtain these estimates in this section.

Another useful feature of maximum likelihood estimates is these estimates are
usually distributed as normal under a wide range of conditions. We can combine this
feature with the approximate standard deviations and construct confidence intervals
for parameters, as well as their point estimators. Again, this feature will be illustrated
in **R** with an example in the present section.

Let us begin with a data example and then use nlm to fit a variety of different
bivariate normal models to it. Table 6.1 lists the 2007 and 2008 US male all-cancer

Table 6.1 US age-adjusted cancer rates for males in 50 states and DC for 2007 and 2008

State	2007	2008
	Rate	Rate
AL	584.5	591.0
AK	526.0	528.3
	. . .	
WI	545.8	514.9
WY	508.9	520.0

Source: CDC

Output 6.2   Read cancer data and produce some summary statistics

```
> cancer <- read.table(file = "Cancer2007_8.dat",
+     header = TRUE, row.names = 1)
> cancer[1 : 3, ]          # look at the first few

     Rate2007 Rate2008
AL     584.5    591.0
AK     526.0    528.3
AZ     459.2    414.3

> cancer[49 : 51, ]        # look at the last few

     Rate2007 Rate2008
WV     602.1    566.5
WI     545.8    514.9
WY     508.9    520.0

> colMeans(cancer)         # some summary statistics

Rate2007 Rate2008
565.6039 548.7373

> sapply(cancer, sd)

Rate2007 Rate2008
42.95529 41.29989

> var(cancer)

          Rate2007 Rate2008
Rate2007 1845.157 1594.973
Rate2008 1594.973 1705.681

> cor(cancer)

          Rate2007  Rate2008
Rate2007 1.0000000 0.8990581
Rate2008 0.8990581 1.0000000
```

age-adjusted rates for each of the 50 states plus DC. Age-adjusted rates take into account the differing demographics of each state. A state with an older population, for example, should not be recording a higher rate of cancer than a younger state simply because of the age differences.

It is always a good idea to print a few of the data values and some summary statistics to verify these are correct. Output 6.2 includes these for the cancer rate data.

Figure 6.6 plots the bivariate data. Three outliers are identified: Arizona (AZ) has very low rates in both years; DC and Nevada are extreme in this bivariate plot, but are not extreme in either of the two years. Multivariate outliers can appear but not be

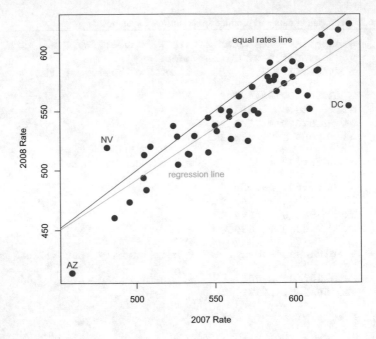

Figure 6.6   US male cancer rates in 2007 and 2008

excessive in any of their marginal components. Other than these three points, there is nothing to indicate a lack of fit to the bivariate normal distribution. Figure 6.6 also contains a 45° line illustrating most of the 2007 rates were higher than those in 2008. The correlation (.889) of the data values is very high across the two years.

Let us fit a bivariate normal distribution to these data. We need an objective function for nlm to evaluate the function we need to maximize. There are five parameters to estimate: two means, two variances, and a correlation. A five-parameter objective function finds the negative log-likelihood for the cancer data appears in Output 6.3. The five parameters in the code are the two means (par[1], par[2]), the two variances (par[3], par[4]), and the correlation (par[5]).

Just before the program ends and returns the value of the negative log-likelihood, the program prints out the value of the parameters, and the value the program is returning. This is a useful habit to get into. In its search for a minimum of the objective function, we will be able to watch the progress of nlm.

Some of the output from the model fitting appears in Output 6.4. The call to nlm includes the hessian=TRUE option producing an estimate of the Hessian matrix.

Most of the output consists of trial parameter values and the resulting negative log-likelihood. These preceded the output given here and have been mostly omitted, except for the last two lines. The next items in the output, in order, are the value of the negative log-likelihood at its minimum, the parameter estimates, the estimated gradient, the estimated Hessian, some information about the computing effort listed under $iterations, and finally an indication of errors.

Output 6.3   Objective function for bivariate normal likelihood

```
        library(mvtnorm)        # library with dmvnorm
        biv5 <- function(par)   # five parameter log-likelihood
                                  function
    {
        cov <- par[5]* sqrt(par[3] * par[4])
        biv5 <- sum(
            -dmvnorm(cancer, mean=c(par[1], par[2]),
                sigma = matrix(c(par[3], cov, cov, par[4]),
                2,2), log = TRUE) )
        print(c(par, biv5))
        biv5
    }
```

Output 6.4   A portion of the output from fitting a bivariate normal distribution

```
nlm(biv5, c(45, 45, 1600, 1600, .8), hessian = TRUE)


      .   .   .

[1]   565.6097533 548.7412240 1702.6278244 1665.0146152 0.8956175 483.2521017
[1]   565.6097533 548.7412240 1702.6278244 1664.8481304 0.8957175 483.2518112
$minimum
[1] 483.2518

$estimate
[1]   565.6097533 548.7412240 1702.6278244 1664.8481304 0.8955175

$gradient
[1]   3.811412e-04 -1.424093e-04 -2.471923e-03  1.959478e-03  3.899459e-05

$hessian
               [,1]          [,2]          [,3]          [,4]          [,5]
[1,]   1.512443e-01 -1.369701e-01 -2.870247e-06  1.632584e-07   0.04117360
[2,]  -1.369701e-01  1.546765e-01  2.345524e-07 -2.677687e-06   0.03584994
[3,]  -2.870247e-06  2.345524e-07  3.015783e-05 -1.888685e-05  -0.08762491
[4,]   1.632584e-07 -2.677687e-06 -1.888685e-05  2.615282e-05  -0.04899606
[5,]   4.117360e-02  3.584994e-02 -8.762491e-02 -4.899606e-02 2361.51979607

$code
[1] 2

$iterations
[1] 58

There were 38 warnings (use warnings() to see them)
```

The estimated means (first two parameters) are the same as those in Output 6.2.
The estimated variances are slightly smaller because these estimates have an n in

the denominator, rather than the familiar $n - 1$ we commonly use. The estimated correlation coefficient is about the same as in Output 6.2.

Much of this output (including the error message) was covered in Sect. 5.7. The gradients are all close to zero indicating an extreme of the function has been found. The warnings arise because `nlm` does not know about the ranges of parameter values, specifically the variances must be positive and the correlation must be between -1 and 1. (Similar warnings were described in Sect. 5.7.) Let us come back to this in a moment, but first, let's show how estimated standard errors can be obtained from the Hessian.

Begin by capturing the output from `nlm`:

```
nlm.out <- nlm(biv5, c(45, 45, 1600, 1600, .8), hessian = TRUE)
```

Verify the output containing the estimated parameter values:

```
> nlm.out$estimate                          # parameter estimates

[1]   565.6097533  548.7412240 1702.6278244 1664.8481304     0.8955175
```

of μ_1, μ_2, σ_1^2, σ_2^2, and ρ, respectively.

This output also captures the Hessian matrix:

```
> nlm.out$hessian                           # estimated Hessian matrix

            [,1]          [,2]          [,3]          [,4]          [,5]
[1,]  1.512443e-01 -1.369701e-01 -2.870247e-06  1.632584e-07    0.04117360
[2,] -1.369701e-01  1.546765e-01  2.345524e-07 -2.677687e-06    0.03584994
[3,] -2.870247e-06  2.345524e-07  3.015783e-05 -1.888685e-05   -0.08762491
[4,]  1.632584e-07 -2.677687e-06 -1.888685e-05  2.615282e-05   -0.04899606
[5,]  4.117360e-02  3.584994e-02 -8.762491e-02 -4.899606e-02 2361.51979607
```

Invert the Hessian matrix,

```
> solve(nlm.out$hessian)                    # invert the Hessian matrix

            [,1]          [,2]          [,3]          [,4]          [,5]
[1,] 33.3874221505 29.5656957245 1.793796e+00 2.400703e+00 -0.0009145817
[2,] 29.5656957245 32.6465638380 1.606956e+00 2.638535e+00 -0.0008967177
[3,]  1.7937963901  1.6069562639 1.015044e+05 8.360972e+04  5.5010045726
[4,]  2.4007031017  2.6385350535 8.360972e+04 1.086530e+05  5.3565794553
[5,] -0.0009145817 -0.0008967177 5.501005e+00 5.356579e+00  0.0007387387
```

to obtain an estimate of the variance matrix of the estimated parameters.

The diagonal elements of the inverse

```
> diag(solve(nlm.out$hessian))              # diagonal elements

[1] 3.338742e+01 3.264656e+01 1.015044e+05 1.086530e+05 7.387387e-04
```

are of most interest to us because these are the estimated variances.

Finally, the square root of these entries

```
> sqrt( diag( solve( nlm.out$hessian )))   # estimated se's

[1]    5.77818502    5.71371716 318.59759219 329.62551825    0.02717975
```

are the estimated standard errors for the five estimated parameters. The parameter estimates are approximately normally distributed with these standard errors so we can easily construct confidence intervals as we show in the following summary.

Let us conclude this section by constructing a summary data.frame of all the results obtained:

```
se <- sqrt(diag(solve(nlm.out$hessian)))
q <- qnorm(.975)                         # normal 95% interval quantile
upper <- nlm.out$estimate + q * se       # upper 95% CI intervals
lower <- nlm.out$estimate - q * se       # lower 95% CI intervals
summary <- data.frame(
    cbind(nlm.out$estimate, se, lower, upper),
    row.names=c("mean1", "mean2", "var1", "var2", "rho"))
colnames(summary)[1] <- "estimate"
print(summary, digits = 3)
```

The resulting summary table is

	estimate	se	lower	upper
mean1	565.610	5.7782	554.285	576.935
mean2	548.741	5.7137	537.543	559.940
var1	1702.628	318.5976	1078.188	2327.068
var2	1664.848	329.6255	1018.794	2310.902
rho	0.896	0.0272	0.842	0.949

The data frame of these summary statistics is a good way to present results in an organized table. In Exercises 6.4 and 6.5, the reader is asked to fit other bivariate normal models to these data.

6.6 Exercises

6.1 See the help file on cor.test to learn about Spearman's ρ and Kendall's τ. These are nonparametric estimators of the correlation coefficient. Nonparametric methods are used when there are outliers or the data may not follow the distribution assumed for the traditional method.

    a. Pick a data set and compute all three estimates of the correlation coefficient.

    b. Add some extreme outliers to the data set and compare the three estimates with those of the original data. Which method appears to be most robust, or insensitive to these introduced outliers?

6.2 Draw plots as given in Figs. 6.2 and 6.3.

a. Contour plots can be produced by creating a square matrix of values of the bivariate normal density function. The bivariate normal is evaluated using dmvnorm in the mvtnorm library. More and more closely spaced points used in this matrix will result in smoother contours in your plot. Use this matrix in the contour program in the graphics library. See the help file for a list of the options available for contour plotting.

b. Obtain images similar to those in Fig. 6.3 using image and persp.

6.3 There are bivariate distributions whose margins are normal but the joint distribution is not bivariate normal. Consider the function generating n bivariate pairs

```
checker <- function(n)      # generates n pairs of
                            # marginal normals
                            # not bivariate normal
{
    checker <- NULL          # start a list
    for (i in 1:n)
      {
        x <- rnorm(2)        # pair of independent
                            # normals
        if(x[1]>0)   x[2] <-  abs(x[2])
            else     x[2] <- -abs(x[2])
        checker <- rbind(checker, x)
      }
    return(checker)
}
```

a. Use the checker program to generate a large number of bivariate pairs. Plot the individual columns of this data.frame and test these using any of the methods described in Sect. 5.4 to see if the separate columns of data are marginally normally distributed.

b. Plot the bivariate pairs to demonstrate the data does not follow a bivariate normal distribution.

c. The bivariate pairs generated in part a. are positively correlated. Write a program in **R** to generate uncorrelated pairs which are marginally distributed as normal but do not follow a bivariate normal distribution. Here is one possible solution: Begin with uncorrelated pairs (X, Y) of bivariate normals and transform these to produce the scatterplot given in Fig. 6.7. The transformation is similar to the folding operation we used in the checker program. The red circle is added to help visualize the transformation is different for observations close to and far from the origin.

d. Use simulation methods to estimate the diameter of the red circle resulting in an uncorrelated bivariate distribution.

6.4 Fit an exchangeable bivariate normal model to the data in Table 6.1. A pair of random variables (X, Y) are said to be exchangeable if the ordered pair (X, Y)

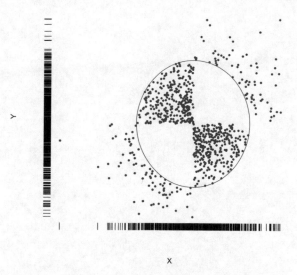

Figure 6.7 Uncorrelated marginal normals which are neither independent nor distributed as bivariate normal

has the same distribution as does (Y, X). This model has three parameters: the same mean for both years' cancer rates, the same variance for both years, and a correlation ρ. Use the Hessian to estimate the standard deviations of the parameter estimates.

6.5 Fit the bivariate normal distribution to the data of Table 6.1 in such a way to remove the chance of `nlm` trying to use an invalid parameter value. Specifically, write an objective function in **R** with five arguments: two mean parameters, the two variances measured on a log scale, and the correlation re-parameterized as

$$\rho = \theta/\sqrt{1+\theta^2}$$

for all values of θ.

6.6 Verify the equivalence of the bivariate normal density function given at (6.1) and the matrix version at (6.5).

6.7 Redraw Fig. 6.4 using the coplot, illustrated in Fig. 3.18. Does this plot help show the conditional segments are also normally distributed? What can you say about the variances inside each slice relative to the variance of the whole sample?

6.8 When $\rho = 0$, show (6.1) and (6.2) can both be written as the product of two standard normal density functions ϕ given at (5.2).

6.9 Why are the ellipses so small in Fig. 6.5? Redraw this figure producing 95 and 99% confidence ellipses for the population. *Hint:* These are obtained by omitting the "$/n$" in (6.11).

Chapter 7
Multivariate Normal Distribution

I N THIS CHAPTER, we generalize the bivariate normal distribution from the previous chapter to an arbitrary number of dimensions. We also make use of the matrix notation. The mathematics is generally more dense and relies on the linear algebra notation covered in Chap. 4. In Sect. 4.5 we pointed out there is a limit on what computations we can reasonably perform by hand. For this reason, we illustrate these various operations with the help of **R**.

The multivariate normal distribution is defined for a vector $x' = (x_1, x_2, \ldots, x_p)$ of p values. Recall from Sect. 4.1 the prime ($'$) notation refers to the transpose of a vector or matrix. The number of dimensions p is a positive integer but otherwise is not restricted in this chapter. This results in a level of abstraction not found in the previous two chapters in which $p = 1$ and 2, respectively. The reader who has studied the material in those chapters and the linear algebra of Chap. 4 should be comfortable with the development here.

The mean of x is a p-tuple vector of values denoted $\mu' = (\mu_1, \ldots, \mu_p)$ and the variance of x is a $p \times p$ symmetric matrix Σ. We will introduce the density function of x. In this chapter, we show how to draw statistical inference on μ and Σ from a data sample.

7.1 Multivariate Normal Density and Its Properties

A useful concept when studying the multivariate normal distribution is the *quadratic form*:

$$x'Ax \tag{7.1}$$

© Springer Nature Switzerland AG 2022
D. Zelterman, *Applied Multivariate Statistics with R*, Statistics for Biology and Health,
https://doi.org/10.1007/978-3-031-13005-2_7

for p-tuple vector x and a square, $p \times p$ matrix

$$A = \begin{pmatrix} a_{11} & a_{12} & \cdots & a_{1p} \\ a_{21} & a_{22} & \cdots & a_{2p} \\ \vdots & & \ddots & \\ a_{p1} & a_{p2} & \cdots & a_{pp} \end{pmatrix}.$$

Notice although (7.1) involves vectors and a matrix, the result is a scalar. If $p = 1$ then (7.1) is

$$x'Ax = a_{11}x^2 .$$

When $p = 2$ then the quadratic form (7.1) can be written as

$$x'Ax = x_1^2 a_{11} + (a_{12} + a_{21})x_1 x_2 + a_{22}x_2^2 .$$

More generally,

$$x'Ax = \sum_{i=1}^{p} a_{ii}x_i^2 + \sum_{i}\sum_{j} a_{ij}x_i x_j .$$

In this chapter, we will also be interested in the special case where the matrix A is symmetric. Recall from Sect. 4.3 the matrix A is symmetric if it is equal to its transpose: $A' = A$. Similarly, we can say the matrix A with entries $\{a_{ij}\}$ is symmetric if $a_{ij} = a_{ji}$ for all valid indices i and j.

In the case where A is a square, symmetric matrix, then we have

$$x'Ax = \sum_{i=1}^{p} a_{ii}x_i^2 + 2\sum_{i<j} a_{ij}x_i x_j .$$

The multivariate normal density function of x can be expressed as a quadratic form $x'\Sigma^{-1}x$ for a square, symmetric, nonnegative definite matrix Σ of variances and covariances. Exercise 4.6 shows a square symmetric matrix is positive definite if and only if every eigenvalue is positive. Similarly, a square symmetric matrix Σ is nonnegative definite if and only if every eigenvalue is nonnegative.

We can now introduce the multivariate normal distribution. The parameters of the *multivariate normal distribution* are the mean vector μ and the variance matrix Σ. The mean vector μ is a p-tuple and Σ is a $p \times p$, symmetric, nonnegative definite matrix of variances and covariances.

The *multivariate normal density function* is

$$f(x \mid \mu, \Sigma) = (2\pi)^{-1/2}\text{Det}(\Sigma)^{-1/2} \exp\left\{-1/2(x - \mu)'\Sigma^{-1}(x - \mu)\right\} \qquad (7.2)$$

When x is a scalar, this expression reduces to the usual univariate density function given at (5.2). Notice the quadratic form in the exponential function. The formula (7.2) may seem rather daunting at first glance. We will not have much need to refer to it because it is available as a programmed feature in **R**. This function is called dvtnorm() and is found in the mvtnorm library.

The vector $x - \mu$ behaves as multivariate normal with mean vector $\mu = 0$ and variance Σ. A property of the multivariate normal variate x is every linear combination of x also has a multivariate normal distribution. Specifically, if A is an arbitrary $q \times p$ matrix, then Ax is a q-tuple behaving as a multivariate normal with mean $A\mu$ and $q \times q$ variance matrix $A\Sigma A'$.

The marginal and conditional distributions of the multivariate normal also behave as multivariate normal. Specifically, let us partition the multivariate normal vector x into a pair of sub-vectors and write

$$x = \begin{pmatrix} x_1 \\ x_2 \end{pmatrix}.$$

The corresponding vector of means has a similar representation:

$$\mu = \begin{pmatrix} \mu_1 \\ \mu_2 \end{pmatrix}$$

and the variance matrix can be partitioned as

$$\Sigma = \begin{pmatrix} \Sigma_{11} & \Sigma_{12} \\ \Sigma_{21} & \Sigma_{22} \end{pmatrix}.$$

The marginal distribution of x_1 (ignoring x_2) behaves as multivariate normal with mean μ_1 and variance matrix Σ_{11}. The conditional distribution of x_1 given the value of x_2 also behaves as multivariate normal with mean

$$\mu_1 - \Sigma_{12}\Sigma_{22}^{-1}(x_2 - \mu_2) \tag{7.3}$$

and variance

$$\text{Var}(x_1 \text{ given } x_2) = \Sigma_{11} - \Sigma_{12}\Sigma_{22}^{-1}\Sigma_{21}. \tag{7.4}$$

These conditional means and variances generalize the bivariate values given at (6.6) and (6.6) respectively. As at (6.6), the conditional variance is independent of the value of x_2 and is smaller than the unconditional variance, Σ_{11}. The conditional mean given at (7.3) is linear in x_2. This linear relationship is the motivation for the multivariable linear regression models described in Chap. 9.

7.2   Inference on Multivariate Normal Means

Suppose we have multivariate normal observations $x_1, x_2, \ldots, x_n$ where $x_i' = (x_{i1}, \ldots, x_{ip})$. We estimate the multivariate mean vector

$$\widehat{\mu} = \overline{x} = n^{-1} \sum_{i=1}^{n} x_i$$

as the component-wise sample averages.

The estimate of the variance matrix Σ is denoted by S and the calculation is analogous to the method used in Sect. 6.3. Specifically, the diagonal elements of S are marginal variances, and the off-diagonal elements are the corresponding covariances.

Usually S will be positive definite. If some components of the data x_i are linearly dependent or there are more observations n than components p, then the matrix S will be singular and have a zero determinant. We calculate $\widehat{\mu}$ in **R** using colMeans(), and S is found using the var() function.

Joint multivariate confidence intervals for the mean vectors μ are constructed as ellipses, generalizing (6.11). Specifically, the $1 - \alpha$ confidence ellipse is the set of all values of μ for which

$$(\widehat{\mu} - \mu)' S^{-1} (\widehat{\mu} - \mu) = \chi^2/n \tag{7.5}$$

where χ^2 is the upper $1 - \alpha$ percentile of the chi-squared distribution with p df.

There is a generalization of the Student t-test for multivariate data. The multivariate t-distribution is available as pmvt() function in **R**, but it is better to describe the test procedure. Specifically, suppose we have two $p-$dimensional multivariate normal samples denoted by $x_1, x_2, \ldots, x_n$ and $y_1, y_2, \ldots, y_m$ with respective population means μ_X and μ_Y. We estimate the means as sample averages, so $\widehat{\mu}_X = \overline{x}$ and $\widehat{\mu}_Y = \overline{y}$. The sample covariance S is estimated as the sample covariance from the pooled sample of $x - \widehat{\mu}_X$ and $y - \widehat{\mu}_Y$.

We want to test the null hypothesis the population means μ_X and μ_Y are equal. One approach is to examine each individual component, marginally, and then perform a correction for the multiplicity of the tests. This approach has some loss of efficiency because of correlations between the individual variables (components of the x's and y's).

Intuitively, the solution is to examine a statistic based on the differences of means $\widehat{\mu}_X - \widehat{\mu}_Y$. Then use the analogy to (7.5) giving rise to the statistic

$$T^2 = (\widehat{\mu}_X - \widehat{\mu}_Y)' S^{-1} (\widehat{\mu}_X - \widehat{\mu}_Y) \tag{7.6}$$

also known as the Hotelling[1] T^2 statistic. Under the null hypothesis of $\mu_X = \mu_Y$ the T^2 statistic behaves as a multiple of the F distribution.

Let us demonstrate the use of this generalization of the two sample t-test in an example from a physiology study. The LASERI data in the ICSNP library is a data frame with 32 measurements made on each of 223 healthy Finnish subjects. The subjects were monitored while in a supine position and then again with their heads elevated on a motorized table. We will concentrate on four measurements and their average differences: average heart rate (HRT1T4); average cardiac output (COT1T4); average systemic vascular resistance index (SVRIT1T4); and average pulse wave velocity (PWVT1T4). Each of these variables is expressed as a difference of the pre- and post-tilt values. Testing equality of means of pre- and post- values is the same as testing whether each of the variables in the data has a zero population mean. More detail on this study and the other variables in the data frame are available in help(LASERI).

The four physiology measurements are plotted in Fig. 7.1 with the axes indicating the zero values. In each of the displays, the zero values seem to occur at or near the center of the data mass so it seems reasonable to test the hypothesis the pre- and post-tilt means are equal. The one-sample Hotelling test for these differences is available in the ICSNP library and gives us

```
> HotellingsT2(LASERI[, 25: 28])

  Hotelling's one sample T2-test

data:  LASERI[, 25:28]
T.2 = 101.6741, df1 = 4, df2 = 219, p-value < 2.2e-16
alternative hypothesis: true location is not equal to c(0,0,0,0)
```

providing considerable evidence the mean measurements are very different in the supine and tilted positions. We conclude tilting the subject results in very different measures.

Exercises 7.1 and 7.2 ask the reader to perform similar tests on multivariate normal means. In Chap. 9 on multivariable regression, we develop a wider set of models for mean parameters of multivariate normally distributed data. The remainder of this chapter discusses models of the multivariate normal variance parameters and tests of adequacy of the multivariate normal distribution as a model for sampled data.

We next introduce a larger example.

7.3   Example: Home Price Index

The Case–Schiller index is a measure of relative home prices in different US cities. This index does not simply look at average prices but, rather, compares the prices of the *same* homes when they were sold at an earlier date. The index for every city

---

[1] Harold Hotelling (1885–1973). US mathematician, statistician, and economist.

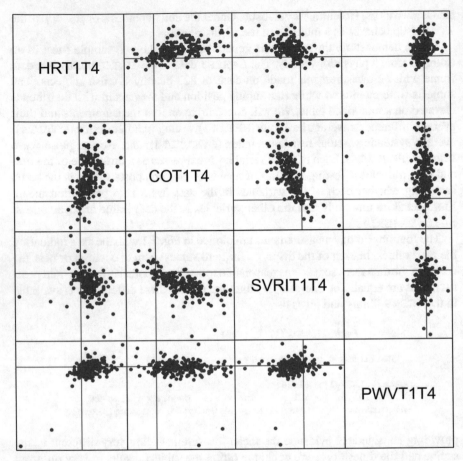

Figure 7.1 Differences in four physiological measures on 225 subjects in the LASERI study. The zero axes are indicated

is standardized at the value of 1.00 in the year 2000. The index is updated monthly but only January values are examined here. Table 7.1 shows these values in several major US cities for the years 2000–11.

The values for the cities are not entirely independent and are subject to identical market forces such as changes in interest rates on mortgages. There was boom in housing prices in 2008 affecting all cities, clearly visible in Table 7.2, but some cities were more affected than others. External forces in the global economy affect all cities as well. In this examination, we will treat the cities as independent of each other and only model the correlation across years within each city.

Table 7.1 The Case–Schiller home price index in January of specified years for several US cities

	Year							
City	2000	2001	2002	2003	...	2009	2010	2011
Phoenix	1	1.0593	1.1161	1.1710	...	1.1713	1.1176	1.0154
Los Angeles	1	1.1088	1.2145	1.4427	...	1.6655	1.7297	1.6988
San Diego	1	1.1754	1.2879	1.5540	...	1.4826	1.5695	1.5703
⋮	⋮	⋮	⋮	⋮		⋮	⋮	⋮
Portland	1	1.0392	1.0813	1.1369	...	1.5380	1.4729	1.3580
Dallas	1	1.0649	1.1176	1.1389	...	1.1260	1.1730	1.1409
Seattle	1	1.0670	1.1179	1.1580	...	1.5438	1.4509	1.3541

Source S&P Dow Jones Indices. Used with permission.

Table 7.2 Log-likelihood tests of nested mean models for home price data

Model	Log-likelihood	Compared to one mean		Compared to previous model	
		Chi-squared	df	Chi-squared	df
One mean	273.12				
Linear	286.99	27.75	1	27.75	1
Quadratic	395.84	245.44	2	217.69	1
Separate	426.77	307.31	10	61.87	7

The data are index values and compare relative change to the baseline value of 1.00 in the year 2000. Similarly, these do not allow a comparison of one city's prices with another but, rather, each city's change from its home prices in the year 2000.

The data values and changes are multiplicative: a value of 1.100 indicates a 10% increase in prices since 2000 for example, so we will take logarithms of these index data in all subsequent examinations of this example. The spaghetti plot of the data appears in Fig. 7.2, with the annual means in red and the values for one extreme city identified.

The means and standard deviations for each year are plotted in Fig. 7.3. The year 2000 data is included with a zero mean and standard deviation of zero. The means (and to a smaller extent, the standard deviations) follow an inverted "U" shape: increasing between 2000 and 2008 and then decreasing in more recent years. In this section, we want to develop models of the correlation structure between the years. In the following sections, we will model $\boldsymbol{\Sigma}$ and $\boldsymbol{\mu}$ separately for the multivariate normal distribution.

The empirical correlation matrix of each year's data with all others is

```
> print(cor(CS), digits = 2)

     2001 2002 2003 2004 2005 2006 2007 2008 2009 2010 2011
2001 1.00 0.80 0.75 0.64 0.53 0.41 0.35 0.33 0.25 0.40 0.45
```

Figure 7.2 Spaghetti plot
of home price data. Annual
means are in red

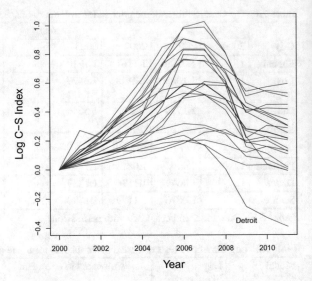

Figure 7.3 Log means (left
scale) and standard
deviations (right scale) of
home price data

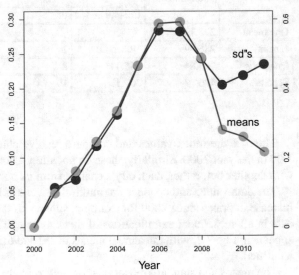

2002	0.80	1.00	0.96	0.88	0.76	0.65	0.58	0.56	0.53	0.60	0.64
2003	0.75	0.96	1.00	0.97	0.87	0.76	0.70	0.68	0.62	0.68	0.71
2004	0.64	0.88	0.97	1.00	0.96	0.87	0.82	0.78	0.66	0.68	0.71
2005	0.53	0.76	0.87	0.96	1.00	0.95	0.91	0.86	0.66	0.62	0.64
2006	0.41	0.65	0.76	0.87	0.95	1.00	0.99	0.93	0.69	0.63	0.62
2007	0.35	0.58	0.70	0.82	0.91	0.99	1.00	0.97	0.74	0.66	0.64
2008	0.33	0.56	0.68	0.78	0.86	0.93	0.97	1.00	0.87	0.79	0.77
2009	0.25	0.53	0.62	0.66	0.66	0.69	0.74	0.87	1.00	0.96	0.94
2010	0.40	0.60	0.68	0.68	0.62	0.63	0.66	0.79	0.96	1.00	0.99
2011	0.45	0.64	0.71	0.71	0.64	0.62	0.64	0.77	0.94	0.99	1.00

Figure 7.4 Autocorrelation
of home price data

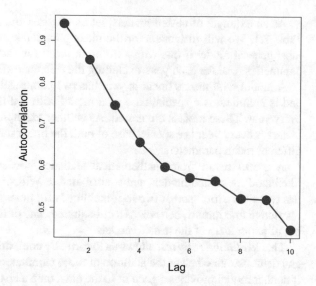

This mass of numbers is not particularly useful to us. One area of multivariate analysis is to model, fit, and interpret different patterns of the covariance matrix Σ. Models for this matrix are the subject of this section.

A more useful summary of this *time series* data is the autocorrelation. The autocorrelation is the correlation between all pairs of years differing by one year, two years, and so on. These differences are referred to as *lags*. More details for time series models are given in Chap. 13.

These autocorrelations are plotted in Fig. 7.4. Adjacent years, with a lag of one, have a very high correlation. Years with a lag of two years are also highly correlated, but a little lower than the one year lag. This monotone pattern continues, with lower correlations as the lag increases between years being compared.

7.4   Maximum Likelihood, Part III: Models for Means

We introduced maximum likelihood estimation in Sects. 5.7 and 6.5. This technique allows us to fit a wider variety of models for which there may not exist software. Specifically, in Sect. 5.7 we show how to write programs in **R** to fit these and in Sect. 6.5, we use the nlm program to extract estimates of parameter estimates. In this section, we will compare two different fitted models.

Suppose we have two or more competing models for our data and would like to choose the best of these. A simple procedure exists if the models follow a specific relationship with each other. Specifically, two models are said to be *nested* if one is a special case of the other.

As an example of nested models, let us consider the home price index given in Table 7.1. We will fit models for the mean parameters for the different years. The most general model is one with a different mean for each year. This model has 11 parameters: one for each year, excluding the reference year 2000.

A model with means linear in year has two parameters (the slope and intercept) and is included as a special case of a model with a different mean parameter for every year. These models are nested. As another example, the model with the same mean for every year is a special case of both the linear model and the model with 11 different mean parameters.

A useful result from mathematical statistics concerns the value of the log-likelihood for nested models and is attributed to Wilks.[2] The approximation specifies twice the difference of two log-likelihoods for nested models, evaluated at their respective maximums, behaves as a chi-squared. The df is the difference in the number of parameters of the nested models.

This *likelihood ratio test* allows us to formally compare two hypothesized models and demonstrate whether the addition of more parameters is worthwhile. Of course, if neither model provides a good fit to the data, then a test of the parameters does not test the adequacy of the models.

Let us work with the home price data given in Table 7.1. The multivariate normal distribution modeling the vector of values for each city has both mean and variance parameters. These will be examined separately: In this section we will fit models to the mean parameters, and in Sect. 7.6 we will examine models for the variance parameters. A more thorough examination of models for means of multivariate normal data is discussed in Chap. 9 on linear regression models.

Begin with a general program evaluating the negative log-likelihood of the home price data. It is best to write a separate function evaluating the model of the means.

This program appears in Output 7.1 and will be called by nlm to maximize the log-likelihood. The variance matrix (vm) is just the empirical variance of the data and is not modeled. Notice how just as this program ends, it prints out the values of all parameters and the likelihood. This is useful for judging the progress being made by nlm and a good habit to get into in similar settings.

This program evaluates the negative log-likelihood of the home price data (CS) but does not specify a model for the means. The model for the means is determined by another function called meanModel specified separately. The function determining the means can easily be changed to accommodate different models, as we will show next.

The meanModel program is a function of two arguments: the parameters (parms) passed to it from nlm and the number of multivariate means (p) required.

Here is a simple example of such a function:

```
meanModel <- function(parms, p)    rep(parms[1], p)
```

---

[2] Samuel Stanley Wilks (1906–1964). American mathematician, worked at Princeton University.

Output 7.1 A general program to evaluate the multivariate normal distribution

```
mvnMean <- function(parms)
# Log-likelihood function to fit means to a multivariate
# normal distribution to CS data
# meanModel is a function to determine the mean
# Requires the mvtnorm library.

{
   n <- dim(CS)[1]                 # sample size
   p <- dim(CS)[2]                 # number of variables

   mu <- meanModel(parms, p)       # mean vector of length p
   resid <-
     CS - t(matrix(rep(mu, n), p, n)) # subtract the mean
   vm <- var(resid)                # the variance of the data
   mvnMean <- sum(dmvnorm(resid, log = TRUE,
          sigma = var(resid)))     # multivariate normal density
   print(c(parms, mvnMean))        # likelihood at this estimate
   -mvnMean                        # return negative to minimize
}
```

This function specifies a model with one mean for all years in the home price data. Specifically, there is only one mean parameter. This function makes p copies of it and returns it as a vector of values.

Using this definition of the meanModel function, we fit a single-mean model with the **R** code

```
oneMout <- nlm(mvnMean, 0, hessian = TRUE)  # capture output
oneMout                                     # print output
```

A portion of the output is as follows:

```
$minimum
[1] -273.1169

$estimate
[1] 0.05061963

$gradient
[1] 4.718004e-06

$hessian
          [,1]
[1,] 32959.48
```

                .   .   .

This output lists the minimum of the negative log-likelihood (−273.1), the estimated value of the single fitted mean (.0506), the gradient (which is very close in value to zero), and the Hessian or curvature of the log-likelihood.

Finally, we compute the reciprocal, square root of the Hessian to obtain an estimate of the standard error of the estimated mean:

```
print(sqrt(1 / oneMout$hessian), 3)          # est'd std error

  [,1]
[1,] 0.00551
```

We are not going to discuss the adequacy of this model except to fit other models for the mean vector and then show how much better these are, relative to increasing the value of the log-likelihood. More detail on fitting regression models, including diagnostics, is discussed in Chap. 9 on multivariate linear regression.

As another example of the means, we can use the function

```
meanModel <- function(parms, p)  parms[1] + parms[2] * (1 : p)
```

to fit a model of the means linear in the year. The two parameters are respectively the intercept (`parms[1]`) and the slope (`parms[2]`) on year. In this model, the year is recorded less than 2000. The effect of this recording is to change the interpretation of the intercept but not the slope.

When we run this new definition of the `meanModel`, it replaces the previous definition of the function. The assignment (<−) operation is best thought of as *replacing* the definition rather than *assigning* a definition. Output 7.2 lists the **R** dialog fitting the linear model and providing parameter estimates.

The call to `nlm` uses the new definition of `meanModel` specifying the mean as a linear function of the year. The initial, starting values for the slope and intercept are both zero. The maximum of the log-likelihood function is 286.99.

A three-parameter quadratic model of the mean can be fitted using

```
meanModel <- function(parms, p)
    parms[1] + parms[2] * (1 : p) / 10 + parms[3] * ((1 : p) ^ 2) / 100
```

In this function, we recode the year as

$$(\text{year} - 2000)/10.$$

The reason for dividing by 10 is to multiply the corresponding parameter estimated values by this amount. Many algorithms will perform better when all parameter values are measured on the same scale, rather than a wide range of values. The interpretation of the parameters needs to be adjusted back when these are reported.

The function fitting a separate mean for every year returns a list of parameter values:

```
meanModel <- function(parms, p)  parms
```

Output 7.2 R dialog fitting a linear model to the home price data

```
> linMout <- nlm(mvnMean, c(0, 0), hessian = TRUE)
> linMout

$minimum
[1] -286.9895

$estimate
[1]  0.06584120 -0.01725947

$gradient
[1] -2.160050e-06 -1.364242e-06

$hessian
            [,1]        [,2]
[1,] 32959.49   29067.81
[2,] 29067.81 118780.37

$code
[1] 1

$iterations
[1] 4

> invhess <- solve(linMout$hessian) # invert hessian matrix
> sqrt(invhess[1, 1])   # est'd std error of intercept

[1] 0.00622018

> sqrt(invhess[2, 2])   # est'd std error of slope

[1] 0.003276581
```

where each of the parameters is the mean for each year.

Let us summarize the log-likelihood of these four nested mean models and the corresponding chi-squared tests in Table 7.2. In this series of models, we see strong evidence each successive model provides a better fit leading up to the model with a separate mean for each year. Our goal is to provide a model with good explanatory value. The model with a different mean for every year fails to provide any intuitive simplification. Specifically, the additional seven parameters make a statistically significant contribution to the model ($\chi^2 = 61.78$; 7df; $p = 0$) but the model offers limited explanatory value.

The quadratic model has fewer parameters, and while statistically not as good as the 11 parameter model, it still provides a good intuitive summary of what we see in Fig. 7.3. That is, relative to the baseline year 2000, home prices increased to around 2008 levels and then declined.

7.5 Inference on Multivariate Normal Variances

The Wishart[3] distribution is the generalization of the (univariate) chi-squared distribution and is used to describe the behavior of an estimated covariance matrix. In Sect. 5.6, the univariate sample variance was distributed as a multiple of the chi-squared distribution. The analogous multivariate sample variance matrix has a distribution known as the Wishart distribution. **R** has functions to calculate the density of the Wishart distribution as well as generate random covariance matrices from a Wishart distribution. (See Table 2.2) Unfortunately, finding cumulative distributions and tail areas from the distribution involves integrating the distribution over a subset of all symmetric, positive definite matrices. For one-dimensional data, the tail area is easily defined. In the case of random matrices, the range of the distribution of all covariance matrices is much more difficult to describe.

Rather than describing the confidence intervals of the whole covariance matrix, we can model the matrix with a small number of parameters. In this section, we will describe patterned covariance matrices having useful interpretations. In Sect. 7.6, we will fit these in **R** and test hypotheses about them.

The *spherical covariance matrix* is so named because all contours of the density function are circular. In order for this to be the case, we must have all zero correlations. The spherical variance matrix is diagonal:

$$\text{Var}\,(X) = \text{Diag}\,(\sigma_1^2,\ \sigma_2^2,\ \ldots,\sigma_p^2) = \begin{pmatrix} \sigma_1^2 & 0 & \cdots & 0 \\ 0 & \sigma_2^2 & \cdots & 0 \\ \vdots & & \ddots & \\ 0 & 0 & \cdots & \sigma_p^2 \end{pmatrix}$$

and the corresponding correlation matrix is a $p \times p$ identity matrix.

Spherical covariance is the simplest pattern. It is the model for mutual independence of all p multivariate normal observations. Saying all multivariate components of the distribution are mutually independent misses the point of modeling such data, however. The model of mutual independence tells us nothing can be learned over p separate marginal analyses of each component of the data.

A special kind of multivariate dependence includes the *exchangeable* model. Exchangeable means every multivariate component behaves the same as the others. An example of this appears in Fig. 1.2 where any one observation is representative of all others.

The exchangeable dependence structure is also the same for every member of the multivariate observation. The result is the exchangeable multivariate normal means and variances as well as every pairwise correlation is the same.

The exchangeable variance matrix is

---

[3] John Wishart (1898–1956). Scottish mathematician and statistician.

$$\text{Var } X = \begin{pmatrix} \sigma^2 & \rho\sigma^2 & \cdots & \rho\sigma^2 \\ \rho\sigma^2 & \sigma^2 & \cdots & \rho\sigma^2 \\ \vdots & & \ddots & \vdots \\ \rho\sigma^2 & \rho\sigma^2 & \cdots & \sigma^2 \end{pmatrix}. \tag{7.7}$$

The diagonal values are all equal to σ^2 and all of the off-diagonals are equal to $\rho\sigma^2$ for some $|\rho| < 1$.

The exchangeable correlation matrix is

$$\text{Corr } X = \begin{pmatrix} 1 & \rho & \cdots & \rho \\ \rho & 1 & \cdots & \rho \\ \vdots & & \ddots & \vdots \\ \rho & \rho & \cdots & 1 \end{pmatrix}. \tag{7.8}$$

In the exchangeable covariance matrix at (7.7) there are two parameters: the variance σ^2 which is the same for all components of X, and the correlations between any pairs of components, ρ. In most cases we have $\rho > 0$ so there is a mutual positive correlation, and (7.7) will be positive definite. In very restrictive cases, we can also have ρ equal to a small negative value even though mathematically (7.7) may no longer be positive definite. What's more, it is difficult to describe a situation where every component is negatively correlated with every other. See Exercise 7.5 for an example of this behavior.

We can also have an exchangeable correlation matrix with different variances. In this case the covariance matrix is

$$\text{Var } X = \begin{pmatrix} \sigma_1^2 & \rho\sigma_1\sigma_2 & \cdots & \rho\sigma_1\sigma_k \\ \rho\sigma_1\sigma_2 & \sigma_2^2 & \cdots & \rho\sigma_2\sigma_k \\ \vdots & & \ddots & \vdots \\ \rho\sigma_1\sigma_k & \rho\sigma_2\sigma_k & \cdots & \sigma_k^2 \end{pmatrix} \tag{7.9}$$

or equivalently,

$$\text{Var } (x_i) = \sigma_i^2$$

and

$$\text{Cov } (x_i, \, x_j) = \rho\sigma_i\sigma_j \text{ for } i \neq j.$$

The variances can all be different. The correlations are the same between all pairs and will also follow (7.8). We will fit the covariance matrix (7.9) to the home price data in Sect. 7.6.

Another commonly encountered patterned covariance matrix appears in observations measured in a temporal or serial manner such as the house-pricing data. We will discuss such time series data in more detail in Chap. 13, but for the present, we can intuitively understand observations closer to each other should be more highly correlated than observations farther apart. If the observations are measured in a uniform fashion (such as every day or every year), then we can expect these correlations to fall off in a prescribed fashion. As an example, we can see this pattern in Fig. 7.4.

The correlation matrix for autocorrelated observations is of the form

$$\text{Corr } X = \begin{pmatrix} 1 & \rho & \rho^2 & \cdots & \rho^{k-1} \\ \rho & 1 & \rho & \cdots & \rho^{k-2} \\ \rho^2 & \rho & 1 & \cdots & \rho^{k-3} \\ \vdots & \vdots & \vdots & \ddots & \vdots \\ \rho^{k-1} & \rho^{k-2} & \rho^{k-3} & \cdots & 1 \end{pmatrix}. \tag{7.10}$$

Specifically, adjacent years have correlation ρ. Years two apart have correlation ρ^2 and so on. This model is only useful when $0 < \rho < 1$. Notice the exchangeable and autocorrelated correlation matrices have the same number of parameters but these have different interpretations and functional forms.

In the next section, we fit patterned variance matrices to the home price data in Table 7.1.

7.6 Fitting Patterned Covariance Matrices

As we see from the summary of fitted models in Table 7.2, the best fitting model for the mean has a separate parameter for every year. Although this model may be the best fitting one, we conclude it lacks a simple message to summarize the data in a succinct manner. By analogy, in Sect. 7.5 we saw the full correlation matrix is more than we need and a simple patterned matrix can go a long way toward providing a simple summary of the data.

Mathematically, we can separate the variances and correlations of the variance matrix Σ. Let σ denote the marginal standard deviations of the multivariate normal x and let R denote the matrix of correlations. Then we can write

$$\Sigma = \text{Diag}(\sigma)\, R\, \text{Diag}(\sigma). \tag{7.11}$$

Equivalently, it is more convenient in **R** to compute this as

$$\Sigma = \sigma\sigma' * R \tag{7.12}$$

where $*$ represents element-by-element multiplication of two matrices.

Ideally, we can choose a functional form of R with a useful interpretation such as any of the different matrices described in Sect. 7.5. Similarly, the vector of variances σ would also be most useful if they followed a prescribed model rather than ranging freely.

Figure 7.5 Detrended plot of home prices

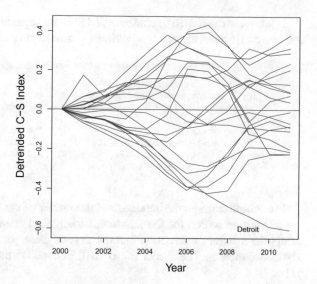

We next fit some models using the home price data. Fig. 7.5 plots the detrended home price data. That is, the mean value for each year has been removed leaving only the annual variability for us to model. Similarly, the mean of all data values is zero for each year so we do not need to consider the multivariate normal mean parameters. As we saw in Fig. 7.2, one unusual city (Detroit) stands out in this figure and is identified. We will model the variances of the data in Fig. 7.5 in this section. Fig. 7.3 demonstrates variances increase up until about 2008 before they decline.

The observations within each city are positively correlated across the years. It is not clear what an appropriate model would be to model this correlation. We can solve this by fitting and then comparing a variety of models.

Next we need general code to allow us to fit a range of models. To do this, break the problem into several small modules to be tested individually before going on to the next step.

Let us begin with code to build the correlation matrix $\boldsymbol{R}$ in (7.11). The exchangeable correlation matrix (7.8) with specified size and ρ is created using

```
exchange.mat <- function(size = 1, rho = 0) # build exchangeable matrix
    matrix(rho, size, size) + (1 - rho) * diag(size)
```

Similarly, the autocorrelation matrix (7.10) can be built with

```
autocorr.mat <- function(size = 1, rho = 0)  # autocorrelation matrix
    rho ^ abs(row(diag(size)) - col(diag(size)))
```

using code attributed to Peter Dalgaard.

Next, we write a shell to compute (7.12) from separate programs (mv.vars and mv.cors) to build the vector of variances σ and correlation matrix R, respectively.

```
cov.model <- function(size, parms)
# shell to fit patterned covariance matrix
#   mv.vars models variances,  mv.cors models correlations
{
  rho <- parms[1]                          # rho is first parameter
  rho <- max(.0001, min(rho, .9999))       # must be between zero and one
  sigma <- sqrt(mv.vars(size, parms[-1]))  # model for marginal st dev's
  sigma %*% t(sigma) * mv.cors(size, rho)  # covariance matrix
}
```

We should consider the iterated, trial parameter values to be passed to this program by nlm in its search for the maximum likelihood estimates of our model. Let us adopt the arbitrary convention that the first of these parameters will always denote the correlation ρ. The model for σ will depend on the other parameters sent by nlm.

In building Σ from trial parameters, nlm does not know ρ must take values between zero and one, so this code enforces the restriction. A similar problem was encountered in Sect. 5.7 when we introduced nlm for obtaining maximum likelihood estimates. Similar adjustments will be made in subsequent code.

The last big step is to compute the log-likelihood of the detrended data (detr). The code in Output 7.3 is called by nlm, builds the covariance matrix cov, and evaluates the multivariate normal log-likelihood logl for the detrended home price data, detr.

The code for fit.cov given in Output 7.3 checks for a singular covariance matrix by flagging situations where the determinant is less than 10^{-30}. The choice of this threshold is arbitrary and was made after watching the printed values from this program. This assures the matrix is positive definite. If the determinant falls below this value, the program adds a large value to the diagonal, making it more positive definite and also penalizing the log-likelihood. The routine ends by printing the parameter values and the log-likelihood so we can judge the progress made by nlm. This is a good practice when attempting to maximize the likelihood using iterative programs such as nlm.

The last step is to create a model for the vector of standard deviations, σ. Figure 7.3 provides strong evidence these are not all the same. We need to make sure values of the parameters passed to us by nlm result in positive values of σ. We can avoid problems by modeling $\log \sigma$ as a function of parameters, because all parameter values will be valid.

The model with a constant variance for all years

$$\log \sigma_i = \beta_0$$

is fitted using the code:.

```
mv.vars <- function(size, parms)  rep(exp(parms[1]), size)
```

Similarly, we have the log-linear model

$$\log \sigma_i = \beta_0 + \beta_1(\text{year} - 2000)$$

and it is fitted by the **R** code

```
mv.vars <- function(size, parms)
   pmin( exp(parms[1] + parms[2] * (1 : size)), # log-linear vars
         rep(10, size))                          # check for overflow
```

checking the σ_i are not too large. The `pmin()` function performs parallel minimums across each element of the vector arguments.

We also fit a quadratic term of the standard deviations on a log scale in order to capture the rising and falling values apparent in Fig. 7.3. This model is

$$\log \sigma_i = \beta_0 + \beta_1(\text{year} - 2000) + \beta_1(\text{year} - 2000)^2 \tag{7.13}$$

and fitted in **R** using

```
mv.vars <- function(size, parms)
   pmin( exp(parms[1] + parms[2] * (1 : size)
         + parms[3] * (1 : size) ^2),           # log-quadratic vars
         rep(10, size))                          # check for overflow
```

We can fit different patterns of covariance matrices by assigning these functional values to `mv.vars` and `mv.cors`. There are two different correlation models (exchangeable and autocorrelation) and three different models for the marginal variances (constant, log-linear, and log-quadratic) for a total of six possibilities.

As an example of fitting one of these six models, we can write

```
mv.vars <- function(size, parms)
   pmin( exp(parms[1] + parms[2] * (1 : size)), # log-linear vars
         rep(10, size))                          # check for overflow
mv.cors <- function (size, rho) exchange.mat(size, rho)  # exchangeable
nlm(fit.cov, c(0.7, -5,  0.2), hessian = TRUE)  # fit the model
```

to fit a log-linear model of standard deviations with an exchangeable correlation matrix.

The fitted values of all six models are summarized in Table 7.3. This table includes the maximized log-likelihood, estimated parameter values, and the corresponding estimated standard errors.

The exchangeable and autocorrelated correlation matrices are not nested so the differences in their log-likelihood values cannot be used as a hypothesis test using the likelihood ratio test. Even so, the likelihood values for the autocorrelated models are much larger, giving good evidence these are better summaries of the data. More formal tests of goodness of fit are described in the following section.

Table 7.3 Fitted parameters, estimated standard errors, and log-likelihoods for variance models of the home price data

Model for σ	Likelihood	$\widehat{\rho}$	SE $\widehat{\rho}$	$\widehat{\beta}_0$	SE $\widehat{\beta}_0$	$\widehat{\beta}_1$	SE $\widehat{\beta}_1$	$\widehat{\beta}_2$	SE $\widehat{\beta}_2$
Exchangeable correlation									
One σ	125.8	0.650	0.079	−3.21	0.22				
Log-linear	149.8	0.673	0.076	−4.74	0.31	0.229	0.034		
Log-Quadratic	180.2	0.707	0.071	−6.65	0.33	0.977	0.089	−0.060	0.007
Autocorrelation matrix									
One σ	256.2	0.927	0.017	−3.39	0.23				
Log-linear	268.7	0.909	0.019	−4.87	0.33	0.197	0.040		
Log-Quadratic	292.1	0.939	0.016	−6.12	0.34	0.807	0.085	−0.050	0.007

Within each of the two types of correlations, the log-linear model has a much larger log-likelihood than the model with a constant standard deviation, and the quadratic model exhibits an even higher log-likelihood. All of these comparisons can be made by differencing the log-likelihoods and treating these as one-half of a chi-squared with one df.

7.7 Tests for Multivariate Normality

Section 5.4 presents many different tests for univariate normality. The variety of these is motivated by all the different ways the sample can appear to deviate from the normal distribution. Most of the tests for multivariate normal described in this section are direct generalizations of those univariate methods. Tests will provide a p-value, quantifying the statistical significance of one deviation from the underlying assumption of normality. The test does not end there, however. After rejecting such a hypothesis, we should also explain how and where the normal model failed.

Visual examinations are among the best tools available. One familiar method is to plot the data in a pairwise scatter plot using `pairs()`. Every pairwise plot should appear to be sampled from a bivariate normal distribution. This is not a universal test of multivariate normality, but it can detect many serious deficiencies in the assumed model. Then again, there is no universal test for all of the possible deviations from this model.

Let us next examine a generalization of the QQ plot. We first need to summarize each multivariate observation as a univariate scalar. This is done by describing each observation in terms of its distance from the multivariate mean.

Define the measure

$$D_i^2 = (Y_i - \overline{Y})' S^{-1} (Y_i - \overline{Y}). \tag{7.14}$$

The D^2 statistic is a popular metric called the *Mahalanobis distance*.[4] This is a convenient way to express the *distance* between an observation Y_i and the multivariate mean $\overline{Y}$. A useful strategy is to plot the scalar D_i^2 values against chi-squared quantiles. Each D_i^2 is a scalar-valued measure of how far the observed value Y_i is from the center of the fitted multivariate normal distribution.

The components of Y_i are correlated and have different variances. For this reason, a simple Euclidean distance would not be appropriate. The S^{-1} sandwiched between the $(Y_i - \overline{Y})$ standardizes the different components to variance one and removes their correlations. See Exercise 7.6 for details. The formula for D_i^2 appears as the exponent of the normal density function given at (7.2) except the mean and variance have been replaced by their estimates. In other words, the likelihood (or value of the density function) of an observation Y_i is approximately proportional to $\exp(-D_i^2/2)$.

The individual D_i^2 are not independent, because all of the observations are used to estimate $\overline{Y}$ and S. However, as approximation when there are many more observations than variable columns, each D_i^2 should behave as independent chi-squares with df equal to the number of data columns.

Let us illustrate the Mahalanobis distances for the candy nutrition values listed in Table 7.4. After reading the data into a data.frame called candy, the Mahalanobis distances are calculated in **R** using

```
mah <- mahalanobis(candy, colMeans(candy), var(candy))
```

where the second and third arguments are the estimated means and variances, respectively.

There are $p = 6$ data columns (calories, fat, saturated fat, carbohydrates, sugar, and sodium), so the ordered Mahalanobis distances from the overall six-dimensional mean are compared to a chi-squared with 6 df. This is only an approximation because we are using estimates of the means and variances as their true values. Nevertheless, even a cursory examination of Fig. 7.6 shows this distribution is reasonable. The two most extreme candy brands are identified by name. In the present example, the identification of extreme brands refers to those most different from the overall average of all others.

All values in Fig. 7.6 appear to fall on the QQ line connecting the upper and lower quartiles of the chi-squared distribution and those of the data. From this plot, we see there is no evidence of a lack of fit, and the data values appear to follow a multivariate normal distribution.

We can create a test of the adequacy of the fit in this figure by converting the Mahalanobis distances from chi-squared values into normal quantiles. In this case, we have

---

[4] Prasanta Chandra Mahalanobis (1893–1972). Indian scientist and statistician.

Output 7.3 Code to evaluate the multivariate normal likelihood for fitting the variance matrix. This program is called by `nlm`

```
fit.cov <- function(parms) # Shell called by nlm
  # Compute the log-likelihood of detrended home price data (detr)
  # Check for positive definite covariance matrix
{
  logl <- 0
  size <- dim(detr)[2]         # width of the detrended data
  cov <- cov.model(size, parms) # the trial built  covariance matrix
  print(det(cov))              # check on trial covariance matrix
  if(det(cov) <= 1.0e-30)      # is the covariance positive definite?
    {
        cov <- cov + diag(size) # adjust the covariance...
        logl <- -1000           #  ... and penalize the likelihood
    }
                               # log multivariate normal density
  logl <- logl + dmvnorm(detr, mean = rep(0, size),
                 sigma = cov, log = TRUE)
  logl <- sum(logl)            # log likelihood of detrended data
  print(c(parms, logl))        # trace the progress of nlm
  -logl                        # return negative log likelihood
}
```

Figure 7.6 QQ plot of Mahalanobis distances of candy nutrition values

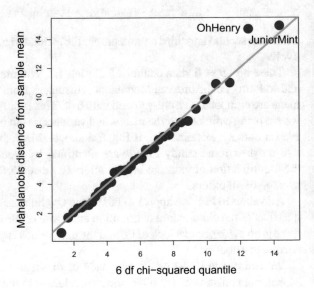

Table 7.4 Nutritional values of popular candy brands

Name	Calories	Fat	Satfat	Carbs	Sugar	Sodium
100 Grand	190	8	5	30	22	90
3 Musketeers	240	7	5	42	36	90
5th Avenue	260	12	5	38	29	120
Almond Joy	220	13	8	26	20	50
Andes Mints	200	13	11	22	20	20
Baby Ruth	275	13	7	39	32	138
Butterfinger	270	11	6	43	29	135
Cadbury Dairy Milk	260	15	9	28	28	0
Charleston Chew	230	6	5	43	30	30
Dove Smooth Milk Choc.	220	13	8	24	22	25
Goobers	200	13	5	20	17	15
Heath Toffee	210	13	7	24	23	135
Hershey's bar	210	13	8	26	24	35
Hershey's Skor	200	12	7	25	24	130
Junior Mints	220	4	3	45	42	35
Kit Kat	207	10	7	26	20	22
M&M's, peanut	250	13	5	30	25	25
M&M's, plain	230	9	6	34	31	35
Milk Duds	230	8	5	38	27	135
Milky Way	240	9	7	37	31	75
Mounds	240	13	10	29	21	55
Mr Goodbar	250	16	7	25	22	50
Nestle Crunch	220	11	7	30	24	60
Oh Henry!	280	17	7	36	32	65
Payday	240	13	3	27	21	120
Raisinets	190	8	5	32	28	15
Reese's Fast Break	260	12	5	35	30	190
Reese's Nutrageous	260	16	5	28	22	100
Reese's Peanut Butter cups	210	13	5	24	21	150
Reese's Pieces	200	9	8	25	21	55
Reese's Sticks	220	13	5	23	17	130
Rolo	220	10	7	33	29	80
Snickers	230	11	4	32	27	115
Symphony	223	13	8	24	23	42
Twix	250	12	7	33	24	100
Whatchamacalit	237	11	8	30	23	144
Whoppers	190	7	7	31	24	100
Zero Candy Bar	200	7	5	34	29	105

Values collected from www.fatsecret.com. Used with permission.

Figure 7.7 Parallel
coordinates plot of candy
nutrition values identifying
the two extremes from
Fig. 7.6

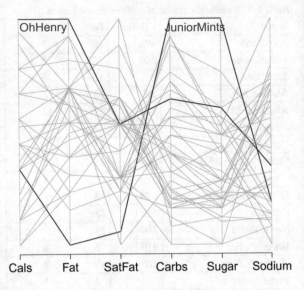

> shapiro.test(qnorm(pchisq(mah, 6)))

            Shapiro-Wilk normality test

data: qnorm(pchisq(mah, 6))
W = 0.9893, p-value = 0.9711

The `pchisq` program converts the Mahalanobis distances (`mah`) into p-values
from the reference chi-squared distribution and then `qnorm` turns this into normal
quantiles needed for the Shapiro–Wilk test. The p-value of the test confirms the good
fit seen in Fig 7.6.

In Fig. 7.7, we present the candy values in a parallel coordinate plot, identifying
the two brands extreme in the Mahalanobis QQ plot of Fig. 7.6. (Parallel coordinate
plots were previously described in Sect. 3.5.) Oh Henry! has the largest calories and
fat content of all brands. Junior Mints are highest in carbohydrates and sugar but also
lowest in fat and very low in saturated fat.

Other tests for the multivariate normal are based on multivariate generalizations
of skewness and kurtosis first described by Mardia (1970). By analogy to (7.14),
define

$$D_{ij} = (Y_i - \overline{Y})'S^{-1}(Y_j - \overline{Y}).$$

We can think of D_{ij} as a Mahalanobis distance between observations Y_i and Y_j.
The *multivariate skewness* is defined as

$$\widehat{\gamma}_3 = N^{-2} \sum_{i \neq j} D_{ij}^3$$

The statistic $N\widehat{\gamma}_3/6$ will behave approximately as chi-squared with $p(p+1)$ $(p+2)/6$ df when sampled from a multivariate normal distribution.

The *multivariate kurtosis* is defined as

$$\widehat{\gamma}_4 = N^{-1} \sum_i D_{ii}^2.$$

The statistic $\widehat{\gamma}_4$ will behave approximately as normal with mean $p(p+2)$ and variance $8p(p+2)/N$. The mardia test includes additional small-sample corrections to approximate the behavior of $\widehat{\gamma}_3$ and $\widehat{\gamma}_4$.

von Eye and Bogat (2004) recommend multivariate skewness $\widehat{\gamma}_3$ as a useful measure of goodness of fit for the multivariate normal. Schwager and Margolin (1982) show the multivariate kurtosis $\widehat{\gamma}_4$ is a good way to test whether multivariate outliers are present in the data. Both of these statistics are programmed in **R** and are available using the mardia function in the psych library. There are also versions in the semTools library.

If we return to the candy data, the **R** commands

```
> require(psych)
> mardia(candy)
```

return, in part,

```
n.obs = 38    num.vars =  6
b1p =  8.59    skew = 54.4   with probability =  0.54
   small sample skew = 60.02  with probability =  0.33
b2p = 44.86   kurtosis =  -0.99  with probability = 0.32
```

and also produce the QQ plot appearing in Fig. 7.6.

From the statistical significance levels given here, we see there is no evidence of extreme multivariate skewness or kurtosis in these data. Tests of skewness and kurtosis generalize the Jarque-Bera test to multivariate data. Another multivariate Jarque-Bera test is examined in Sect. 13.2 as a test of normality of residuals in a multivariate regression model.

Another test of the multivariate normal distribution is a generalization of the Shapiro–Wilk test for the QQ plot. The packages mvnormtest and mvShapiro Test both include a multivariate Shapiro–Wilk test.

The code and output for the candy data of Table 7.4

```
> library(mvnormtest)
> mshapiro.test( t(candy) )

        Shapiro-Wilk normality test

data:  Z
W = 0.8755, p-value = 0.0005544
```

indicates a poor fit to the multivariate normal distribution. The `mshapiro` program expects the data to be organized as variables in rows and cases in columns, so we must transpose the data matrix using the `t` function.

Let us see if we can identify the source of this problem by examining the individual QQ plots for each of the variables in these data. Fig. 7.8 lists these and includes the individual p-values of the Shapiro–Wilk tests. Sugar and fat values approach statistical significance but their joint effect should be diminished when we take into account the multiplicity of these six hypothesis tests. That is, there is no one stand-out variable demonstrating a lack of fit. However, when taken collectively, the multivariate Shapiro–Wilk test indicates an overall deficiency. This is often the case with multivariate analyses of data: Overall outliers or lack of fit may not be apparent in marginal analyses of the same data.

As a final method of testing for multivariate normality, let us describe the *energy test*. The energy test is programmed in the library of the same name. Additional mathematical details are described in Székely and Rizzo (2005).

The energy test begins by standardizing the multivariate observations Y_i by their sample means and variance S. Specifically,

$$Z_i = S^{-1/2} \left(Y_i - \overline{Y} \right) \tag{7.15}$$

transforms a multivariate normal sample Y_i into a multivariate sample with zero means and zero covariances.

Recall (see Exercise 4.6) the matrix square root is not unique, so there is no unique way to perform this transformation. Briefly, the Z_i are linear combinations of the multivariate data values for each observation and can be interpreted as the square root of the Mahalanobis distances.

The energy test compares the Euclidean distances between the transformed Z_i and randomly sampled, uncorrelated multivariate normal random variables. The energy test can be written as

$$\text{Energy statistic} = 2A - B - C$$

Here, B is the average Euclidean distance between the transformed Z_i, and C is the average distance between observations made on a simulated multivariate random sample X_i with zero means and identity covariance matrix. The A term is the average distance between the X's and the Z's. Intuitively, this statistic has a

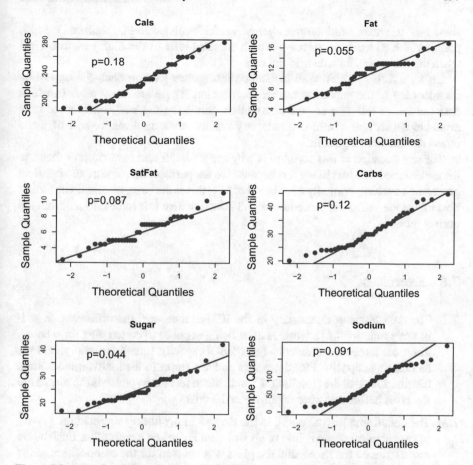

Figure 7.8 Univariate QQ plots for the candy data

large value if the distance between the observed and simulated values is greater than the distances within either the data values or the simulated values.

The energy test performed on the candy data:

```
> library( energy )
> mvnorm.etest( candy )
```

```
        Energy test of multivariate normality: estimated parameters

        data:  x, sample size 38, dimension 6, replicates 999
        E-statistic = 1.1793, p-value = 0.7638
```

In this case, there were 999 replicated random samples X_i. The energy test does not indicate a lack of fit to the multivariate normal distribution. In Exercise 7.7, we show how to create and interpret *energy residuals* related to this statistic. We also point out the `MissMech` package which contains tests of the multivariate normal when there are missing values in the data.

Let us end this section with the same message we gave in Sect. 5.4 on testing for adequacy of the univariate normal distribution. There are many ways in which data can fail to follow a normal distribution. Similarly, there are many good tests available which may return contradictory results: some indicate a good fit while others demonstrate a poor fit.

The real question in this scenario is why are we interested in testing for the fit to the normal model? Most likely it is because we are performing some other statistical procedure requiring normally distributed data. If this is the case, we should be asking how robust the statistical procedure is and how sensitive it is to deviations from the normal model.

7.8   Exercises

7.1   The data frame `pulmonary` in the ICSNP measures the difference in pulmonary function in 12 workers after being exposed to cotton dust for 6 hours. There are three measurements: forced vital capacity, forced expiratory volume, and closing capacity. Plot these data and test for fit to the multivariate normal distribution. Use the Hotelling T^2 statistic to test the hypothesis the means are the same before and after exposure to the dust.

7.2   The data frame `bottle.df` in the `Hotelling` library summarizes a study of the chemical composition of six different Heineken beer bottles. Each bottle was examined ten times, and the glass was assayed for the composition of the elements manganese, barium, strontium, zirconium, and titanium.

    a.   Examine the data using plots to identify outliers. Identify any remarkable outliers or abnormalities. Test the data for multivariate normal distribution, both marginally and within each of the six bottles.

    b.   Apply the Hotelling test to examine whether the multivariate normal means are the same across the six bottles. Is there evidence the variance matrices are all the same?

7.3   Find the correlation matrix of the OECD PISA academic score data in Table 1.2. Is this suggestive of an exchangeable correlation? Fit this model for the correlation matrix. What is the estimated value of the off-diagonal elements? What does this value tell you? Other examinations of these data appear in Exercises 2.9 and 8.9.

7.4   Consider the home price data given in Table 7.1.

    a.   All index values are relative to the value 100 for every city in the year 2000. Does this motivate examining the logarithms of these data?

b. Find the mean index value for each year, over all cities, to see the national trend. Plot these values. Is there evidence of a real estate "boom" or "bust?"

c. Subtract this national, annual trend from each city's values to identify outliers. Test the adequacy of the multivariate normal model.

7.5 Describe a situation where multivariate data is collected and every component is *negatively* correlated with every other. Can this happen in practice?

7.6 Show how the S^{-1} in the sandwich of (7.14) corrects for the different variances. Specifically, write a program in **R** to compute the Z_i defined at 7.15. Use **R** to show the variance of these transformed values is an identity matrix. *Hint*: Use the program for calculating the matrix square root given in Sect. 4.5.6.

7.7 Let us look into the details of the energy test and develop a set of residuals for it. Let Z_i be the normalized data values defined at (7.15) and let Y_j ($j = 1, \ldots, n$) be a set of random multivariate normal values with zero means and identity covariance matrix. Then define

$$A_i = \text{Average } ||Z_i - Y_j|| \text{ over all } j$$
$$B_i = \text{Average } ||Z_i - Z_j|| \text{ over all } j \neq i$$
$$C = \text{Average } ||Y_i - Y_j|| \text{ over all } i \text{ and } j \ (i \neq j)$$

where $|| \cdot ||$ is the Euclidean length defined at (4.4), and $||Z - Y||$ is the Euclidean distance between the vectors Y and Z.

a. Interpret the statistics A, B, and C in simple terms.

b. Define the *energy statistic residuals* as

$$\text{Energy residual}_i = 2A_i - B_i - C$$

Write a program in **R** to calculate the energy residuals for a given set of data.

c. The energy residuals defined in this manner are functions of random values Y and will not be the same every time you generate them. Show for large sample sizes n, the energy statistics have high correlation with the Mahalanobis distances on the data.

7.8 The data in Table 7.5 lists rates of student obesity in different regions of New York State for 2010–2012, excluding New York City.

a. Display these data in a manner to identify trends and/or outliers. Are the rates different in the two different grades?

b. Test for multivariate normality. Does the Mahalanobis distance identify the same outliers you found in part a.?

c. Fit a multivariate normal distribution to these data with different means and variances but an exchangeable correlation matrix. What is your estimate of the mutual correlation between the four different rates? Interpret this finding.

Table 7.5 Percentages of obese students in upstate regions of New York State, 2010–2012

	Elementary schools		Middle and high schools	
Region	Overweight	Obese	Overweight	Obese
Central NY	16.8	18.6	17.5	20.7
Finger Lakes	16.0	17.0	16.7	19.5
Hudson Valley	15.2	16.1	16.9	16.6
Nassau-Suffolk	15.8	17.3	16.4	16.1
New York-Penn	16.3	17.5	16.4	20.8
NorthEastern NY	16.0	16.9	16.6	19.2
Western NY	15.2	17.1	17.1	19.8

Source https://health.data.ny.gov/

7.9   Write a program in **R** to calculate the autocorrelation function of the home price data plotted in Fig. 7.4.

7.10 There are *robust* estimators of the parameters of the multivariate normal distribution. Robust estimators are described in terms of their *breakdown*. Breakdown is the percentage of observations to wander off to infinity without greatly affecting the estimator.

   a. Describe the breakdown properties of a sample mean versus the sample median for a univariate sample.
   b. The `cov.rob` program in the MASS library performs robust estimation of the multivariate normal mean and variance parameters by identifying and using only those observations closest to the center of the data as measured by their Mahalanobis distance. Use `cov.rob` to estimate parameters of the numeric, demographic parameters in the LASERI data. How different are the estimates we obtain from `var`?
   c. Try perturbing a fraction of the observations in LASERI by a huge amount and see how this affects the estimates. What percent of the observations can be changed before the estimates from `cov.rob` break down? How well do conventional estimators work under these circumstances? Also consider using the `cov.trob` program to estimate parameters of a long-tailed multivariate t-distribution.

7.11 Table 7.6 lists the percentage of Americans with disabilities, by age, according to the US Census. Fit a multivariate normal distribution to these data with separate models for the means and variances. As with rates in general, it may be useful to do all of the model fitting after taking logs of the data.

   a. Some rates are much higher than others and some disabilities increase faster with age. Fit separate models for the means of each disability, assuming all rates are independent. Use nested models to see if different slopes for each disability are better than one slope for all.

Table 7.6 Percentage of Americans with disabilities, by age

Disability	Age		
	65–74	75–84	85+
Vision	16.5	18.2	24.9
Hearing	34.9	40.6	48.1
Cognitive	22.6	28.0	39.1
Ambulatory	63.6	65.2	72.8
Self-care	20.2	26.9	42.4
Independent living	34.0	47.2	68.7

Source Wan and Larsen (2014)

b. Describe a correlation structure for these data over age. Do the rates across ages appear dependent? Does this dependence appear exchangeable or auto-correlated?

7.12 In this exercise we consider two types of *banded* correlation matrices in which correlations are all zero if they are beyond a certain distance from the diagonal. Let us define elements $\{\sigma_{ij}\}$ of the matrix Σ with subscripts i and j equal to $1, 2 \ldots, p$. The *banded exchangeable correlation* matrix is of the form

$$\sigma_{ij} = \begin{cases} 1 & \text{for } i = j \\ \rho & \text{for } \mid i - j \mid \leq k \leq p \\ 0 & \text{for } \mid i - j \mid > k \end{cases}$$

where correlations are zero between sequential observations if they are separated by more than k observations.

Similarly, the *banded autocorrelation matrix* is of the form

$$\sigma_{ij} = \begin{cases} 1 & \text{for } i = j \\ \rho^{\mid i - j \mid} & \text{for } \mid i - j \mid \leq k \leq p \\ 0 & \text{for } \mid i - j \mid > k \end{cases}$$

a. Write programs in **R** to build these two matrices for specified parameters ρ and k. Your code will be similar to the one used for `exchange.mat` and `autocorr.mat` in Sect. 7.6.
b. Fit these correlation matrices to the home price data and build a table similar to Table 7.3. Is there evidence these banded correlations fit better or worse than the correlations used in the table?
c. Examine the home price data and test the adequacy of the multivariate normal distribution. Can you find other remarkable cities in addition to Detroit?

Chapter 8
Factor Methods

THE PREVIOUS CHAPTER described inference on the multivariate normal distribution. Sometimes this is more than we actually need. The multivariate distribution is used as a basis of modeling means and covariances. The covariances describe the multivariate relationship between pairs of individual attributes. In this chapter, we go further and describe methods for identifying relationships between several variables concurrently. In the following chapter, we will use regression methods to model the means.

In this chapter, we want to express a multivariate setting in a smaller number of dimensions. Some measured variables will appear to act together in near-unison behavior, while others will seem to act independently. The aim of this chapter is to develop methods to identify and characterize these relationships. In some situations, we may already have an understanding of these relationships and can be able to direct the analyses.

As with other statistical methods, it remains our responsibility to interpret the results the computer provides. It is not good enough for us to say the software identified several variables appearing to act in parallel. We also need to explain this conclusion in terms of our knowledge of the original data. This final step is often overlooked and is needed to complete the data analysis.

Consider the data in Table 1.5 of investment recommendations. Every row sums to 100%, so we immediately see some reduction in dimension. In the following section, we will demonstrate a much greater reduction in dimensionality with little loss of the variability of the original data.

As with many statistical methods, we need to be concerned with *scalability*. That is, does the method slow down or fail when applied to huge datasets. As an example, if there are too many variables or too many observations then the `pairs()` plot will not be useful. If there are simply too many plotted data points then the computing will become slow. This is a common difficulty in the analysis of such large datasets. Some statistical procedures easily scale up, however. Scalable methods include principal components (Sect. 8.1) and factor analysis (Sect. 8.5) because these only rely on the correlation matrix of the variables but not the sample size. Of course, these will also slow down or fail if there are too many variables.

© Springer Nature Switzerland AG 2022
D. Zelterman, *Applied Multivariate Statistics with R*, Statistics for Biology and Health,
https://doi.org/10.1007/978-3-031-13005-2_8

8.1 Principal Component Analysis

It is reasonable to think of the multivariate normal as a football-shaped ellipse containing most of the population. It would be useful to describe the orientation of the football with its long axis. This long axis directs us to look at the largest orientation, or, in statistical terms, the axis with the largest variability. There are other directions for describing the orientation of our football, as well, and these are at right angles to the longest axis.

Principal components analysis is the identification of linear combination of variables providing the maximum variability. The first principal component has the greatest variability. The second component has the maximum variability among all linear combinations orthogonal to the first. The third principal component is orthogonal to both the first and second, and so on for further components. In other words, principal components analysis reduces a large number of multivariate variables into a relatively small number of linear combinations of these, used to account for much of the variability in the data. Variables with the greatest variance will typically dominate the analysis. So in practice, the principal components analysis is often performed on the correlation matrix. (There are exceptions to this general rule, as we will point out.) The correlation provides the appropriate scaling so all variables can be compared on an equal footing. Similarly, in much of the following description of principal components analysis, we can interchangeably make use of the correlation and covariance matrices.

To perform a principal components analysis, we begin with a multivariate random vector $x = (x_1, x_2, \ldots, x_p)$ with mean μ and covariance Σ. For the moment, it is not necessary to assume x has a multivariate normal distribution.

Consider p different linear combinations of x which we write out as

$$
\begin{aligned}
y_1 &= w_1' x = w_{11}x_1 + w_{12}x_2 + \cdots + w_{1p}x_p \\
y_2 &= w_2' x = w_{21}x_1 + w_{22}x_2 + \cdots + w_{2p}x_p \\
&\ \ \vdots \qquad\qquad \vdots \\
y_p &= w_p' x = w_{p1}x_1 + w_{p2}x_2 + \cdots + w_{pp}x_p
\end{aligned}
\tag{8.1}
$$

for suitable multipliers w_{ij} resulting in p new random variables denoted by $y_1, y_2, \ldots, y_p$, referred to as the *principal components* of x.

The weights w_{ij} are also called *loadings* because they explain how much each of the original observations x_i contribute to each of the principal components. The loadings w_i in (8.1) are chosen so the y_i have the largest possible variances and are mutually uncorrelated.

For each $i = 1, \ldots, , p$ the variances of y_i can be expressed as

$$
\text{Var } y_i = w_i' \, \Sigma \, w_i \ .
\tag{8.2}
$$

These variances can be made arbitrarily large by multiplying w_i by a large scalar. To avoid this ambiguity, we restrict the loadings w_i to have unit length and require $w_i' w_i = 1$.

The second criteria is to make the y_i mutually uncorrelated, so we set

$$\text{Cov}\,(y_i, y_j) = w_i'\, \Sigma\, w_j = 0 \tag{8.3}$$

for all $i \neq j$ both between 1 and p.

The goal, then, is to make the variances in (8.2) as large as possible and have all of covariances in (8.3) equal to zero.

In order to achieve this end, we first notice the objective functions in (8.2) and (8.3) are concerned with the Σ matrix and not the means μ of x. The means of x can then be assumed to be zero. In Chap. 9, we will model the means.

We usually don't know Σ and will need to estimate it using the sample variance matrix S. Nothing in this formulation requires us to assume x has a multivariate normal distribution.

The solution to maximizing the variances of orthogonal principal components is to examine the pairs of eigenvalues (λ_i) and eigenvectors (e_i)

$$(\lambda_1, e_1),\ (\lambda_2, e_2),\ \ldots,\ (\lambda_p, e_p)$$

where $\lambda_1 \geq \lambda_2 \geq \cdots \geq \lambda_p \geq 0$ are the ordered eigenvalues of S. In Sect. 4.5.3, we explain the `eigen()` function in **R** calculates eigenvectors e_i, all have unit length, and are mutually orthogonal.

If the weights w_i in (8.1) are replaced by the respective eigenvectors e_i then the estimated variances of the principal components y_i are maximized with respect to the estimated covariance matrix S, and these y_i are uncorrelated. The details of this assertion are verified in Exercise 8.1 but will not be proved here.

The estimated variances satisfy

$$\widehat{\text{Var}}\, y_i = e_i'\, S\, e_i = \lambda_i\,. \tag{8.4}$$

To show the estimated (y_i, y_j) are uncorrelated, we begin by recalling the eigenvector Eq. (4.8), so

$$S\, e_j = \lambda_j\, e_j$$

for every $j = 1, 2, \ldots, p$.

If we multiply this equation on the left by e_i and use (8.3) then we have

$$\widehat{\text{Cov}}\,(y_i, y_j) = e_i'\, S\, e_j = \lambda_j e_i'\, e_j = 0$$

because the eigenvectors e_i and e_j are mutually orthogonal for $i \neq j$.

What does all of this say? We began with p dimensional multivariate observations x. At (8.1) we re-expressed these as a different set of p dimensional observations

y which are linear combinations of the original x's. In a way, nothing has been lost or gained. These principal components $y = \{y_i\}$ are mutually uncorrelated so this makes them easier to manage, but more difficult to interpret.

The first of these, y_1, has the largest variance, λ_1. Second and subsequent components have smaller variances, so the first principal component captures the largest amount of variability in the data. The second component y_2 describes the largest amount of variability left over from y_1 because y_1 and y_2 are uncorrelated.

We can use (8.4) to say the i–th principal component y_i captures

$$ t_i = \lambda_i \Big/ \sum_{j=1}^{p} \lambda_j. \tag{8.5} $$

fraction of the total variability.

If t_1 in (8.5) is a substantially large fraction, then we have reduced a p-dimensional problem down to one dimension with little loss of information or variability. Similarly, if t_1 and t_2 were both large fractions, then we would have a two-dimensional summary of the data with little variability omitted. A *scree plot* examines the ordered values of λ_i. This figure allows us to visualize how many principal components are needed to reasonably summarize the data. This plot will be illustrated in the following example.

8.2   Example 1: Investment Allocations

Now we can work out an example in **R**. Consider the investment recommendation data appearing in Table 1.5. Every financial management firm has a set of recommended percentages in each of eight different investment types. These sum to 100%, so there is a lower dimensional data summary than what is presented.

The program `princomp` computes eigenvalues and eigenvectors, and presents these in a suitable format. See Exercise 8.1 to verify these numerical values are indeed the same. The command line and the output appear in Output 8.1. The `summary` statement describes the eigenvalues and the estimated cumulative proportion of the total variance explained for each principal component.

The **R** command

```
pc <- princomp(invest)
```

captures all the output from the principal components program.

The `summary(pc)` in the top half of Output 8.1 provides a simple explanation of the contributions of each principal component. The standard deviations are given by $\sqrt{\lambda_1} \geq \sqrt{\lambda_2} \geq \cdots \geq \sqrt{\lambda_8}$ where the λ's are the eigenvalues of the covariance matrix. From this output we also see the first two principal components account for over 80% of the variability in the data. These contributions are calculated at (8.5).

Output 8.1 Command and output for principal components analysis of the financial recommendation data

```
> pc <- princomp(invest)
> summary(pc)

Importance of components:
                          Comp.1    Comp.2    Comp.3     Comp.4     Comp.5
Standard deviation     14.976263 7.4764087 6.3540720 3.44766464 2.64881614
Proportion of Variance  0.646986 0.1612404 0.1164641 0.03428767 0.02023912
Cumulative Proportion   0.646986 0.8082264 0.9246905 0.95897819 0.97921731
                          Comp.6       Comp.7       Comp.8
Standard deviation     2.2348600 1.464974785 0.2528154516
Proportion of Variance 0.0144075 0.006190821 0.0001843721
Cumulative Proportion  0.9936248 0.999815628 1.0000000000

> pc$loadings

Loadings:
      Comp.1 Comp.2 Comp.3 Comp.4 Comp.5 Comp.6 Comp.7 Comp.8
USst   0.706  0.521 -0.182 -0.154         0.188        -0.356
Fst                  0.734 -0.249  0.476  0.196        -0.348
Dst          -0.188 -0.135  0.840  0.286  0.163        -0.359
USb    0.114 -0.716 -0.413 -0.398         0.123        -0.352
Fb    -0.109         0.315  0.136 -0.800  0.221  0.224 -0.364
Db                               -0.161 -0.257 -0.887 -0.340
Alt   -0.686  0.410 -0.372 -0.166  0.149  0.208        -0.353
Cash                             -0.852  0.376 -0.356
```

Subsequent principal components contribute much lower amounts. In other words, much of the variability within the original data can be explained by only two derived values. It remains for us to identify these and explain them in simple terms. To do this, we look at the factor loadings.

The `pc$loadings` shows the estimated eigenvector loadings w_{ij} in (8.1). Several of these are printed as blanks. Omitted values are not zero but are close to zero in value and should be ignored. Similarly, only the largest (absolute) loadings are important to us. The eigenvectors of the covariance matrix provide the omitted values but these are often unnecessary.

In the case of the first principal component, the two largest loadings are .706 for US stocks (`USst`) and −.686 for alternative investments (`Alt`). We can ignore the other much smaller loadings for this component. These two important loadings of the first principal component are then about equal for US stocks and alternatives but opposite in magnitude. In other words, the first principal component is roughly the difference between the recommended allocations to these two investment choices. This principal component makes up almost 65% of the variability in the original data.

If we again look at Output 8.1, we see the loadings for the second estimated principal component are almost entirely made up of the recommendations for US

Figure 8.1 Scree plot for
the investment
recommendations

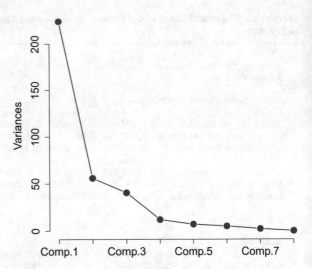

bonds (USb). This component is orthogonal to the first because it is made up of different information.

The scree plot for these data appears in Fig. 8.1. Specifically, this figure plots the ordered eigenvalues $\lambda_1 \geq \lambda_2 \geq \cdots \geq \lambda_8$ of the sample covariance matrix S. This figure was obtained using the command

```
screeplot(pc, col = "red", pch = 16,
    type = "lines", cex = 2, lwd = 2, main = "")
```

This figure shows that most of the variability is contained in the first principal component. Together, the first two principal components explain almost 81% of the variability in the original data and have a simple interpretation. The remaining components represent smaller contributions and can be ignored as background noise.

Another useful graphical method to help interpret the first two principal components is called the *biplot*. Fig. 8.2 plots the estimated loadings of the first two principal components using arrows to indicate their direction. We can create this figure using `biplot(pc)` in **R**.

The actual details for producing this figure are

```
pc <- princomp(invest)
biplot(pc, col = c(2,3), cex = c(.75, 1.5), cex.lab = 1.25,
    xlim=c(-.45, .45),
    xlab = "First principal component",
    ylab = "Second principal component")
```

where `col=` sets all colors and `cex` changes the fonts: smaller fonts for observations and larger for the principal components. The `xlim` option is used here because some of the text labels run outside the plot limits.

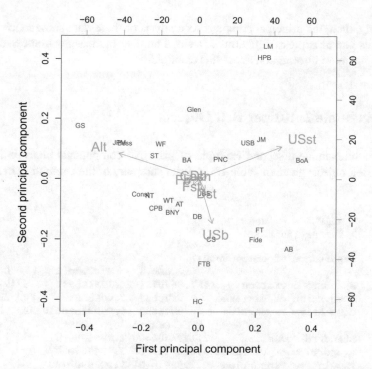

Figure 8.2 Biplot of the first two principal components of the investment recommendations, data appearing in Table 1.5

The US stocks USst and alternative investments Alt in Fig. 8.2 point in almost opposite directions along the x-axis. The allocation to US bonds USb is nearly at right angles to both of these and parallel to the y-axis. These three arrows illustrate our interpretation. The first component is the difference between US stocks and alternatives, in nearly a straight, horizontal line along the first component x-axis with very little change along the vertical, second component y-axis. The second component is made up almost entirely of US bonds and appears as an almost vertical line in this figure. The loadings for the other types of investments (cash or foreign stocks and bonds) play almost no role in the principal components analysis, and their presence is lost in a jumble in the figure's center.

Finally, the biplot includes the names of the individual financial firms, located at their positions along these two principal components. A few notable stand-outs are worth mentioning. On the far left is GenSpring (GS) whose recommendations were very high in alternatives (45%), few US stocks (13%), and an average number of US bonds (23%). On the far right is Bank of America (BoA) whose recommendations were largely US stocks (53%), an average number of bonds (28%) and no alternative investments.

Briefly, then, the principal components analysis of these data show much of the variability can be expressed in terms of a small number of measurements. See Exercise 8.1 for more information about this example.

8.3   Example 2: Kuiper Belt Objects

Let us now examine a second example of principal components analysis for the Kuiper Belt objects given in Table 1.3. A brief summary of the computing in **R** is as follows:

```
> KuiPC <- princomp(Kuiper)
> summary(KuiPC)

Importance of components:
                          Comp.1         Comp.2        Comp.3
Standard deviation     467.8570721 20.198455940 7.1584977540
Proportion of Variance   0.9978853  0.001859904 0.0002336135
Cumulative Proportion    0.9978853  0.999745186 0.9999788000
                          Comp.4        Comp.5
Standard deviation     2.139420e+00 2.705506e-01
Proportion of Variance 2.086634e-05 3.336962e-07
Cumulative Proportion  9.999997e-01 1.000000e+00
```

From this, we see 99.8% of the variability is explained in the first principal component. On the surface, this appears to be a remarkable reduction in the dimensionality of the problem.

The loadings

```
> KuiPC$loadings

Loadings:
         Comp.1 Comp.2 Comp.3 Comp.4 Comp.5
mag                                   0.999
albedo           0.876  0.480
diameter -0.999
axis                          -0.995
Year             0.479 -0.872
```

indicate that this first principal component is simply the diameter of the Kuiper object.

This finding can be explained by noting the standard deviations of the individual measurements

```
> sapply(Kuiper, sd)

      mag     albedo   diameter      axis       Year
 1.720651  27.379290 486.254960  2.595953  20.746331
```

are all very different. By far, the largest of these is the diameter.

A better approach, then, is to record all of these values on the same scale. The principal components should be obtained from the correlation matrix in most cases. The instruction in **R** is to use the `cor=TRUE` option as in this dialog:

```
> KuiPCc <- princomp(Kuiper, cor = TRUE)
> summary(KuiPCc)


Importance of components:
                          Comp.1      Comp.2      Comp.3
Standard deviation      1.7868751   1.1360500   0.6719163
Proportion of Variance  0.6385845   0.2581219   0.0902943
Cumulative Proportion   0.6385845   0.8967065   0.9870008
                          Comp.4       Comp.5
Standard deviation      0.219666359  0.129394388
Proportion of Variance  0.009650662  0.003348582
Cumulative Proportion   0.996651418  1.000000000
```

The first two principal components account for almost 90% of the variability. The biplot for this appears in Fig. 8.3, and the corresponding loadings are

```
> KuiPCc$loadings


Loadings:
          Comp.1 Comp.2 Comp.3 Comp.4 Comp.5
mag        0.538 -0.194 -0.188 -0.161  0.782
albedo    -0.463  0.405  0.446 -0.493  0.425
diameter  -0.546        -0.216  0.671  0.451
axis       0.109  0.785 -0.608
Year       0.432  0.424  0.591  0.529


                 Comp.1 Comp.2 Comp.3 Comp.4 Comp.5
SS loadings         1.0    1.0    1.0    1.0    1.0
Proportion Var      0.2    0.2    0.2    0.2    0.2
Cumulative Var      0.2    0.4    0.6    0.8    1.0
```

The first principal component of the Kuiper objects is approximately

$$\text{Magnitude} + \text{Year of discovery} - \text{Albedo} - \text{Diameter}$$

and the second component is almost entirely the axis.

We are working with the correlation matrix, not the covariance, so all measures have been divided by their standard deviations. The objects on the right side of the biplot are brighter, more recently discovered, less reflective, and smaller. Objects on top are farther away. The opposite is true for objects appearing on the right or bottom of Fig. 8.3.

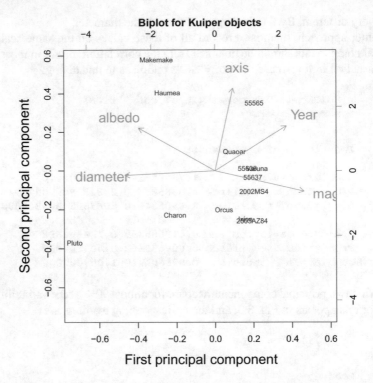

Figure 8.3 Biplot of the first two principal components of the Kuiper objects, data appearing in Table 1.3

Why did we need to scale the Kuiper objects and use the correlation in order to obtain a reasonable principal components analysis while the investment recommendations examined in the previous section provided an acceptable summary using the original data? The answer is the investment recommendations were already measured on the same scale as percentages of the total. The multivariate data for the Kuiper objects were all different, and these were measured on different scales. The general rule then is to perform principal components analysis on the scaled (correlation) matrix.

8.4   Example 3: Health Outcomes in US Hospitals

For the third example of a principal components analysis, Table 8.1 lists outcome data on US hospitals, as reported by Medicare. There are 16 variables measured. After deleting those cases with missing data, there are 1,906 hospitals remaining. This dataset is also available online.[1] As an example of the scalability of principal

---

[1] See: https://data.medicare.gov/.

Table 8.1 Variables in Medicare data on US hospitals

Variable name	Measurement
SDeathN	Number of surgical deaths
SDeathR	Rate of surgical deaths
LungN	Number of collapsed lungs
LungR	Rate of collapsed lungs
ClotN	Number of clots
ClotR	Rate of clots
SplitN	Number of split incisions
SplitR	Rate of split incisions
CutsN	Number of cuts
CutsR	Rate of cuts
HADeathN	Number of heart attack deaths
HADeathR	Rate of heart attack deaths
HFDeathN	Number of heart failure deaths
HFDeathR	Rate of heart failure deaths
PDeathN	Number of pneumonia deaths
PDeathR	Rate of pneumonia deaths

components, there is little difficulty analyzing these data but a `pairs()` plot is not useful.

Principal components analysis proves to be a useful approach for starting the statistical examination of such a large dataset. The main benefit comes from reducing the large dataset to a 16×16 covariance matrix. Of course, much can be lost in this reduction, but the benefit is we can easily identify some overall patterns without lengthy computing times.

The scree plot for these data appears in Fig. 8.4. This figure gives strong evidence that there is only one component to be used to summarize this large dataset. We examine the loadings of this first principal component (rounded to two digits):

```
> round(phosp$loadings[ , 1], digits = 2)

  SDeathN  SDeathR    LungN    LungR    ClotN    ClotR   SplitN   SplitR
     0.34     0.00     0.38     0.02     0.36     0.07     0.35    -0.03
    CutsN    CutsR HADeathR HADeathN HFDeathR HFDeathN  PDeathR  PDeathN
     0.38     0.00    -0.11     0.33    -0.07     0.34    -0.07     0.30
```

These loadings are chiefly composed of equal weighting of eight measures, each with weights in the range of .3 to .38. These measures are `SDeathN`, `LungN`, `ClotN`, `SplitN`, `CutsN`, `HADeathN`, `HFDeathN`, and `PDeathN`. In every case, these variables represent the *number* of adverse events recorded and none of the measures of *rates*. This suggests that the rate values are generally not useful in discriminating between the different hospitals. Instead, the numbers of

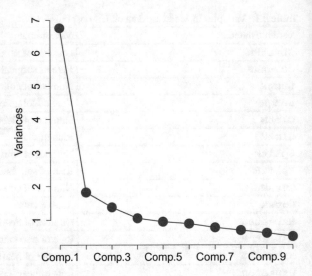

Figure 8.4 Screeplot for the US hospital data

events are more representative of the size of the hospital than anything else. The principal components analysis, then, suggests we also need a variable indicating the size of the hospital, and this single measure might be the best summary of the variability of the hospitals in these data.

8.5   Factor Analysis

Factor analysis is a method for identifying groups of variables (or *factors*) whose actions appear to work in parallel. Within a single factor, several measured variables within every individual are highly correlated, whether positively or negatively. Other variables may seem to act independently of all others. The aim of factor analysis is to identify and interpret these groups of factors. We will also need to estimate the appropriate number of factors needed to model the data. As with principal components, we do not have to assume the data follow a multivariate normal distribution.

Let us begin with an example from medicine. Hemangioma is the most common of all childhood cancer diagnoses. It appears as a lump of blood vessels on the skin. If left untreated it usually resolves within a few years. Some parents opt for surgical removal. The data in Table 8.2 is from a registry of surgically treated infants along with measurements on several genetic markers thought to be related to the disease. The age, measured in days, is the infant's age at the time of the surgery. The age, then, represents how long the infant was exposed to the tumor. It was hypothesized exposure to the tumor might influence the magnitude of the expression of some of these genes over time. A cursory examination of these data reveals several extreme outliers.

Table 8.2   Age, in days. and expression of genetic markers for infants who were surgically treated for hemangioma

Age	RB	p16	DLK	Nanog	C-Myc	EZH2	IGF-2
81	2.0	3.07	308975	94	6.49	2.76	11176
95	6.5	1.90	70988	382	1.00	7.09	5340
95	3.6	3.82	153061	237	0.00	5.57	6310
165	1.9	3.74	596992	88	0.00	2.47	7009
286	2.6	5.17	369601	282	12.23	1.63	7104
299	2.9	5.76	1119258	177	8.76	3.51	9342
380	1.9	2.40	214071	45	5.76	1.41	3726
418	7.1	3.38	69511	265	1.17	3.07	8039
420	6.4	3.37	81457	659	1.88	3.87	12583
547	6.4	4.05	64348	336	0.78	4.76	6505
590	1.8	5.15	164881	2012	35.65	9.45	32722
635	6.7	2.67	126016	3072	0.00	4.35	11763
752	1.8	3.28	567858	127	4.13	1.00	10283
760	7.3	0.92	43438	698	1.77	3.32	11518
1171	1.8	6.56	716260	392	12.92	2.90	13264
1277	1.3	0.05	94	15	0.36	3.83	30
1520	4.0	2.79	31125	454	0.62	2.33	1163
2138	0.5	0.00	2331	33	0.03	0.17	66
3626	4.2	4.24	560208	340	5.43	1.36	21174

Data courtesy of Dr. Deepak Nayaran

The model for factor analysis is as follows. Suppose y is a p-dimensional random vector with mean μ and covariance matrix Σ. The means μ are removed from y so we only model the random components of the observations. The idea is to see how well we can express the p-dimensional random vector $y - \mu$ as linear combinations of a relatively smaller number of m *factors* f and their respective *loadings* Λ plus a randomly distributed error ϵ.

Mathematically we write

$$\underset{(p \times 1)}{y - \mu} = \underset{(p \times m)}{\Lambda} \underset{(m \times 1)}{f} + \underset{(p \times 1)}{\epsilon} \tag{8.6}$$

In linear regression (covered in Chap. 9), we know the values of the m explanatory variables. In (8.6), the choice of explanatory variables are not known to us and must be determined. The value of m is specified by us in the program fitting this model.

Estimating the loadings Λ and factors f is not possible without some additional assumptions. Among these assumptions, both the unobservable factors and errors have zero means. Further, these are all assumed to be mutually and jointly uncorrelated.

Neither (8.6) nor the subsequent derivation given below needs to specify a multivariate normal distribution. Briefly, (8.6) suggests the centered data $y - \mu$ can be expressed as a product of lower-dimensional factors and loadings plus a small amount of random error ϵ.

Specifically, we need to assume:

$$\mathrm{E}f = 0 \quad \text{and} \quad \mathrm{Cov}(f) = \mathrm{E}ff' = I, \tag{8.7}$$

$$\mathrm{E}\epsilon = 0 \quad \text{and} \quad \mathrm{Cov}(\epsilon) = \mathrm{E}(\epsilon\epsilon') = \Psi = \mathbf{Diag}(\Psi_1, \Psi_2, \dots, \Psi_p). \tag{8.8}$$

In addition, the factors f are uncorrelated with the errors ϵ:

$$\mathrm{Cov}(f, \epsilon) = 0. \tag{8.9}$$

Together, these assumptions are sufficient for us to fit the model (8.6).

These assumptions can also be used to describe an alternative form for the factor analysis model. If we begin at (8.6), then we can write

$$(y - \mu)(y - \mu)' = (\Lambda f + \epsilon)(\Lambda f + \epsilon)'$$
$$= \Lambda f(\Lambda f)' + \epsilon(\Lambda f)' + \Lambda f \epsilon' + \epsilon\epsilon'.$$

Using the three assumptions (8.7), (8.8), and (8.9), we can then express the covariance matrix Σ of y as

$$\mathrm{Cov}(y) = \mathrm{E}(y - \mu)(y - \mu)'$$
$$= \Lambda\mathrm{E}(ff')\Lambda' + \mathrm{E}(\epsilon f')\Lambda' + \Lambda\mathrm{E}(f\epsilon') + \mathrm{E}(\epsilon\epsilon')$$
$$= \Lambda\Lambda' + \Psi \tag{8.10}$$

demonstrating the equivalence of two formulations of the factor analysis models at (8.6) and (8.10).

In **R** we perform a factor analysis using `factanal(x, factors=m)` where x is the data arranged in the usual fashion as columns of variables and rows for observations. The m parameter specifies how many factors we want **R** to fit. Usually we try to fit a relatively small number of factors (at most three or four) because of the difficulty of their interpretation. There is also a formal statistical hypothesis test performed in `factanal()` testing whether m factors are adequate or not.

A factor analysis of the hemangioma data appears in Output 8.2 using three factors. The hypothesis test at the bottom of this table indicates the eight measures (age and seven genetic markers) can be summarized as a three-dimensional measurement, plus a small amount of random error. We examine the three-factor loadings to see (`C.Myc`, `EZH2`, `IGF-2`) collectively appear to work together in the first factor. The second factor is almost entirely the `DLK` marker. The third factor is almost represented by the `RB` marker. Age plays almost no part, contrary to our original hypothesis about the length of time the tumor burden is carried by the patient.

Output 8.2 ends with a hypothesis test indicating three factors are adequate to explain these data ($p = .33$).

Output 8.2 Factor analysis for the hemangioma data

```
> factanal(hemangioma, factors = 3)


Call:
factanal(x = hemangioma, factors = 3)

Uniquenesses:
   Age    RB    p16    DLK Nanog C.Myc  EZH2 IGF.2
 0.962 0.035 0.292 0.005 0.616 0.005 0.491 0.254

Loadings:
       Factor1 Factor2 Factor3
Age                    -0.171
RB             -0.173   0.962
p16     0.382   0.745
DLK             0.971  -0.211
Nanog   0.475           0.391
C.Myc   0.931   0.280  -0.225
EZH2    0.614  -0.115   0.345
IGF.2   0.767   0.350   0.188

               Factor1 Factor2 Factor3
SS loadings      2.226   1.750   1.365
Proportion Var   0.278   0.219   0.171
Cumulative Var   0.278   0.497   0.668

Test of the hypothesis that 3 factors are sufficient.
The chi square statistic is 8.03 on 7 degrees of freedom.
The p-value is 0.33
```

A more thorough analysis of these data would require we additionally research the roles of these identified genetic markers and then try to understand why they appear to linked, as we identified in this statistical analysis. Some of these topics are addressed in the following section. Additional examination of this example is continued in Exercise 8.4.

Factor analysis is a powerful tool. As with many statistical methods, it also requires us to do our homework to interpret the results of the computer output. Historically, it has been well known that this method can yield misleading conclusions, and a small change in the data values can bring about further chaos. Armstrong [1967] presents an educational and elementary case of misuse of factor analysis.

8.6 Confirmatory Factor Analysis

The topics, principal components, and factor analysis covered so far in this chapter, are useful because these methods are *unsupervised*. From these analyses, we can learn about topics such as the hemangioma study without any special knowledge about the function of the genetic markers involved, or even why these specific markers were measured. Similarly, we didn't need any specific background in investments, astronomy, or health outcomes in order to perform the other statistical analyses already covered in this chapter. The downside of these methods is the resulting models may not make sense to somebody with the specialized background in any one of these topics.

Suppose, instead, we *do* have some background knowledge of the subject and want to use this in model building. Or maybe we want to test a theory about the variables collected in our data. After all, data on the specific variables was collected because we already had strong feelings about how these measures work together. Such an approach to the statistical examination is considered *supervised* because it incorporates our *a priori* understanding of the subject matter.

As an example, let us begin with a factor analysis of the hamburger data given in Table 1.6. We first try running `factanal` with two, and then three factors. Output 8.3 contains excerpts of the output from **R**.

The loadings of Factor 1 and 2 are almost identical in both of these factor analyses. Specifically, loadings for Factor 1 are chiefly `CalFat`, `Fat`, and `SatFat`. The loadings for Factor 2 are almost entirely `Carbs`, in both cases. The loadings for Factor 3 are all small and we interpret this to be mostly noise.

If we only concentrate on the *p*-values in Output 8.3, then we might conclude two factors are just barely adequate in summarizing the data. The p-value is .065 for two latent variables and .7 for three. We already noted the third factor does not have a reasonable interpretation beyond a measure of noise in the data. The message in this example, so far, is we cannot rely entirely on *p*-values to identify the correct model, and we must also work at interpreting the output carefully. But does the model make sense?

This unsupervised analysis assumes we know nothing about nutrition. Our examination relies entirely on the statistical methods to teach us how the variables in the data work together.

Instead, it is easy to gain some basic knowledge about nutrition and then incorporate this into our model. We know ground beef contains almost no carbohydrates and very little sodium. Salt is added to the recipe. Carbs come chiefly from the bun, or maybe the secret sauce. In other words, salt and carbohydrates are conceptually detached from the ground beef in the hamburger and added separately.

The `lavaan` package in **R** contains a number of useful routines which allow us to specify the functional form we want the factor analysis to take. Such *confirmatory factor analysis* methods allow us to incorporate our knowledge of the form of the model and then estimate the parameters. (The closely-related topic of path analysis discussed in Sect. 8.7 also uses programs in `lavaan`).

Output 8.3 Selected output from a factor analysis for the hamburger data

```
> library(stats)
> burger <- read.table(file = "burger.txt", header = T)
> factanal(burger[, -1], factors = 2)   #  Omit burger number

                . . .

Loadings:
          Factor1 Factor2
CalFat    0.964    0.230
Cal       0.755    0.606
Fat       0.950    0.303
SatFat    0.912   -0.121
Sodium    0.634    0.347
Carbs              0.997
Protein   0.717   -0.111
                . . .

Test of the hypothesis that 2 factors are sufficient.
The chi square statistic is 14.7 on 8 degrees of freedom.
The p-value is 0.0652


> factanal(burger[, -1], factors = 3)   # Now try three factors

                . . .

Loadings:
          Factor1 Factor2 Factor3
CalFat    0.960    0.226  -0.126
Cal       0.752    0.611
Fat       0.949    0.301
SatFat    0.940   -0.131   0.308
Sodium    0.654    0.348   0.248
Carbs              0.980
Protein   0.724   -0.117
                . . .

Test of the hypothesis that 3 factors are sufficient.
The chi square statistic is 1.43 on 3 degrees of freedom.
The p-value is 0.699
```

Output 8.4 contains a brief confirmatory factor analysis program (cfa) to incorporate our understanding about the nutritional content of the hamburger data.

Let us model two latent variables, labeled meat and added. The added factor is a linear combination of sodium and carbohydrates with weights to be estimated. Models in cfa are expressed as text using the string = ~ to show the relationship between these factors and their components. The cfa program fits the model and summary prints derived statistics.

Among the output we see the weights for the components of the two latent variables meat and added. The first component has a weight fixed at 1 and the remaining components can be tested for statistical significance. In the paragraph headed

Output 8.4 Confirmatory factor analysis for the hamburger data

```
> library(lavaan)
> burger_model <-
        " meat =~  CalFat + Cal + Fat + SatFat + Protein
          added =~  Sodium + Carbs  "
> fit <- cfa(model = burger_model, data = scale(burger))
> summary(fit, fit.measures = TRUE)


        .    .    .


Latent Variables:
                    Estimate  Std.Err  z-value  P(>|z|)
  meat =~
    CalFat            1.000
    Cal               0.927    0.076    12.194    0.000
    Fat               1.034    0.030    34.716    0.000
    SatFat            0.844    0.096     8.772    0.000
    Protein           0.630    0.129     4.895    0.000
  added =~
    Sodium            1.000
    Carbs             0.442    0.218     2.026    0.043

Covariances:
                    Estimate  Std.Err  z-value  P(>|z|)
  meat ~~
    added             0.652    0.185     3.522    0.000

Variances:
                    Estimate  Std.Err  z-value  P(>|z|)

        .    .    .


    meat              0.929    0.220     4.213    0.000
    added             0.716    0.340     2.109    0.035
```

`Latent Variables`, we see every component of the two factors is statistically significant. That is, the components appear to be correctly expressed and all provide a large contribution to each of the two latent variables. The two factors `meat` and `added` are not orthogonal but the fitted model presented here provides a lot of confirmation of our understanding of nutrition brought to the analysis.

There are several messages we can learn from the two examinations of the burger data given in this section. The unsupervised examination given in Output 8.3 is not too far from the model we fitted using confirmatory factor analysis using a rudimentary knowledge of nutrition. Which of these is easier to interpret? Does the unsupervised model come close to the supervised model we fit using confirmatory factor analysis?

Confirmatory factor analysis does not prove a model is correct but, rather, shows whether a model is plausible. We also see factor analysis is fragile in the sense there may be many other possible equally well-fitting models for the data located not too far from the one obtained using unsupervised model building.

8.7 Path Analysis

Path analysis is a class of models used to illustrate the directed dependencies among a group of variables. Often, these dependencies are expressed as weights of a latent variable. This family of models includes multiple regression (described in Sect. 9.2), factor analysis (Sect. 8.5), discriminant analysis (Sect. 10.5), and canonical correlations (Sect. 14.2).

The use of directed dependencies (as opposed to correlation) is to imply a causal direction. The direction is understood when one measurement precedes another so the causal direction is understood. Our understanding of the underlying data allows us to make such assumptions. Path analysis does not allow us to say two latent factors cause each other, for example.

A good feature of path analysis is it allows us to create our own latent variables, much as we did in confirmatory factor analysis. Factor analysis creates latent variables but leaves it up to us to interpret the various loadings. Path analysis and confirmatory factor analysis allow us to describe the structure of these factors and then estimates the factor loadings for us. A nice feature of path analysis is the graphical representation we can create in **R**. In this section, we continue the use of the confirmatory factor analysis program `cfa` in the `lavaan` library, introduced in the previous section.

As an example, let us examine the `mtcars` data in **R**. This is a set of physical measurements on 32 cars. The list of variables included is given in Table 9.1 and analyzed in greater detail in the following chapter.

To start with a simple example, let us examine the regression of miles per gallon `mpg` in response to horsepower `hp` in the following **R** code:

```
model <- "mpg ~ 1 + hp"
fit <- cfa(model, data = mtcars)
semPaths(fit, rotation = 2)
```

The `lavaan` library contains a number of useful programs to fit and draw path analyses. The text in `model` expresses the example model, including an intercept similar to the notation we use in `lm`. The `cfa` program fits the model, and also produces output similar to the `lm` program for linear models but allows for more flexibility, as we will show in other examples later in this chapter. The `semPaths` program draws the figure:

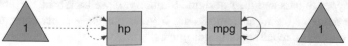

Observed variables (hp and mpg) are given in boxes. The arrow pointing toward miles per gallon indicates the causal direction: horsepower is a strong determinant of the miles per gallon. The triangles are variable means or model intercepts, always taking the value 1. The circular arrows pointing back to the observed variables remind us that these have their own variances.

Output 8.5 Path analysis for the car data and selected output. This program produces Fig. 8.5

```
> library(lavaan)
> library(semPlot)
> sc <- scale(mtcars, center = TRUE)          # standardize the columns
> car.model <- 'eng =~ hp + cyl + disp + carb # engine, latent variable
                drv =~ gear + drat + am        # drive train, latent variable
                eng + drv ~ mpg + wt + qsec'   # total experience
> fit <- cfa(car.model, data=sc, std.lv=TRUE)
> semPaths(fit,title=FALSE, curvePivot = TRUE, layout = "spring")
> summary(fit)
. . .
```

```
    Latent Variables:
                     Estimate  Std.Err  z-value  P(>|z|)
      eng =~
        hp            0.192     0.053    3.634    0.000
        cyl           0.213     0.056    3.826    0.000
        disp          0.208     0.055    3.795    0.000
        carb          0.128     0.046    2.790    0.005
      drv =~
        gear          0.433     0.087    4.964    0.000
        drat          0.409     0.088    4.665    0.000
        am            0.471     0.088    5.343    0.000

    Regressions:
                     Estimate  Std.Err  z-value  P(>|z|)
      eng ~
        mpg          -0.847     0.636   -1.331    0.183
        wt            2.768     0.902    3.068    0.002
        qsec         -1.884     0.572   -3.292    0.001
      drv ~
        mpg           1.051     0.538    1.954    0.051
        wt           -0.738     0.483   -1.527    0.127
        qsec         -0.931     0.304   -3.067    0.002

    . . .
```

A deeper examination of the mtcars data asks us to recognize the purpose it was collected. We are probably less interested in individual characteristics and measurements but rather look to these data as a means of distinguishing and comparing different types of cars and their designs. Similarly, if we look back at Table 9.1 we recognize many of the measurements are beyond our daily experience, unless, of course, we work on repairing or building cars.

A small amount of understanding of how cars operate allows us to guide the construction of meaningful models. We can construct latent variables made up of groups of related variables whose individual measurements are less important than their collective effect. The first of these we will refer to as the *engine*. The variables measuring engine characteristics include horsepower (hp), number of cylinders (cyl), displacement (disp), and number of carburetors (carb). None of these measurements by themselves are particularly useful to a driver or readily appreciated, but together reflect our intuitive understanding as these contribute to the engine.

Another group of variables we will refer to collectively as the *drive train*, the mechanism transferring the output of the engine to the motion in the wheels. As with the engine, the individual measurements of the drive train are not of interest to us, but collectively act together. The variables measured on the drive train include the number of forward gears (gear); the rear axle ratio (drat); and the type of transmission (automatic/manual) (am).

The remaining variables, not associated with the engine or the drive train include empirical measurements, easily experienced in our day-to-day life as a driver of the car, namely, miles per gallon (mpg); weight (wt); and acceleration, as measured by the 1/4 mile time (qsec).

The program to fit this path analysis model is given in Output 8.5. We begin by standardizing all of the columns in mtcar data to have zero mean and unit variance. This is accomplished using the scale program in **R**. We remove the means because we are looking for effects of one measurement on another, not estimating one set of values. The variances are also standardized so we can interpret effect sizes. Also, the estimation of parameters in path analysis is numerically more stable if all variables have comparable variances.

The car.model variable has text listing the relationships between the columns in the data. Specifically, the pair of symbols = ~ is used to list the components of a latent variable. In the present example, there are two latent variables: engine (eng); and drive train (drv). These two latent variables are combined to explain the three empirical variables (weight, miles per gallon, and 1/4 mile times.)

The model is fitted in cfa, the output is captured in the variable fit, and the path figure given in Fig. 8.5 is produced by semPaths. A portion of the output from cfa is given in Output 8.5. Specifically, this includes estimated regression coefficients, standard errors, and tests of statistical significance for the components of both latent variables, as well as the effect of these latent variables on each of the empirical variables. Overall, there appears to be a good fit although the drive train latent variable has negligible effect on the car's weight, as we might expect.

The circles in the path diagram Fig. 8.5 represent the two latent variables, engine and drive train. Each of these is identified by its respective components. The empirical measurements (miles per gallon, 1/4 mile time, and weight) are related to each other but only to the remaining measurements except through the two latent variables. The triangles (representing means and intercepts) were removed when we standardized the data.

To summarize this section, path analysis allows us to create latent variables whose composition we can construct through our knowledge of the underlying data. The

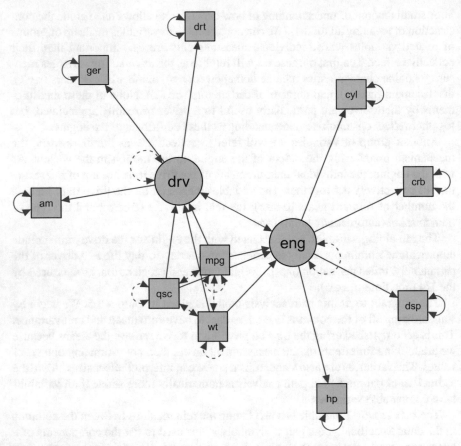

Figure 8.5 Path diagram of car data with two latent variables: engine and drive train. This figure was produced by the program in Output 8.5

path figure is a nice way to convey this structure to an audience without the need for mathematical equations. The downside is we need this intimate knowledge of our data. In the case of cars, we interact with these on a daily basis so this is not asking too much of us. This process is almost the opposite of factor analysis in which the program identifies the latent factors but requires us to interpret these.

8.8   Structural Equations and Latent Growth Modeling

A further generalization to confirmatory factor analysis and path analysis includes modeling different relationships between observed variables and constructed latent variables. These methods include methods to analyze repeated measurements with models for measuring underlying trends. The lavaan package has capabilities allowing us to build more complex models than illustrated in Outputs 8.4 or 8.5.

We will illustrate these methods using the home price index data also modeled in Sect. 7.3 with multivariate normal distribution. Briefly, this data describes a relative index of changes in home prices in 20 different US cities, for each of the years 2000–2011. All values are indexed in the year 2000 equal to 1 for all cities. These data are plotted here in Fig. 8.6 and also appeared earlier as Fig. 7.2.

We added two variables from US Census data: population in 2000 and the percent change in population over 2000–2011. The population only covers the city proper and not the surrounding suburbs. It is not clear using these values alone whether people have moved into or out of the surrounding suburbs or else there was migration to (or from) much further away. These two demographic variables will be used to model the price changes.

There was a price bubble leading to extreme values in 2007 followed by a large decline in the following years. We will separately model the price trends before and after the year 2007. Detroit is a standout as those home prices fell most dramatically.

We will model these data using a combination of correlated latent variables and explanatory variables. As with confirmatory factor analysis and path analysis, we choose our models based on their interpretation. The **R** code and some of the output appears in Output 8.6. The corresponding path diagram is given in Fig. 8.7.

As we saw in Output 8.5, we specify models in lavaan using a character variable. The pair of operators = ~ is used to define a latent variable. In the present example of home prices, we write

```
demo =~ growth + pop00
```

Figure 8.6 Spaghetti plot of home price data. Annual means are in red

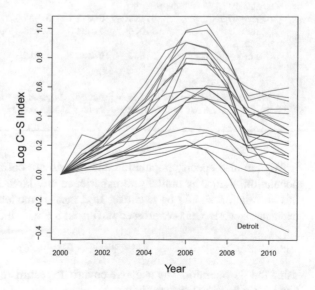

to create the latent variable measuring demographics (demo) which is constructed from the population growth rate and the population in 2000.

Output 8.6 Latent growth analysis of home prices and selected output This program produces Fig. 8.7

```
> library(lavaan)
> library(semPlot)
> model <-                          # latent slope, up to 2007
    "pre07 =~  1*X2001 + 2*X2002 + 3*X2003 + 4*X2004 + 5*X2005 +
              6*X2006 + 7*X2007
                                # latent slope and intercept after 2007
    post07 =~  1*X2008 + 2*X2009 + 3*X2010 + 4*X2011
    post07i=~  1*X2008 + 1*X2009 + 1*X2010 + 1*X2011
    demo =~ growth + pop00      # latent demographics
    growth ~~ pop00             # residual covariance
    post07 ~ demo  "            # regression of latent variables
> fit <- growth(model, data=scale(home[,-1]))
> summary(fit)
  . . .


Regressions:
                  Estimate  Std.Err  z-value  P(>|z|)
  post07 ~
    demo           -0.111    0.076   -1.467    0.142

Covariances:
                  Estimate  Std.Err  z-value  P(>|z|)
 .growth ~~
   .pop00          -0.322    0.213   -1.513    0.130
  pre07 ~~
    post07i         0.115    0.046    2.507    0.012
    demo            0.045    0.031    1.456    0.145
  post07i ~~
    demo            0.500    0.249    2.011    0.044

      . . .

> semPaths(fit, edge.color = "blue", layout = "spring",
          color = list(lat = "pink", man = "lightgreen", int = "tan1"))
```

We can also specify population and growth are correlated. If a city has a large population, then it is unlikely to experience any large change in growth. That is, this correlation should be negative. In lavaan models, this correlation between explanatory variables is expressed in Output 8.6 with the line

$$growth \ \text{~~} \ pop00$$

using the ~~ operator. The negative covariance estimate between these variables in Output 8.6 confirms our suspicion.

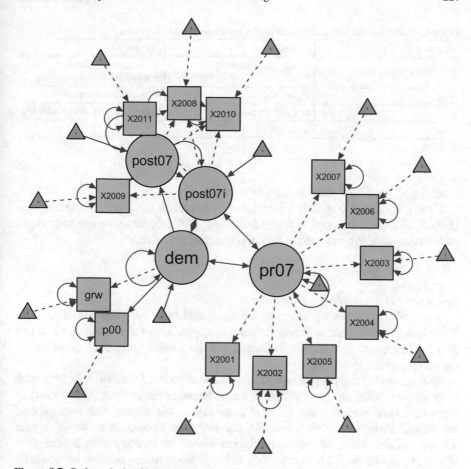

Figure 8.7 Path analysis of latent growth for home prices

To create a slope, we can't simply specify a model by adding together the price index values for the years 2001–2007. Instead, the definition

```
pre07 =~  1*X2001 + 2*X2002 + 3*X2003 + 4*X2004 + 5*X2005 +
          6*X2006 + 7*X2007
```

creates a latent slope for pre-2007 price changes specifying the linear weights given to each of these years' values. The pre-2007 slope has no corresponding intercept because the index values were standardized so all 2000 values are equal to zero.

The post–2007 slope was specified in a similar manner as the pre-2007 slope. The model for changes in home prices after 2007 needs an intercept and this is expressed as

```
post07i=~  1*X2008 + 1*X2009 + 1*X2010 + 1*X2011
```

Table 8.3 Notation and interpretation of model operators used in `lavaan`

Operator	Definition	Interpretation
= ~	define latent variable	is measured by these components
~	regression	between latent variables
~~	residual covariance	between explanatory variables
~ 1	intercept	

requiring all post-2007 years to have equal weights.

Finally, we can also specify a regression model relationship between latent variables. Specifically, the slope in prices following 2007 may partly be due to changes in demographics. We can specify this in our model by writing

```
post07  ~   demo
```

making use of the single ~ operator.

A list of the various operators in `lavaan` and their interpretation appears in Table 8.3. The `semPaths` function needs to appear after the `summary()` in our **R** code. The use of `semPaths` in Output 8.6 show how to add different colors to the various nodes in the figure.

The message of this chapter is principal components and factor analysis are useful tools for identifying groups of variables whose behavior can be described as working together. Latent variables are a useful summary in this regard. The examples of investment allocations, Kuiper belt objects, and gene expression allow us to gain a better understanding of complex subjects whose multivariate data is otherwise left to experts in the field. The models built by the software need to be carefully interpreted and these interpretations might be either misleading or obvious to those with specialized knowledge. On the other hand, even a rudimentary knowledge of nutrition or how cars operate, guides us toward meaningful models reflecting our understanding of the subject.

8.9 Exercises

8.1 a. In the biplot of Fig. 8.2, notice Legg Mason (LM) and Harris (HPB) appear at the top and Highmount (HC) appears at the bottom. Why is this the case? What does the second principal component in the vertical axis represent?

b. Use **R** to find the eigenvalues and eigenvectors of the correlation matrix of the investment recommendation data of Table 1.5. Show the eigenvectors represent the variances of the principal components of the correlation matrix with the code

```
sqrt(eigen(cor(invest))$values)
```

and verify these are same the values obtained from principal components using the code

```
princomp(invest, cor = TRUE)
```

8.2 The `Harmon23.cor` data in the `datasets` package is a correlation matrix of eight physical measurements made on 305 girls between the ages of seven and 17.

a. Perform a factor analysis of these data using the command

```
factanal(factors = m, covmat = Harman23.cor)
```

where m is the number of factors.
b. Vary the number of factors to find an adequate fit of the model and interpret the resulting factor loadings.
c. Does the principal component analysis produce different conclusions when the correlation matrix (`cor = TRUE`) option is used? Which analysis do you prefer?

8.3 Consider a principal component analysis on the data appearing in Table 1.4. This table lists rates of individual cancer types (and overall rates) for each of the 50 US states plus DC.

a. Begin by examining the standard deviations of each cancer type, including the overall rates.
b. Perform a principal components analysis on these data and look at the biplot. Interpret the loadings on the first two principal components. Are these heavily weighted towards the largest standard deviations found in part a?
c. Repeat the principal components analysis on the scaled correlation matrix of the cancer rate data. How do you interpret this biplot?
d. Which analysis do you find more useful: the scaled or unscaled principal components analysis for these data?

8.4 How robust is the factor analysis procedure against outliers in the data?

a. Examine the marginal distributions of genetic markers in the hemangioma data of Table 8.2. Which of these appear to be normally distributed? Identify both large and small outliers. Are there transformations of the form (5.5) making these distributions more normal-looking?
b. Repeat the factor analysis along the lines of the method described in Sect. 8.5. Are your conclusions the same or how do these differ? Which conclusions do you prefer?

8.5 Examine the `USJudgeRatings` data in the `datasets` library. These data contain the ratings of 43 US Superior Court judges by attorneys. Each of the judges is evaluated on each of 12 attributes such as demeanor, preparation for trial, sound rulings, and the number of contacts each attorney had with the judge. See the **R** help file for more information on this dataset.

   a. Examine the pair-wise scatterplot for these data (with the `pairs` command) to show some variables are very highly correlated.
   b. Perform a principal components analysis for these data. The first two components explain 94% of the variability. The second component is almost entirely the number of contacts, and the first component is essentially all other variables, all given the same weight. Interpret this result.

8.6 Six different tests of intelligence and ability were administered to 112 people. The covariance matrix (but not the original data) of the test results is given in `ability.cov` in the `datasets` library. The six tests are called general, picture, blocks, maze, reading, vocabulary, and reading. More information is given in the **R** help file.

   a. Perform a factor analysis on the covariance matrix with

```
factanal(factors = 2, covmat=ability.cov)
```

Use the loadings to identify those variables grouping together within the first two factors. Interpret these factors.
   b. Perform a principal components analysis using the covariance matrix

```
summary(pc <- princomp(ability.cov))
pc$loadings
```

and identify the variables making the largest contributions to the first two principal components. How do you interpret these principal components?
   c. Do you think it more is appropriate to examine the covariance or the correlation in a principal components analysis of these data?
   d. The `cov2cor` function efficiently converts covariances into correlation matrices. That is,

```
ability.cor <- cov2cor(ability.cov$cov)
princomp(ability.cor)
princomp(ability.cor)$loadings
```

obtains the correlation and performs the principal components analysis. Examine the loadings and interpret the first two principal components. Compare this data summary with parts a and b. How do these differ? How are they similar?

8.7 The academic score data appears in Table 1.2 and is examined in Exercise 2.5.

   a. Perform a principal components analysis of these data. Notice the first principal component accounts for much of the variance. What do the factor

Table 8.4 Rates of mechanistic causes of death for 50 states

State	All	Cut	Drown	Fall	Fire	Firearm	MotorVeh	Poison	Suffocate
AL	74.5	1.0	2.0	4.2	2.1	16.9	19.4	14.1	5.3
AK	87.1	NA	5.1	6.1	1.7	18.8	8.7	21.8	7.9
AZ	72.0	1.1	1.6	11.9	0.7	14.2	12.4	17.7	5.5
⋮	⋮	⋮	⋮	⋮	⋮				
WI	57.8	0.7	1.3	14.4	0.8	8.1	9.9	12.3	5.1
WY	84.5	NA	1.3	9.5	NA	16.7	21.0	16.7	7.2

Source National Vital Statistics System, http://www.cdc.gov/nchs/deaths.htm

     loadings suggest? Do the loadings differ if you use the covariance matrix or the correlation matrix?

  b. Look at the correlation matrix of these data. What does the correlation matrix suggest about these data? Is this consistent with conclusion of the principal components analysis of part a and Exercise 2.5?

8.8 Table 8.4 lists the rates of mechanistic (as opposed to natural) causes of death, by state, for the years 1999–2010, as reported by the Centers for Disease Control. Rates are per 100,000 persons and include both accidental and intentional. There are a number of NA's listed where estimates are unreliable due to small numbers. Consider replacing these NA's with a small number such as .2.

  a. Plot the data and identify any remarkable states. Explain these. In which states do deaths following falls seem unusually frequent?

  b. Perform a principal components analysis. Should the "All" category be included in this? Show states with high rates of motor vehicle deaths also have high rates of mortality associated with firearms. Poisoning is also important but does it seem to be independent of these other two causes?

8.9 The `tree` dataset in the `datasets` library has three measurements on each of 31 black cherry trees: girth (diameter, in inches, measured at breast height); height in feet; and timber volume in cubic feet.

  a. Draw a `pairs()` plot to identify strong correlations and any outliers.

  b. Perform a principal components analysis of these data. Use the biplot to show how the first principal component captures the strong correlation in part a. Again, identify any outliers in these data.

8.10 A psychological study was conducted at Northwestern University on 160 subjects. Each subject was assessed on a variety of standard psychological measures. Then each subject was shown one of four different movies (comedy, horror, nature, and documentary) and then assessed again. The variable `affect` in the `psych` library contains these data. Look at the help file to see details on the variables, published references, and several summary displays of these data in **R**. Develop a few displays of your own for these data and interpret your findings.

8.11 The Synthetic Aperture Personality Assessment (SAPA) Project is a web-based psychological data collection.[2] A subset of the data is available in **R** as bfi in the psych library. This subset contains data on three demographic variables and 25 personality items submitted by 2800 volunteers. As examples of these items, we have:

- I know how to comfort others.
- I waste my time.
- I make friends easily.

Each item is rated on a scale of 1 to 7, on whether the respondent feels he or she agrees with the statement a lot, disagrees a lot, or falls somewhere in between. See the bfi help file for more details.

a. Use the complete.cases() command to remove individuals in bfi with any missing values.
b. Use factor analysis to group together items of a similar nature. Try to interpret the nature of items clustering together. This is a useful exercise in psychology. The chi-squared test of the adequacy of the number of factors may not be appropriate with such a large sample size.
c. Identify those questions having a preponderance of extreme agree and/or disagree responses. Similarly, identify suspected outliers such as persons who appear to respond in an extreme fashion. That is, persons who tend to strongly agree and or disagree with a majority of the questions.

8.12 Table 8.5 summarizes oil consumption in the largest importing and exporting nations for the year 2011. Consumption is expressed both as a daily figure and per capita. These are expressed in barrels (bbl) and cubic meters. The ratio of production to consumption is given as well.

Perform a principal components analysis on these data and draw the scree plot and biplot. How does the biplot group similar nations together? Does this analysis confirm our knowledge of the economies of these nations?

8.13 The bodyfat data frame in the TH.data library lists 10 anthropomorphic measurements made on 71 healthy women. A key feature of these data is the method of measuring their total body fat with great precision but also at great cost. Use principal components to summarize these data. Show the data can be well summarized using only two principal components.

---

[2] You can learn more and take the assessment at: https://sapa-project.org/.

Table 8.5 Statistics on oil consuming nations in 2011

Nation	Daily consumption		Population	Annual per capita		Production /
	1000 bbl	1000 meter^3	in millions	bbl	meter^3	consumption
United States	18,835.5	2994.6	314	21.8	3.47	0.51
China	9,790.0	1556.5	1345	2.7	0.43	0.41
Japan	4,464.1	709.7	127	12.8	2.04	0.03
India	3,292.2	523.4	1198	1.0	0.16	0.26
Russia	3,145.1	500.0	140	8.1	1.29	3.35
Saudi Arabia	2,817.5	447.9	27	40.0	6.40	3.64
Brazil	2,594.2	412.4	193	4.9	0.78	0.99
Germany	2,400.1	381.6	82	10.7	1.70	0.06
Canada	2,259.1	359.2	33	24.6	3.91	1.54
South Korea	2,230.2	354.6	48	16.8	2.67	0.02
Mexico	2,132.7	339.1	109	7.1	1.13	1.39
France	1,791.5	284.8	62	10.5	1.67	0.03
Iran	1,694.4	269.4	74	8.3	1.32	2.54
United Kingdom	1,607.9	255.6	61	9.5	1.51	0.93
Italy	1,453.6	231.1	60	8.9	1.41	0.10

Source US Energy Information Administration

8.14 Perform a principal component analysis on the housing cost data in Sect. 3.3. Plot the loadings on each of the two principal components. Interpret this figure. *Hint:* The first component is roughly the sum or housing and rents and can be interpreted as the cost-of-living. The second component is roughly the difference and can be interpreted as whether renting or buying makes better sense, economically.

Chapter 9
Multivariable Linear Regression

L INEAR REGRESSION is probably one of the most powerful and useful tools available to the applied statistician. This method uses one or more variables to explain the values of another. Statistics alone cannot prove a cause and effect relationship, but we can show how changes in one set of measurements are associated with changes of the average values in another.

Notice how this approach is different from principal components analysis. In principal components, all variables are associated with each other and the statistical analysis attempts to uncover groups of variables varying together. In contrast, in linear regression, the data analyst specifies which of the variables are to be considered explanatory and which are the responses to these. This process requires a good understanding of the data. Sometimes we have a cause and effect relationship where some conditions are under our control. More often, we have jointly observed data and we want to express the behavior of some variables for given conditions of the others. A cause and effect relationship is difficult to demonstrate. The interested reader is referred to Pearl (2009) for a detailed description of the issues involved. Some topics of causality are introduced in Sect. 14.3

The methods in this chapter assume linear relationships between all the dependent and independent variables. In Sect. 10.7, we consider regression tree models for non-parametric settings where we can assume monotone, but not necessarily linear, relationships between these variables.

Let us begin by considering the mtcars dataset in the datasets package. This data.frame contains 11 measurements on each of 32 model cars available in 1973 to 4. These 11 measurements are listed in Table 9.1.

Some characteristics could be considered *design features* not be readily observed unless one were to open the hood, or perhaps dismantle an assembly and count the teeth on the various gears. These design features include the number of cylinders, displacement, rear axle ratio, "V" arrangement of cylinders, number of forward gears, and the number of carburetors.

© Springer Nature Switzerland AG 2022
D. Zelterman, *Applied Multivariate Statistics with R*, Statistics for Biology and Health,
https://doi.org/10.1007/978-3-031-13005-2_9

Table 9.1 Measures on 32 cars in the mtcars dataset

Name	Definition	Design or empirical
mpg	Miles/(US) gallon	E
cyl	Number of cylinders	D
disp	Displacement (cu.in.)	D
hp	Gross horsepower	E
drat	Rear axle ratio	D
wt	Weight (lb/1000)	E
qsec	1/4 mile time	E
vs	Cylinders form a "V" or are in a straight line	D
am	Transmission (0 = automatic, 1 = manual)	D
gear	Number of forward gears	D
carb	Number of carburetors	D

Other features in this list are *empirical* and readily experienced by a driver. This list includes the miles per gallon, horsepower, weight, and quarter-mile time. The casual driver would not know the exact weight or horsepower, of course, but in relative terms, these would be experienced in comparison to other cars with markedly different values. In this example, we will classify the type of transmission (manual or automatic) as a design feature, although it might be considered an empirical feature, as well.

In this chapter, we will develop mathematical models using the design features to explain differences in the empirical features. The mean value of each empirical feature is modeled as a linear function of all the design features. The multivariable approach is to do this for all empirical features and then examine whatever is left over from the modeling process, i.e., the residuals). These multivariate residuals are used to determine if the empirical features remain correlated after having taken into account the linear effects of the design features.

9.1   Univariate Regression

The goal of linear regression is to attempt to explain the different values of one variable in terms of others. This idea is not to predict but rather to make a statement about the typical or mean value under specified conditions.

To begin, let's build a linear regression to explain the miles per gallon (mpg) values from the design features. The plan is not to predict mpg values but rather, attempt to reasonably explain the values we have already observed. There is a danger of extrapolation: We cannot make any intelligent statement about combinations or values that are beyond the range of our experience. Within the range of observed data, we will be able to say something about which design features are more closely associated with mpg values.

We denote by Y_i a random variable with a distribution depending on a vector of known explanatory values x_i. The functional form is

$$Y_i = \beta' x_i + e_i \tag{9.1}$$

where the independent, normally distributed errors e_i have zero means and constant variances σ^2. The regression coefficients β are parameters needed to be estimated from the observed data (y_i, x_i). In the present example, y_i is the observed, empirical feature (such as mpg) of the i-th car, and x_i is the vector of values of all the design features of each car.

The linear model of one variable in terms of another is motivated by the properties of the multivariate normal distribution with conditional mean and variance given at (6.6) and (6.7), respectively. Specifically, the conditional means of the Y_i are linear in the explanatory variables, and the conditional variances are independent of the values of the explanatory variables.

Least squares methods are used to obtain fitted parameter values $\widehat{\beta}$ estimating β. Also useful are *fitted values*

$$\widehat{Y_i} = \widehat{\beta}' x_i$$

or the estimated mean values anticipated by model (9.1).

The estimated parameters $\widehat{\beta}$ are those values minimizing the sum of squared residuals $\sum r_i^2$ where the residuals are the observed differences between the observed and expected values

$$r_i = y_i - \widehat{\beta}' x_i .$$

Similarly, the $\widehat{\beta}$ are often referred to as least square estimates. Plots of the residuals r_i are instrumental in identifying lack of fit and deviations from the assumed linear model (9.1) as we will illustrate in this chapter.

In **R**, we can fit a linear regression, and also capture the residuals, estimated regression coefficients $\widehat{\beta}$, and fitted values. These appear in Output 9.1. This Output lists, in respective columns, the estimated regression coefficients $\widehat{\beta}$, their standard errors, t-test statistics, and p-values testing the null hypothesis the corresponding population coefficient (β) is zero. The asterisks indicate the level of statistical significance.

In this table of parameter estimates, we see the number of cylinders (cyl) and weight (wt) provide a great amount of explanatory value in describing mpg values. The number of carburetors (carb) has limited value, and the transmission type (am: automatic or manual) makes a minimal contribution. The estimated coefficients for cylinders and weight are negative because, intuitively, larger engines and heavier cars will get fewer miles per gallon.

Output 9.1 Output from the linear model fitting mpg values

```
> library(datasets)
> univ <- lm(formula = mpg ~ cyl + wt + am + carb, data = mtcars)
> fit <- univ$fitted.values
> resid <- univ$residuals
> summary(univ)

Call:
lm(formula = mpg ~ cyl + wt + am + carb, data = mtcars)

Residuals:
    Min      1Q  Median      3Q     Max
-4.5451 -1.2184 -0.3739  1.4699  5.3528

Coefficients:
             Estimate Std. Error t value Pr(>|t|)
(Intercept)  36.8503     2.8694   12.843 5.17e-13 ***
cyl          -1.1968     0.4368   -2.740   0.0108 *
wt           -2.4785     0.9364   -2.647   0.0134 *
am            1.7801     1.5091    1.180   0.2485
carb         -0.7480     0.3956   -1.891   0.0694 .
---
Signif. codes:  0 '***' 0.001 '**' 0.01 '*' 0.05 '.' 0.1 ' ' 1

Residual standard error: 2.5 on 27 degrees of freedom
Multiple R-squared: 0.8502,    Adjusted R-squared: 0.828
F-statistic:  38.3 on 4 and 27 DF,  p-value: 9.255e-11
```

The analysis of variance (ANOVA) expresses the total sum of squares:

$$\sum (y_i - \overline{y})^2 = \sum (\overline{y} - \widehat{y}_i)^2 + \sum r_i^2 . \tag{9.2}$$

The total sum of squares of the observed y_i about their average $\overline{y}$ is the total amount of variability in the dependent variable. This amount can be partitioned into the sum of squared values of the observed values about the fitted values plus the sum of squared residuals. The sum of squared residuals was minimized in order to estimate $\widehat{\beta}$. The sum of squared residuals is referred to as the *error sum of squares* or the *unexplained sum of squares*.

The sum of squares about the fitted values $\widehat{y}_i$ is the amount of variability attributed to knowing the explanatory variables x_i. This is often called the *explained* or *model sum of squares*. Ideally, we want the model sum of squares to be large relative to the error sum of squares. This difference is usually expressed as a ratio, or more specifically, the *F-statistic* given at the end of Output 9.1.

How did we decide on this subset of all design features to use in explaining the mpg values? It helps to have a good understanding of the nature of the data. In this case, we all have a basic understanding of how a car works. A little trial and error identified number of cylinders, weight, automatic/manual, and number of carburetors as useful. Useful explanatory variables are generally identified by extremely small p-values. The table of fitted coefficients in Output 9.1 prints *'s to guide our attention toward those most highly statistically significant explanatory variables.

For every parameter (coefficient) in the regression model, **R** provides an estimated value and a standard error of each estimate. The t value is the ratio

$$t\,value = Estimate/Std.Error$$

The corresponding statistical significance of this t–statistic appears under Pr[>|t|]. This tests the null hypothesis the true, underlying population parameter is actually zero. A small p-value for this test indicates the strong relationship between the variables could not have happened by chance alone.

The regression model with fitted parameter values is

$$mpg = 36.85 - 1.20\,cyl - 2.48\,wt + 1.78\,am - .75\,carb + error. \qquad (9.3)$$

In other words, increasing the cylinders, weight and number of carburetors all result in decreased estimates of the miles per gallon. The difference between manual and automatic transmissions is less than 2mpg, and not statistically significant. For a range of values within those contained in these data, given a set of values of cylinders, weight, transmission type, and number of carburetors, this last expression can be used to give a reasonable estimate of the average miles per gallon of a car with those characteristics. Ultimately, (9.3) is easily interpreted and agrees with our intuition about factors influencing mpg.

Output 9.1 includes an estimate of 2.5 for the standard deviation of the errors associated with the linear model. That is, the fitted model at (9.3) estimates the mpg with a standard deviation of about 2.5. To appreciate the value of the regression, let us compare this value to the standard deviation of the marginal mpg values,

```
> sd(mtcars$mpg)

[1] 6.026948
```

illustrating the much higher variability associated without the use of the linear model.

We should always examine the residuals of the fitted model. The plot of residuals and fitted values is given in Fig. 9.1. The marginal distributions are displayed as rug fringes. A few unusual values are identified in this plot.

The rug fringe along the left marginal axis shows the residuals from this fitted model appear normally distributed. There are no extreme poorly fitting observations in the data. The three cars identified by name in the plot are notable. All three have high miles per gallon, as expected by the fitted model. Two models (Volvo 142E and Datsun—now Nissan 710) have much lower mpg than expected. The Toyota Corolla has much higher gas mileage than anticipated by the fitted model. The model assumptions seem to be reasonable in this example. In such plots we look for evidence of outliers, trends not accounted for by the model and nonconstant variability of the residuals.

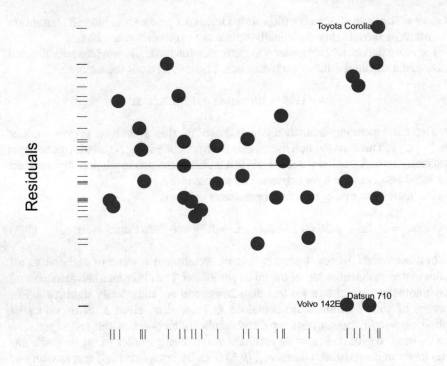

Fitted values

Figure 9.1 Fitted and residual values for the linear regression model (9.3) of mpg data

Let us end this section with a brief discussion of the options **R** offers us in performing linear regression.

We use the `formula` = parameter to specify the linear model to be fitted. The notation

        mpg ~ cyl + wt

for example, is shorthand for the model

$$\text{mpg} = \beta_0 + \beta_1\,\text{cyl} + \beta_2\,\text{wt}$$

where the tilde ($\sim$) takes the role of the equal sign in the formula.

To specify a model without an intercept β_0, we would write

        mpg ~ cyl + wt - 1

or equivalently

```
mpg ~ 0 + cyl + wt.
```

There are other options you can read about using `help(formula)` in **R**.

In addition to `lm()`, the `glm` and `aov` programs have a similar syntax. The `aov` program will be demonstrated in the following section. GLM is the abbreviation of *generalized linear model* and will be illustrated here.

To illustrate the use of `glm`, we can write

```
> univ.glm <- glm(formula = mpg ~ cyl + wt + am + carb , data =
  mtcars)
> summary(univ.glm)
```

This produces output similar to what you obtain using `lm`.

As with `lm`, the `glm` routine allows us to capture statistics about the fitted parameter values appearing in the output. Corresponding to Output 9.1, we can also write

```
> tt <- summary(univ.glm)
> print( tt$coefficients, digits=4)

            Estimate Std. Error t value  Pr(>|t|)
(Intercept)  36.850     2.8694  12.843 5.172e-13
cyl          -1.197     0.4368  -2.740 1.075e-02
wt           -2.478     0.9364  -2.647 1.339e-02
am            1.780     1.5091   1.180 2.485e-01
carb         -0.748     0.3956  -1.891 6.941e-02
```

In this code, the variable `tt` contains a data frame with the values produced in `glm` and printed by `summary(univ)`. The variable `tt$coefficients` contains the values produced by `summary`. We can then obtain separate values for the *t*-statistics and their *p*-values, for example, in addition to the estimated regression coefficients.

9.2 Multivariable Regression in **R**

The popularity of linear regression cannot be understated. It stands to reason there are methods generalizing to more than one dependent variable. Such multivariable regression methods build upon the univariate linear regression of the previous section and then follow up with the principal components analysis described in Sect. 8.1. There are also multivariable analogies to the ANOVA called the *multivariable analysis of variance* or MANOVA, but this is not in common use today. See Hand and Taylor (1987) for more on the multivariate analysis of variance.

Multivariable linear regression is performed in two steps. First, we perform separate, univariate linear regressions for each of the dependent variables y and capture the residuals for each of these regressions. Each separate regression provides the estimated regression coefficients, regardless of how the various dependent variables are correlated with each other.

The second step is to perform principal components or factor analysis on the residuals to see if there is additional information in the dependent variables, after having corrected for the effects of the explanatory x variables. We use graphical methods to check model assumptions and examine residuals for outliers and lack of fit.

The best way to illustrate the multivariable linear regression is to work through two examples in detail. In this section, we examine the characteristics of cars in the mtcars dataset also examined in the previous section. In the following section, we will examine a much larger dataset taken from a health survey.

In the mtcars example, Table 9.1 identifies the variables we classified as *design features* and those described as *performance features* to be experienced by the owner.

We build a multivariable linear regression by explaining each of the empirical features (mpg, hp, wt, qsec) from the design features (cyl, disp, am, drat, carb, vs, gear). Four separate linear regressions for these empirical features were fitted using

```
univ.mpg <- aov(mpg ~ cyl + disp + am + carb , data = mtcars)
summary(univ.mpg)

univ.hp <- aov( hp ~ cyl + drat + am + gear + carb, data = mtcars)
summary(univ.hp)

univ.wt <- aov( wt ~ cyl + disp + drat + am + carb, data = mtcars)
summary(univ.wt)

univ.qsec <- aov( qsec ~ cyl + disp + drat + vs + am + gear, data =
  mtcars)
summary(univ.qsec)
```

producing four separate, marginal ANOVA's.

The fitted models are

$$mpg = 30.19 - 0.657cyl - 0.0180disp + 3.599am - 1.19carb + error$$
$$hp = -100. + 27.7cyl - 3.98drat + 3.16am + 13.4gear + 13.8carb + error$$
$$wt = 3.77 - 0.231cyl + 0.006659disp - 0.263drat - 0.647am + 0.195carb + error$$
$$qsec = 26.3 - 0.804cyl + 0.000770disp - 0.362drat + 1.05vs - 1.38am$$
$$-0.623gear + error$$

The choice of explanatory variables is not the same in each of these regressions. These were chosen using a little trial and error to include only those with both intuitive explanatory value and statistical significance. The residuals from the four separate regressions can be captured and combined into a single data.frame:

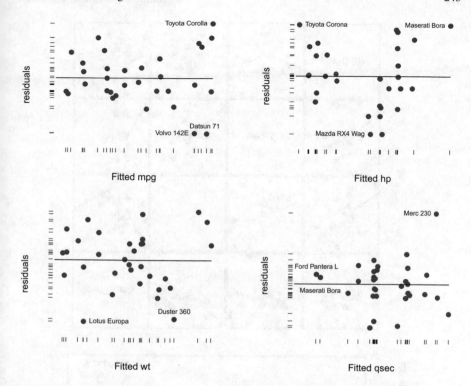

Figure 9.2 Fitted and residual values from four marginal linear regressions of car data

```
> car.res <- cbind( univ.mpg$residuals, univ.hp$residuals,
+                   univ.wt$residuals, univ.qsec$residuals)
> colnames(car.res)<- c("mpg_res", "hp_res", "wt_res", "qsec_res")
> car.res <- data.frame(car.res)
> print(car.res, digits=2)

                mpg_res  hp_res  wt_res  qsec_res
Mazda RX4       -1.2058 -52.749  0.0626    0.1024
Mazda RX4 Wag   -1.2058 -52.749  0.3176    0.6624
Datsun 710      -5.2311  26.952  0.2200   -0.3860

     . . .                 . . .

Maserati Bora    1.4107  46.675 -0.3407    0.2332
Volvo 142E      -5.2054  30.181  0.4665   -0.3118
```

Four separate, marginal plots of fitted and residuals are given in Fig. 9.2. A number of unusual and remarkable cars are identified by name. These are typically either economy makes (Toyota, Duster, and Datsun) or else large, luxury models (Maserati, Lotus, or Mercury).

A multivariate examination of these residuals begins with the matrix scatterplot presented in the top panel of Fig. 9.3. This figure includes the loess smoothing and does not identify any strong correlations between residuals not explained by the linear models. (See Fig. 3.16 for details on how we draw this figure in **R**.)

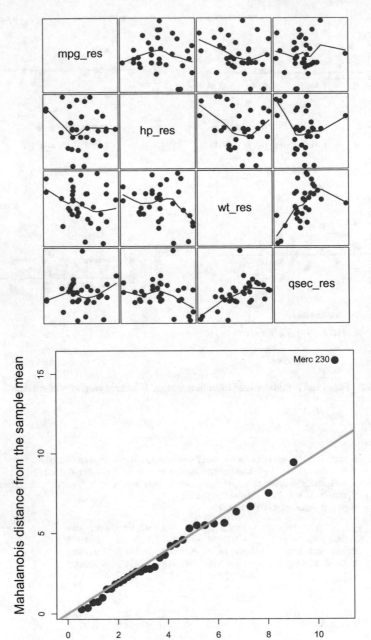

Figure 9.3 Scatter plot of residual values of car data with loess smooth (top panel) and QQ plot of Mahalanobis Distances (bottom panel)

We can also perform a series of tests for the multivariate normal distribution of the residuals. The bottom panel of Fig. 9.3 is a QQ plot of the Mahalanobis distances from the centroid for the four-dimensional residuals. The clear outlier (Mercury 230) is identified by name. The plot of univariate residuals in Fig. 9.2 identified this car model as having an unusually large quarter-mile time.

Formal statistical tests for the multivariate normal behavior of the residuals reflect what is observed in the QQ plot. Specifically, the code

```
> library(mvnormtest)
> mshapiro.test( t( car.res))

    Shapiro-Wilk normality test

data:  Z
W = 0.8389, p-value = 0.0002403
```

yields a *p*-value of 0.0002 indicating a poor correspondence to the multivariate normal distribution.

We can omit the single observation with the largest Mahalanobis statistic in its residual:

```
> mah <- mahalanobis(car.res, colMeans(car.res), var(car.res))
> outi <- match(max(mah),mah)    # index of outlier
> mshapiro.test( t( car.res[-outi,] ))

Shapiro-Wilk normality test

data:  Z
W = 0.9232, p-value = 0.02877
```

The fit to a multivariate normal distribution improves slightly, but is still suspect.

The next step in this multivariable linear regression is to perform a principal components analysis on these residuals. The object of this examination is to see if there is any additional information remaining between the four dependent variables (mpg, hp, wt, qsec) after accounting the linear effects of the explanatory variables (cyl, disp, drat, vs. am, gear, carb).

The principal components analysis in **R** is

```
> print(prcomp(car.res, scale = TRUE), digits = 3)

Standard deviations:
[1] 1.312 1.061 0.885 0.607

Rotation:
            PC1    PC2    PC3     PC4
mpg_res   0.160 -0.864 0.277   0.388
hp_res    0.426  0.400 0.798   0.146
wt_res   -0.658  0.230 0.106   0.709
qsec_res -0.600 -0.199 0.524  -0.571
```

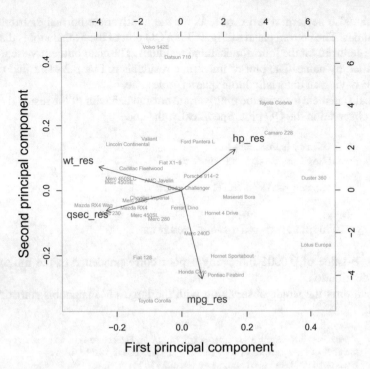

Figure 9.4   Principal component biplot of the residuals from the car data

In the list of ordered standard deviations, we see all four principal components are comparable in magnitude; the largest is just slightly twice the size of the smallest. We interpret the loadings here to mean the residuals of hp, wt, and qsec are all highly correlated with each. The mpg residuals are independent of these three.

The biplot for the first two principal components

```
biplot(prcomp(car.res, scale = TRUE), cex = c(.6, 1.2),
    col = c(3, 4), cex.lab=1.5,
    xlab = "First principal component",
    ylab = "Second principal component")
```

is given in Fig. 9.4.

The loadings of the first principal component show the residuals of weight and quarter second times are positively correlated with each other and negatively correlated with hp residuals. The second principal component is composed almost entirely of the mpg residuals showing these are independent of the other three.

In summary, the four individual linear regressions appear to capture much of the useful information about the four dependent variables. There are a few remarkable outliers. What is left over are residuals for mpg which appear independent of the other three sets of residuals.

9.3 A Large Health Survey

In this section, we examine a large dataset and use it to further illustrate the uses of multivariable linear regression. The Behavior Risk Factor Surveillance System (BRFSS) is a large initiative sponsored by the Centers for Disease Control (CDC) in Atlanta, Georgia. This is a telephone survey of individuals living in the largest metropolitan areas concerning their health, health behaviors, and individual risk factors. The survey is weighted towards reaching individuals who might not be easily identified in a traditional, straightforward sample. We will examine data from the survey taken in the year 2010. More details on these questions, other health-related questions, and surveys from other years are available on the SMART (Selected Metropolitan/Micropolitan Area Risk Trends) website.

Table 9.2 lists a number of survey items selected from the total. The items themselves form two separate types of measurements: behavioral and health outcomes. As examples, a report of binge drinking is a behavioral measure, and a report of asthma is a health outcome. Some of these measures are not clearly one or the other such as BMI or health coverage. We will classify both of these measures as behavioral to simplify the discussion.

The object of the data analysis is to see if we can identify the behavioral risk factor's effects on the associated health outcomes. These associations are aggregate for cities, not individuals, so we can only infer properties of populations. For example, we cannot infer the people who regularly see a dentist are less likely to have missing teeth, but rather, populations with large numbers of people seeing dentists are also populations with fewer missing teeth.

As another example of the shortcomings of this cross-sectional data, we are unable to tell if those individuals with asthma are more or less likely to be binge drinkers. Instead, we can only say something about the rates of asthma in cities with high levels of binge drinking. One person is the binge drinker, but a different person in the same city develops asthma. Finally, the data examined here is only for one year (2010), so we are unable to determine if binge drinking has any long-term health effects or if binge drinking is on the rise.

The dataset is too large for examining all possible pairs of scatter plots using `pairs()`. Instead, Fig. 9.5 plots `pairs()` for only those variables considered as outcomes. There are several highly correlated pairs of outcomes, including the perception of general health with each of having a heart attack, diabetes, and loss of any permanent teeth.

Let us illustrate how multivariable linear regression methods can help summarize the various patterns occurring in this dataset. We begin by performing separate linear regressions for each of the eight outcome variables using all 10 of the behavioral measures as explanatory variables.

The first examination asks which of these behaviors is associated with each of the different health outcomes. The second analysis asks how each of the health outcomes is related to each other after having corrected all of the behavioral measures.

Table 9.2 The subset of the BRFSS dataset summarizes the percentage of respondents answering positively to these items in each of 192 US metropolitan areas. Every variable is classified as either behavioral (B) or health outcome (O)

Variable name	Description	Outcome or Behavior
Binge	Regular binge drinking	B
Asthma	Reporting asthma	O
HeartAt	Ever had a heart attack	O
Colonosc	Adults 50+ who ever had a colonoscopy	B
Diabetes	Any diagnosis of diabetes	O
PregDia	Pregnancy related diabetes	O
PreDia	Pre-diabetic or borderline diabetes	O
Disability	Limited activities due to disability	O
Exercise	Any exercise in the past month	B
Coverage	Any healthcare coverage	B
GeneralH	Self-reported general health of good or better	O
FluShot	Adults 65+ having a flu shot in the past year	B
Dentist	Visited a dentist in the past year	B
Teeth	Any permanent teeth extracted	O
BMI	BMI under 25 (not overweight)	B
PSA	Men 40+ with a PSA screen over the past year	B
Smokers	Current smokers	B
PAP	Women 18+ with a Pap test over the past 3 years	B

Source http://apps.nccd.cdc.gov/BRFSS-SMART/

The separate linear regression for each of the eight health outcomes regressing on all of ten explanatory variables results in an 11×8 matrix of regression coefficients (including the intercepts). A simple way to examine all of these coefficients is to produce a *heatmap*, as in Fig. 9.6. The regression coefficients with the greatest statistical significance are in white, and those less so are in yellow, with red indicating no statistical significance. The heatmap() program reorganizes the rows (behaviors) and columns (outcomes) in order to visually group together regression coefficients with similar significance values. Heatmaps are discussed again in Sect. 11.3.

The red/yellow color pattern only indicates statistical significance of the estimated regression coefficient. These do not all correspond to good or bad health patterns because the explanatory variables are not all indicative of the same direction. Frequent binge drinking is (presumably) a bad health behavior and visiting a dentist is a good

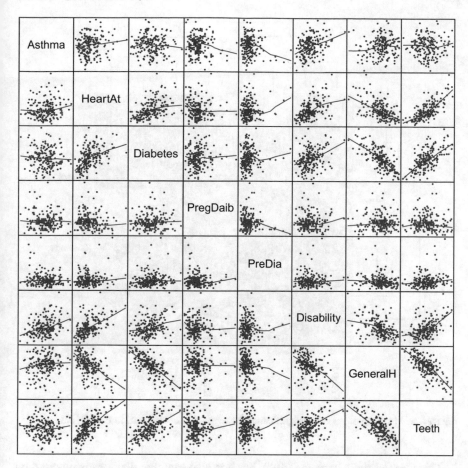

Figure 9.5   Matrix scatter plot and smooth fit of BRFSS health outcome variables

behavior. So in these two examples, positive regression coefficients can have opposite interpretations. Similarly, smoking is highly correlated with any reported disability, but it is not clear from the heatmap whether this correlation is positive or negative. Further, it is not obvious why these two variables should be highly correlated.

The eight separate regressions create eight vectors of residuals. These different residuals represent the eight different health outcomes for each of 192 metropolitan areas after having corrected for each of the 10 behavioral measures.

The `corrplot()` of the residuals appears in Fig. 9.7. (The `corrplot()` was described in Sect. 3.5.1.) Again, these are not the correlations between the various health outcomes in Table 9.5, but, rather, the correlations of the eight health outcomes after having corrected for each of the 10 behavioral measures. The largest correlation is between the diabetes residuals and self-reported general health residuals. We interpret this to mean the relationship between diabetes and general health at the population level is not accounted for by any of the behavioral measures.

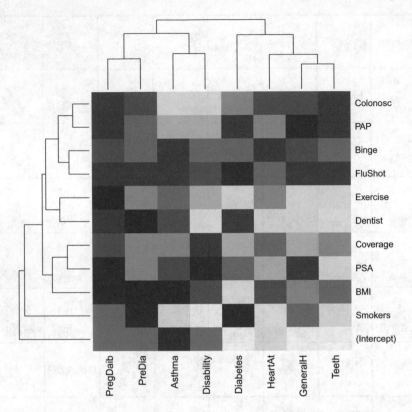

Figure 9.6 Heatmap of statistical significance for regression coefficients in BRFSS data

This correlation is large (-0.493), but it is also true that diabetes is reported by less than 9% of those surveyed. That is, the strong correlation may only reflect a small portion of those affected in the population. Similarly, there is also a large correlation (0.44) between the residuals of those reporting a heart attack and those reporting loss of adult teeth. Heart attacks were reported by only 4.3% of those surveyed. In both of these examples (diabetes and heart attack), strong correlations only occur in small segments of the population.

The largest correlation we can identify among the residuals is a large negative and intuitive relationship between those of disability and perception of general health, after having corrected for all of the explanatory behavioral variables in the dataset. The "any disability" question is reported by 21.3% of those surveyed and is experienced by a larger portion of the population than either diabetes or heart attack.

A scatter plot of "any disability" and "reported general health" is given in Fig. 9.9, both as raw data and as residuals after correcting for all of the behavior variables. These separate plots will again reinforce the difference between these different concepts. Noticeably, the residual plot is given on a smaller scale than the original data. In both plots, Huntington, West Virginia exhibits a high level of individuals with a

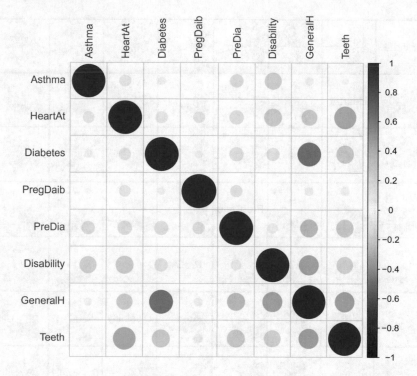

Figure 9.7 `corrplot` of residuals for individual linear refressions in BRFSS data

disability and low levels of individuals with self-reported good or excellent general health. On the basis of the 2006 BRFSS survey, the CDC listed Huntington as one of the most unhealthy cities in the US.

In contrast, Fayette, Arkansas appears to have a high level of self-reported health as a residual, after having corrected for health behaviors. This city does not appear unusual in the original, raw data. Fayette is a university town with an unusually large percentage of citizens with Masters and Ph.D. degrees. The Fayette metropolitan area includes Bentonville, home to many well-paid executives at the Walmart corporate headquarters.

A pairwise scatter plot of the eight sets of residuals is given in Fig. 9.8. There does not appear to be any obvious deviation from the assumption of a multivariate normal distribution. (See Exercise 9.2 for more details.) A principal components analysis of the residuals from these individual regressions completes the multivariate analysis. A portion of this analysis appears in Output 9.2.

From the standard deviations, we see the first few components contain most of the variability. In this case, the residual for loss of `Teeth` has almost all of the weight in the first component and seems to be independent of all other residuals. Similarly, the second component is almost entirely composed of the `Disability` residual. The third component is the `GeneralH` residual.

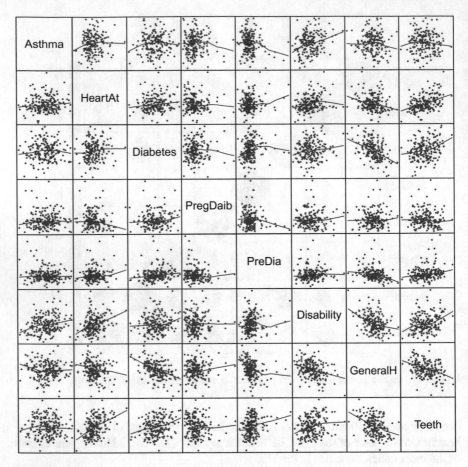

Figure 9.8   Matrix scatter plot and smooth fit of BRFSS residuals

The biplot of this principal component analysis appears in Fig. 9.10. The largest contributors to health residuals appear to be loss of permanent teeth and the presence of a disability. These two outcomes, after having corrected all of the behavior variables, are orthogonal to each other and appear to offer a large amount of explanatory value to the residuals from the multivariate regressions.

In summary, the multivariate regression of the large health survey yields a number of useful summary measures. Behavior variables such as having seen a dentist recently is a good explanatory measure of health outcomes, and the perception of one's health is a single stand-out determinant of other health outcomes across cities. Two cities appear as outliers at opposite ends of the health scale. Tooth loss and having any disability remain highly variable even after taking into account the effects of the explanatory variables.

Output 9.2   Principal components analysis for BRFSS residuals

```
Standard deviations:
[1] 4.609 2.943 2.057 1.727 1.127 0.839 0.740
[8] 0.476

Rotation:
                  PC1       PC2       PC3       PC4
Asthma        0.0138   0.25499   0.17051  -0.9437
HeartAt       0.1009   0.02420   0.03981  -0.0453
Diabetes      0.1101   0.05205  -0.35152  -0.1134
PregDaib     -0.0070   0.00653   0.00677   0.0142
PreDia        0.0530  -0.00957  -0.08155   0.0738
Disability    0.2926   0.85581   0.30301   0.2882
GeneralH     -0.2549  -0.26160   0.84547   0.0591
Teeth         0.9078  -0.36152   0.18012  -0.0473

                  PC5       PC6       PC7        PC8
Asthma       -0.0619   0.0341  -0.09833  -0.019658
HeartAt      -0.0794  -0.9342   0.31974  -0.065046
Diabetes      0.9171  -0.0713   0.01803   0.046964
PregDaib      0.0610   0.0912   0.08302  -0.990321
PreDia       -0.0282  -0.3118  -0.93550  -0.108811
Disability    0.0707   0.0409  -0.01358   0.016743
GeneralH      0.3727  -0.0595  -0.07430   0.017944
Teeth        -0.0174   0.1010   0.00252   0.000187
```

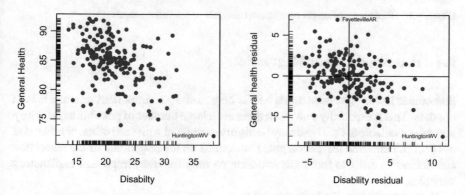

Figure 9.9   Scatterplot of disability and general health, both as raw data, and as residuals corrected for all of the behavioral measures

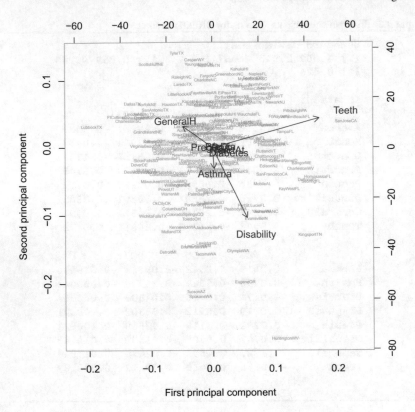

Figure 9.10 Biploty for principal components analysis of BRFSS residuals

9.4 Penalized Linear Regression

Sometimes linear regression needs a little help to show us important relationships in our data. This is especially true when there are a large number of possible explanatory variables available to us. These may be highly correlated with each other, or otherwise not useful. Penalized regression puts restrictions on the magnitude of the regression coefficients in order to focus our attention on only the most important explanatory variables.

In vector notation, the linear model is

$$y = \beta' X$$

for response values $y = (y_1, \ldots y_N)$ and matrix of explanatory values X.

The regression coefficients β are obtained by minimizing the sum of squared residuals

$$||y - \beta' X||^2 \tag{9.4}$$

where

$$||z|| = \left(\sum z_i^2 \right)^{1/2}$$

is the Euclidean norm, given in (4.4).

When there are many explanatory variables, we can force the overall vector β to be small by charging a penalty to (9.4) for large values of $||\beta||$. Specifically, we can find the value of β to minimize

$$||y - \beta'X||^2 + \epsilon_1 ||\beta||^2$$

for some small value $\epsilon_1 > 0$. This is called *ridge regression* and represents a compromise between minimizing the sum of squared residuals and also minimizing the magnitude of β.

Another common approach is to penalize the sum of squared residuals by the sum of absolute β's. That is, we find β to minimize

$$||y - \beta'X||^2 + \epsilon_2 \sum |\beta_i|$$

for a small value $\epsilon_2 > 0$. This approach is called *least absolute shrinkage and selection operator*, abbreviated as *lasso regression*.

A good compromise between these two approaches is *elastic-net regression* which incorporates both penalties, in different ratios. The **R** program glmnet() (in the library of the same name) fits a model by finding the value of β which minimizes

$$1/N \ ||y - \beta'X||^2 + \lambda \left\{ (1 - \alpha) \ ||\beta||^2 / 2 \ + \ \alpha \sum_i |\beta_i| \right\} \tag{9.5}$$

When $\alpha = 0$ in (9.5) we have ridge regression and $\alpha = 1$ gives the lasso estimate. The value of $\lambda > 0$ varies the magnitude of the penalty term. The usual approach is to pick one α between 0–1 and fit many models by varying λ. By default, the glmnet() program fits a range of 100 values of λ from most restrictive to least restrictive.

Before we go any further, let us return to the BRFSS data as an example. The variables in this data set and their names are summarized in Table 9.2. To illustrate penalized regression we will build a model of self-reported health (GeneralH) as a linear function of all other variables in the data. The code and some output is given in Output 9.3.

A basic **R** program fit the BRFSS data is given in Output 9.3. The data is read and formatted, separating the outcome (GeneralH) variable from all others which will be used as explanatory values. The value of alpha = 1 corresponding to lasso is the default option for glmnet.

This code fits the model and produces a plot similar to the one at the top of Fig. 9.11. The corresponding plot for alpha = 0 and ridge regression is given in the bottom half of Fig. 9.11. We added a small number of labels to these plots

Output 9.3 Program to fit elastic-net regression to the BRFSS data with selected output

```
library(glmnet)
BRFSS<-read.table("BRFSS.txt", header=TRUE, row.names = 1)
genh <- BRFSS$GeneralH            # general health is the outcome
expl <- as.matrix(BRFSS[, -11])   # everything else is explanatory
fit <- glmnet(x = expl, y = genh) # lasso model is the default
plot(fit)                         # plot beta's
coef(fit, s = .75)                # print one set of  beta's

(Intercept) 77.9945565503
Binge          .
Asthma         .
HeartAt        .
Colonosc       0.0009948497
Diabetes      -0.5324319878
PregDaib       .
PreDia         .
Disability     .
Exercise       0.0294418159
Coverage       0.0219660262
FluShot        .
Dentist        0.1456234150
Teeth         -0.0621013539
BMI            .
PSA            .
Smokers        .
PAP            .

print(fit)
    Df  %Dev  Lambda
1    0  0.00 2.79700
2    2 11.89 2.54900
3    2 21.81 2.32200
4    2 30.04 2.11600
5    2 36.88 1.92800
6    3 42.80 1.75700
     .   .    .
71  17 77.82 0.00415
72  17 77.82 0.00378
```

for clarity using text(), using **R** code not given here. There are many options
in glmnet to plot other measures but this is enough to introduce us to elastic-net
regression.

Figure 9.11 plots the values of the fitted β values for lasso (on top) and ridge
regression (bottom). The horizontal axes in this figure are the values of $\sum |\beta_i|$ also
referred to as the L_1-norm. These two figures present the β in fitted models from
the most restricted to least penalized, left to right.

Ridge regression keeps all of the explanatory variables in the model but tends to
shrink less important β's toward zero. At the left side of Fig. 9.11, ridge regression
forces all β's to be close to zero. As ridge regression becomes less restrictive, from
left to right, we see diabetes and pre-diabetes emerge as important determinants of
self-reported general health. Having had a heart attack is also important but becomes
less so as the restrictions on the model are reduced.

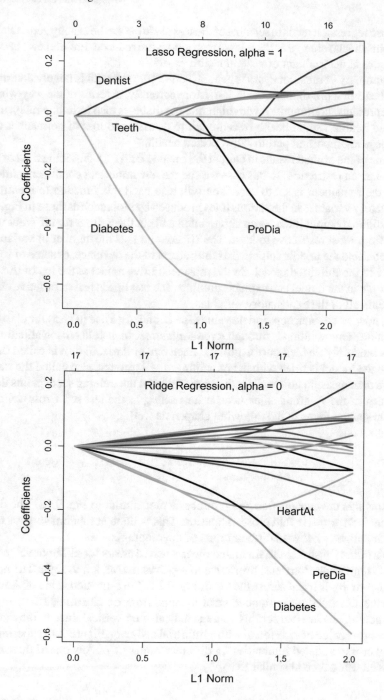

Figure 9.11 Estimated lasso and ridge regression parameters to model self-reported health

Lasso regression tends to set most of the less useful β's to be exactly zero. Diabetes and dental health emerge as these lasso restrictions are reduced. Pre-diabetes becomes an important determinant of general health as well.

A summary of these analyses is general self-reported health is largely determined by diabetes or a pre-diabetic condition. More correctly, in terms of the way what the data represents, communities with high rates of diabetes also have low rates of self-reported health. Dental health (recent visit to dentist, and loss of permanent teeth) also plays an important part in self-reported health.

Some of the printed results in Output 9.3 include `coef()` providing a set of fitted β for a given restriction. In this case we see the few important coefficients fitted by lasso, the remainder is set to zero. You will also need this function to identify the explanatory variables in the various lines produced by plots such as those in Fig. 9.11.

Additional output includes an abbreviated table at the bottom for different values of λ, from most restrictive to least. The `Df` column lists the number of variables in the model and the middle column lists the percent of the deviance, or sums of squares relative to the full fitted model. So the most restrictive model at the top of this table has no β's in the model and explains nothing. The last line is least restrictive enough to include all of the explanatory variables.

So, how do we pick appropriate values for α and λ to use in (9.5) for elastic-net regression? One solution is through *cross-validation*. In n-fold cross-validation, the data is randomly divided into n groups. Each one of these, in turn is called the test set and the model is fitted with the remaining $n - 1$ groups, also called the training set. We then measure how well the fitted model from the training set explains the test set. Each of the n groups then takes a turn acting as the test set. Cross-validation appears several times in the following chapter as well.

The **R** code

```
cv.lasso <- cv.glmnet(x = expl, y = genh)
plot(cv.lasso)
```

performs this cross-validation and produces a plot similar to Fig. 9.12. The default is to perform $n = 10$ fold cross-validation. This is done at random so your results will vary slightly between different runs of the program.

This figure illustrates the simulated mean squared errors for different values of λ in lasso regression from least restrictive to most restrictive, left to right. The number of non-zero β's is listed across the top of Fig. 9.12. The estimated value of λ to minimize the simulated mean squared error is found from `cv.lasso$lambda.1se` and a confidence interval for this value is indicated by vertical lines in the figure.

The best choice of α is found with a little trial and error. Figure 9.13 superimposes several cross-validated summaries for different values of α. Any one of these can be produced using **R** code similar to

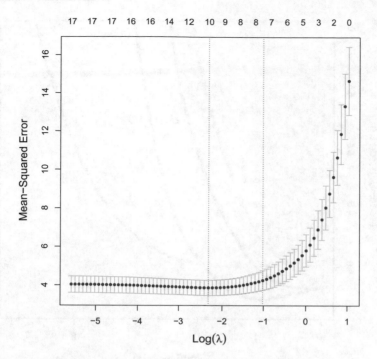

Figure 9.12 Cross-validated mean squared errors for lasso

```
cv13   <- cv.glmnet(x = expl, y = genh, alpha = 1/3)
plot(log(cv13$lambda), cv13$cvm, type = "l")
```

In Fig. 9.13, we see the value of α to produce the smallest estimated mean squared error is nether lasso ($\alpha = 1$) nor ridge ($\alpha = 0$) but some combination of the two, close to $\alpha = 1/3$, for the present example.

In summary, elastic-net regression is useful for constructing parsimonious linear models, especially when there are a large number of explanatory variables available to us. The glmnet program and library offer a large suite of diagnostic tools to work in these big-data settings. Cross-validation is useful in choosing just the right mix of restriction and quality of model fit. Finally, elastic-net regression is also a special case of the support vector machine, described in Sect. 10.6.

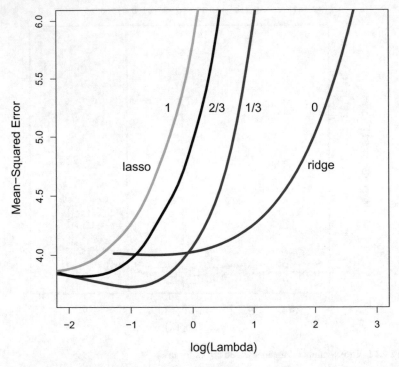

Figure 9.13 Cross-validated mean squared errors for different values of α

9.5 Exercises

9.1 Table 1.1 lists some cost of living statistics for each of the 50 states plus DC.
   The three costs are apartment rents, costs of houses, and the cost of living
   index. Perform a multivariable linear regression to explain these three metrics
   in terms of the state populations and average incomes. Are these explanatory
   variables useful for each of the cost variables? Capture the residuals from the
   three separate linear regressions and perform a principal component analysis. Is
   there anything left over what the regressions fail to capture? Are there outliers
   to be noted?
9.2 Test the BRFSS residuals for multivariate normality using the tests introduced
   in Sect. 7.7. Are the outliers highlighted in Fig. 9.9 large enough to lead us to
   question multivariate normality using these tests? Do the tests have markedly
   different outcomes if we delete the residuals from these two cities?
9.3 The Medicare Current Beneficiary Survey (MCBS) is an ongoing, representative, nation-wide survey of all persons who were Medicare recipients during
   any part of the current year. The data in Table 9.3 reports all healthcare goods
   and services purchased directly by the Medicare recipient. Recipients were
   contacted by telephone to assess their (self-reported) disability status. Physical

Table 9.3 Personal healthcare expenditures by Medicare patients, listed by functional status for the years 1992–2007

Year	All	No disability	Any physical limitation	Any IADL limitation	1–2 ADL's	3–6 ADL's
1992	6,550	2,980	3,468	5,770	7,373	17,058
1993	7,063	3,101	3,841	6,240	7,949	18,782
1994	7,730	3,355	3,783	6,396	8,349	22,994
⋮	⋮	⋮	⋮	⋮	⋮	⋮
2005	13,218	7,577	8,975	12,363	16,489	33,663
2006	14,448	8,847	9,520	14,353	17,759	34,751
2007	14,842	7,664	10,009	15,641	17,725	38,809

Source MCBS

disabilities were classified as essential activities of daily living (ADL) such as bathing, dressing, eating, and as instrumental activities of daily living (IADL) such as preparing meals, shopping, or answering the telephone. Another examination of these data appears in Exercise 13.4.

a. Fit separate linear regressions using the year as the explanatory variable. Choose your dependent variables (disability categories) carefully because some of these include others. Do discontinuous jumps occur in the annual expenditures? These may be attributed to policy changes.

b. Plot the residuals for each regression by year and comment on any apparent lack of independence from one year to the next.

c. Does a principal component analysis reveal any remarkable years?

9.4 Table 9.4 lists the annual number of coal miners and the number of deaths for the industry as reported by the US Department of Labor. The deaths and numbers of workers have decreased dramatically during the time period covered by these data. In Fig. 9.14, we see the death rate is falling faster than the number of miners. Perform a multivariable regression using year as the explanatory variable. Consider taking logs of the two response variables. What additional information would you like to see in order to draw useful conclusions from this data analysis?

9.5 Elston and Grizzle (1962) present the data in Table 9.5 on measurements of Ramus (jaw) bones on 20 boys at four different ages. The explanatory variable is age. We should expect correlations of the four measurements within each boy.

a. Fit a regression model using Age as the explanatory variable. Examine residuals graphically and identify outliers. Does a principal components analysis provide additional insights?

b. Are the variances the same at every age?

Table 9.4 Coal mining workers and fatalities by year

Years	Miners	Fatalities
1900	448,581	1,489
1901	485,544	1,574
1902	518,197	1,724
⋮	⋮	⋮
2010	135,500	48
2011	143,437	21
2012	137,650	20

Source MSHA

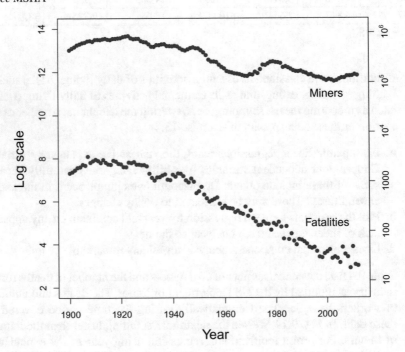

Figure 9.14 Annual number of US coal miners and fatalities, on a logarithmic scale

9.6 Many investors in stocks are looking for dividends to be paid out of future profits. Table 9.6 lists a number of the largest technology companies and information of their financial status, as of September 2010. The outcome variables to explain are current and future dividends. See what models you can develop from market capitalization, net cash, and cash flow. You can also create new measures as non-linear functions of other explanatory variables such as the ratio of cash flow and market capitalization.

Table 9.5 Measures of jaw bones on 20 boys at four different ages

	Age in years			
	8	8.5	9	9.5
1	47.8	48.8	49.0	49.7
2	46.4	47.3	47.7	48.4
3	46.3	46.8	47.8	48.5
⋮	⋮	⋮	⋮	⋮
19	46.2	47.5	48.1	48.4
20	46.3	47.6	51.3	51.8
mean	48.7	49.6	50.6	51.5

Source Elston and Grizzle (1962)

Table 9.6 Characteristics of several high-tech companies as of September 2010. Dollar amounts are in $Million

Company	Market cap	Net cash	2009 cash flow	Cash flow as % of cap	Cash+cash flow as % of cap	Current dividend rate	Dividend at 60% payout
Adobe	$17,254	$1,370	$1,118	6.48%	14.42	0.0%	3.9%
Amazon	66,336	5,070	3,293	4.96	12.61	0.0	3.0
Apple	252,664	45,800	10,159	4.02	22.15	0.0	2.4
Cisco	125,246	23,700	10,173	8.12	27.05	0.0	4.9
Dell	24,153	8,800	3,906	16.17	52.61	0.0	9.7
eBay	31,361	6,720	2,908	9.27	30.70	0.0	5.6
Google	153,317	30,300	9,316	6.08	25.84	0.0	3.6
Hewlett-Packard	90,280	6,400	13,379	14.82	21.91	0.8	8.9
Intel	105,625	22,100	11,170	10.58	31.50	3.4	6.3
Microsoft	219,195	38,450	24,073	10.98	28.52	2.1	6.6
Oracle	127,578	9,914	8,681	6.80	14.58	0.8	4.1
Qualcomm	67,370	2,870	7,172	10.65	14.91	1.8	6.4
Symantec	11,793	1,040	1,693	14.36	23.17	0.0	8.6
Texas Instruments	30,560	3,557	2,643	8.65	20.29	1.9	5.2
Yahoo!	19,132	7,230	1,310	6.85	44.64	0.0	4.1

Source StreetAuthority (www.StreetAuthority.com) and David Sterman
Used with permission

9.7 Stepwise regression automates the model-building process. The program

```
library(datasets)
library(MASS)
data(mtcars)
univ <- lm(mpg ~ cyl + disp + hp + drat + wt + qsec +
           vs + am + gear + carb, data = mtcars)
backward <- stepAIC(univ)
summary(backward)
```

begins with a linear model containing all of the explanatory variables and removes one at a time. This *backward stepwise regression* allows every explanatory a chance to contribute to the model and uses AIC to eliminate not making a significant contribution.

The AIC is equal to twice the log-likelihood, less than 2 times the numbers of parameters. Unlike the likelihood, AIC charges a "penalty" for every parameter in the model, forcing every parameter to make a contribution to the model. AIC was developed for times series models with many parameters and is described in Sect. 13.2.

Does the final fitted model from this program coincide with our intuition? What are the advantage and disadvantages of having the computer decide on the model for us?

9.8 The program

```
influence(univ)
```

produces a large number of diagnostics for the regression model. These include $hat which is a measure of the influence each observation has on its fitted value. The $coefficients estimates how much each estimated regression coefficient is changed when each observation is omitted, and the model is refitted. Omitting each observation, in turn, is a method called the *jackknife*. Similarly, $sigma estimated the change in estimated standard deviation of the residuals changes when this observation is jackknifed.

Plot some of these diagnostics for the mtcars data. Are influential observations also those with unusually large residuals?

9.9 Examine glmrob in the robustbase library, to perform *robust* linear regression. Does the robust fitted model in the mtcars data differ from the least squares regression model we fitted here? A larger set of data on more recent cars is available as car.test.frame in the rpart library.

9.10 The data in Table 9.7 is a record of forest fires in Montesinho Park, located in northeast Portugal. The variables X, Y refer to map coordinates in the park. The character valued weekday and month of the fire may not be useful. The variables FFMC, DMC, DC, ISI each refer to specific elements of the Forest Fire Weather Index, a method used to determine the risk of forest fires based on specified conditions. Atmospheric conditions at the time of the fire

Table 9.7 Areas and conditions of burn in forest fires in Montesinho Park

	X	Y	month	day	FFMC	DMC	DC	ISI	temp	RH	wind	rain	area
1	7	5	mar	fri	86.2	26.2	94.3	5.1	8.2	51	6.7	0	0.00
2	7	4	oct	tue	90.6	35.4	669.1	6.7	18.0	33	0.9	0	0.00
3	7	4	oct	sat	90.6	43.7	686.9	6.7	14.6	33	1.3	0	0.00
					· · ·			· · ·					
515	7	4	aug	sun	81.6	56.7	665.6	1.9	21.2	70	6.7	0	11.16
516	1	4	aug	sat	94.4	146.0	614.7	11.3	25.6	42	4.0	0	0.00
517	6	3	nov	tue	79.5	3.0	106.7	1.1	11.8	31	4.5	0	0.00

include temperature, relative humidity, wind speed, and amount of rain. The data appears in the UCI database and available at

http://archive.ics.uci.edu/ml/datasets/Forest+Fires

The outcome variable we want to explain is the area of the burn, measured in hectares. These values are highly skewed with many zero values. You might want to transform these as $\log(1 + area)$. Taking logs twice, i.e. $\log(1 + \log(1 + area))$ produces a clear mixture of a normal population and a point mass at zero.

There are a number of explanatory variables and not all of these may be useful in explaining the areas of the burns. Perform restricted linear regressions and prepare figures similar to Fig. 9.11 for these data. Identify the largest contributors to area of burn as wind speed and rain, presumably contributing to lightening strikes.

Chapter 10
Discrimination and Classification

I F WE HAVE multivariate observations from two or more identified populations, how can we characterize them? Is there a combination of measurements to clearly distinguish between these groups? It is not good enough to simply say the mean of one variable is statistically higher in one group in order to solve this problem, because the histograms of the groups may have considerable overlap making the discriminatory process only a little better than guesswork. To think in multivariate terms, we do not use only one variable at a time to distinguish between groups of individuals, but rather, we use a combination of explanatory variables.

The difference between discriminant analysis and principal component analysis is in discriminant analysis, we begin by knowing the group membership. In the discriminant analysis, we try to identify linear combinations of several variables used to distinguish between the groups. In principal components, by contrast, it is not clear if there are separate groups. If principal components identify groups, then there is no confirmatory step because we may not be aware of separate groups a priori. Similarly, in the following chapter on clustering methods, we assume there are groups within the data but do not identify these in advance.

10.1 Logistic Regression

The reader may already be familiar with the univariate discriminant method called *logistic regression* in which we use regression methods to distinguish between two different groups. This classification criterion is based on a probabilistic statement about the group membership of each observation. Let us begin with a brief review of this method with a small example and demonstrate advances useful in situations with many explanatory variables in the following section.

© Springer Nature Switzerland AG 2022

D. Zelterman, *Applied Multivariate Statistics with R*, Statistics for Biology and Health, https://doi.org/10.1007/978-3-031-13005-2_10

Table 10.1 Mortality of beetles exposed to various doses of an insecticide

Dead	15	24	26	24	29	29
Alive	35	25	24	26	21	20
Number exposed N_i	50	49	50	50	50	49
Exposure dose	1.082	1.161	1.212	1.2 58	1.310	1.348
Mortality rate	0.30	0.49	0.52	0.48	0.58	0.59

Source Plackett (1981), p. 54

In linear logistic regression, we assume group membership is expressible as a binary-valued response, $y = 0$ or 1, conditional on a vector of explanatory variables x. The data on the i-th observation is then (y_i, x_i). The model is expressed as a probability statement about the distribution of a future observation y and any arbitrary value of x. This model gives us a mathematical statement of the probability of $y = 0$ or 1 for any given value of x.

Table 10.1 is a simple example of the type of data lending itself to this analysis. In this experiment, there were six large jars, each containing a number of beetles and a carefully measured, small amount of insecticide. After a specified amount of time, the experimenters examined the number of beetles still alive. We can calculate the empirical death rate for each jar's level of exposure to the insecticide. These are given in the last row of Table 10.1 using

$$\text{Mortality rate} = \frac{\text{Number died}}{\text{Number exposed}}.$$

How can we develop statistical models to describe this data? We should immediately recognize the outcomes for each individual insect are binary-valued: alive or dead. We can probably assume these events are independent of each other. The counts of alive or dead insects within each jar should then follow the binomial distribution. There are different probabilities of mortality between the jars. The goal of logistic regression in this example is to model these different probabilities as a function of the level of insecticide exposure.

There are six separate and independent binomial experiments in this example. The N_i parameters for the six binomial models are the number of insects in the i-th jar. Similarly, the p_i parameters represent the mortality probabilities in the i-th jar. The aim is to model the p parameters of these six binomial experiments. Any models we develop for this data will need to incorporate something about the various insecticide dose levels to describe the mortality probability p_i in the i-th jar.

The alert reader will notice the empirical mortality rates given in the last row of Table 10.1 are not monotonically increasing with increasing exposure levels of the insecticide. Despite this remark, there is no reason for us to fit a non-monotonic model to these data.

Output 10.1 Program and selected output to fit models to data in Table 10.1

```
bugs <- read.table(file = "beetle.txt", header = TRUE)
bugs$lived <- bugs$N - bugs$died
resp <- cbind(bugs$died, bugs$lived)      # create paired response values
resp                                      # check response values

     [,1] [,2]
[1,]   15   35
[2,]   24   25
[3,]   26   24
[4,]   24   26
[5,]   29   21
[6,]   29   20

  glm(resp ~ dose, family = binomial, data = bugs)  # logit is default link

Coefficients:
(Intercept)         dose
     -4.898        3.964

  glm(resp ~ dose, family = binomial(link = probit), data = bugs) # fit
    probit

Coefficients:
(Intercept)         dose
     -3.064        2.479

  newb <- binomial(link = "identity")        # create a new family with
    identity
  glm(resp ~ dose, family = newb, data = bugs) # fit linear

Coefficients:
(Intercept)         dose
    -0.7137       0.9820
```

The program in Output 10.1 fits three models to these data. In the notation of generalized linear models, we need to specify the `link` function connecting the linear predictor $x'\beta$. The initial temptation is to model p as a linear function of dose, x but this may lead to parameter estimated outside the permissible range $0 \le p \le 1$. This `identity` link is discouraged and `glm()` will rightfully warn you against its use for binary-valued data. In Output 10.1, we specifically need to create a new family to allow such a link function.

The model of logistic regression is the default for `glm()`. This link is based on the model

$$\log(p(x)/(1 - p(x))) = \log\left(\frac{\Pr[\, y = 0 \mid x\,]}{\Pr[\, y = 1 \mid x\,]} \right) = \beta'x \qquad (10.1)$$

or the log-odds for $y = 0$ versus $y = 1$ is a linear function of the explanatory variables x.

We interpret each β parameter as the log-odds change in $\Pr[Y = 1]$ for each unit change in the corresponding explanatory variable x. Logistic regression makes no assumption about the distribution of the explanatory variables x.

We can solve (10.1) for $Pr[\,Y = 1\,]$ in terms of x:

$$p(x) = \Pr[\,Y = 1 \mid \beta'x\,] = \exp(\beta'x)\big/\{1 + \exp(\beta'x)\}.$$

Another popular link is the *probit* for which

$$p = \Phi(\beta'x) \tag{10.2}$$

where Φ is the cumulative normal distribution function.

The parameter vector β is estimated using maximum likelihood and we perform statistical inference on it, much as we did in the previous chapter on linear regression models. Intercepts are typically included in these regression coefficients. The estimated parameters are given in Output 10.1

These three fitted models are plotted in Fig. 10.1. The observed data is plotted as dots in *red*. There are several points we can make by looking at this figure. The first of these is the logit and probit models are almost identical, except at the extreme ends of their range. As with any model, extrapolation beyond the observed data is a cardinal sin. Similarly, in practice, it is almost impossible to distinguish between

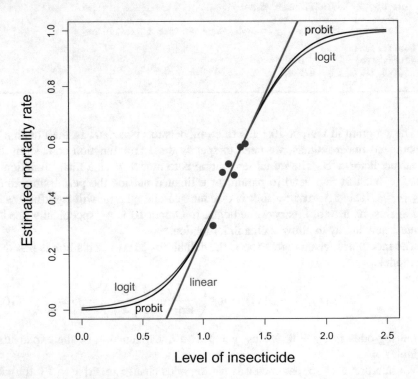

Figure 10.1 Fitted models for the insecticide data in Table 10.1. The empirical rates are plotted in *red*

the logit and probit models. The probit model approaches its limits of 0 and 1 a little faster than the logit model. In the center of the model, where all of the data is located, all three models coincide and are virtually identical. Even so, the use of the linear model is discouraged.

10.2 Penalized Logistic Regression

The approach here has many parallels to the penalized linear regression covered in Sect. 9.4. In linear regression, the process of least squares estimation makes no restriction on the number or magnitudes of the regression coefficients in the model. Similarly, penalized regression prevents us from fitting models with many, large-valued coefficients when a few small coefficients might offer an equally good summary of the data. This is the approach taken in this section. Namely, to place similar restrictions on the estimated logistic regression coefficients in (10.1).

We begin by continuing the idea of maximum likelihood estimation discussed in Sects. 5.7, 6.5, and 7.4. Sometimes, especially in large data sets, the maximum likelihood can run astray and needs some help on our part. In this section, we introduce some common methods to reign it in.

The observed data is (N_i, x_i, y_i) for $i = 1, 2, \ldots, n$. The y_i are independent observations, each from a binomial (N_i, p_i) distribution. In the previous section, the N_i were the number of bugs in each of the jars. In this section, will we take all $N_i = 1$.

The $p_i = p_i(x)$ parameters are connected to the linear predictor $\beta' x_i$ through the link function. That is,

$$\text{link}(p_i) = \beta' x_i$$

usually taken to be the logit given at (10.1) or the probit, defined at (10.2).

If all of the $N_i = 1$ then joint probability of the observed data is

$$\prod_{i=1}^{n} p_i^{y_i} (1 - p_i)^{1-y_i}$$

and the deviance (sometimes also called the likelihood or the log-likelihood) is the logarithm of this function,

$$\Lambda = \sum_{i=1}^{n} y_i \log(p_i) + (1 - y_i) \log(1 - p_i) .$$

The likelihood Λ depends on the value of the regression coefficients so we usually write $\Lambda(\beta)$. The β are estimated by maximizing Λ. These maximum likelihood estimates $\widehat{\boldsymbol{\beta}}$ are obtained by `glm()` and their estimated standard errors are the curvature of the log-likelihood, as we explained in Sect. 6.5.

This covers the details of fitting the logistic (or probit) regression model introduced in the previous section. When there are only a few explanatory variables then this generally runs smoothly. But when there are many possible x's available to us then model fitting can get messy. For example, if some of the explanatory variables are highly correlated with each other then the estimated β's can become huge and cancel each other out resulting in a lack of useful interpretation. We fix this situation by adding a restriction to the likelihood Λ.

Specifically, the restricted likelihood for binary-valued data is

$$\Lambda - \lambda \left\{ (1 - \alpha) \, ||\boldsymbol{\beta}||^2 / 2 \, + \, \alpha \sum_i \, |\beta_i| \right\} \tag{10.3}$$

with a close analogy to the restricted objective in (9.5) for linear regression.

A value of $\alpha = 1$ gives us lasso regression, by penalizing large values of $\sum |\beta_i|$ and $\alpha = 0$ is called ridge regression by restricting $\sum \beta_i^2$. All coefficients remain in the regression model but shrink toward zero in ridge regression. Conversely, in lasso, some of the regression coefficients are set to exactly zero.

The value of $\lambda > 0$ controls the amount of restriction relative to the maximum of the likelihood Λ. Values of α between 0 and 1 are more flexible and referred to as elastic regression. We won't give many more details because much of this was covered in Sect. 9.4 including the implementation in **R**.

We will give an example of restricted logistic regression in data on the diagnosis of breast cancer from biopsy data. A small portion of these data is given in Table 10.2. These data contain 30 covariate measurements on biopsy from 569 women. The first two columns of data are identifying the subject number and the diagnosis, classified as either malignant (M) or benign (B). We will see which of the 30 biopsy values are useful in explaining the binary-valued diagnosis.

Table 10.2 A portion of the breast cancer diagnostic data. Source: UCI database

	id	diagnosis	radius_mean	...	symmetry_worst	fractal_dimension_worst
1	842302	M	17.99	...	0.4601	0.11890
2	842517	M	20.57	...	0.2750	0.08902
3	84300903	M	19.69	...	0.3613	0.08758
567	926954	M	16.60	...	0.2218	0.07820
568	927241	M	20.60	...	0.4087	0.12400
569	92751	B	7.76	...	0.2871	0.07039

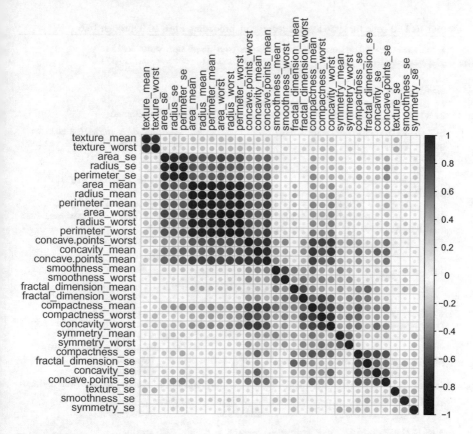

Figure 10.2 The measures of the breast cancer data displayed in a `corrplot`

A `corrplot` given in Fig. 10.2 reveals several of the measurements have large positive correlations. Similarly, any regression method will uncover many redundancies and only a few biopsy values will be needed. There are very few negative correlations among these data.

The code to produce this figure is

```
bc <- read.csv("breast_cancer_diagnosis.csv", header = TRUE,
        na.strings = c("",NA))
corrplot(cor(bc[ , -1 : -2]), order = "hclust")
```

where the biopsy variables have been reordered and grouped together using hierarchical clustering. Hierarchical clustering is described in Sect. 11.1.

An examination of the logistic regression for these data in **R** appears in Output 10.2. The code begins with the usual, unrestricted approach we might take to

Output 10.2 **R** code for lasso logistic regression, producing Figs. 10.3 through 10.6

```
# unrestricted logistic regression in glm does not work well:
glm(diagnosis == "M" ~ . , family = binomial, data = bc[, -1])

...

Warning messages:
1: glm.fit: algorithm did not converge
2: glm.fit: fitted probabilities numerically 0 or 1 occurred
bcX <- as.matrix(bc[,-c(1, 2)])            # explanatory variable matrix
bcY <- bc$diagnosis == "M"                 # binary values outcome values
library(glmnet)
lasso <- cv.glmnet(bcX, bcY, family = "binomial", alpha = 1)
plot(lasso, cex.lab = 1.25)                # cv est'd lambda: Fig.10.3
plot(lasso$glmnet.fit, "lambda", lwd = 3,
     cex.lab = 1.25)                       # plot global fit: Fig. 10.4
ext <- sort(lasso$glmnet.fit[2]$beta[,100])[c(1,30)] # identify two extremes
text(c(-8.4, -8.4), ext, labels = names(ext))
(lmin <- log(lasso$lambda.min))            # best cross-validated log
                                             lambda

[1] -6.353895

lines(rep(log(lmin), 2), c(-4000, 2000), lwd = 2, col = "tomato3")

#  Plot in a narrow range around cv estimate of lambda: Fig. 10.5
lamrange <- exp( lmin + (-20 : 20)/10)     # narrower range for lambda
lasso2 <- glmnet(bcX, bcY, family = "binomial", alpha = 1,
                lambda = lamrange)         # fit models win this range
plot(lasso2, "lambda", cex.lab = 1.25, lwd = 2)   # produce Fig. 10.6
lines(rep(lmin, 2), c(-1000, 1000), lwd = 2, col = "seashell3")
(extreme <- sort(lasso2$beta[,40])[c(1, 29, 30)]) #  identify extreme beta's

fractal_dimension_se        smoothness_se       concave.points_se
         -1301.9727             251.3955                 363.6058

text(c(-5.8, -5.8), y = extreme, labels = names(extreme))
```

perform logistic regression using `glm`. The corresponding error messages are reproduced here and warn us this is not a useful approach.

The code

$$\text{diagnosis == "M" ~ .}$$

specifies the binary outcomes are determined by the TRUE or FALSE values whether
the `diagnosis` value is M (malignant) or not. The logit link is the default option.
The code `~ .` sets the logit link equal to a linear combination of all remaining
variables in the data.

The remainder of Output 10.2 contains the **R** code to perform a lasso logis-
tic regression. The lasso restriction minimizes $\sum |\beta_i|$ and corresponds to $\alpha = 1$
in (10.3).

The `glmnet` library contains programs to fit restricted, generalized linear models.
Specifically, the `cv.glmet` program uses cross-validation to estimate an optimal

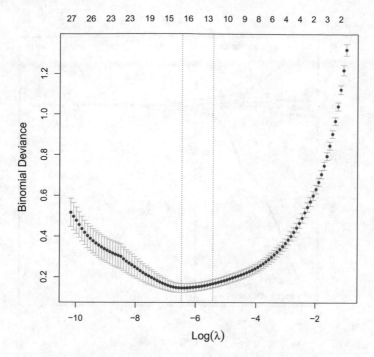

Figure 10.3 Cross-validated estimation of λ in lasso logistic regression for breast cancer data

value of λ to minimize the deviance in (10.3). We print this value (-6.35) in Output 10.2. The plot in Fig. 10.3 illustrates the behavior of the deviance function for different values of λ, also on a log scale. See Sect. 9.4 for a discussion of cross-validation in restricted regression.

The estimated values of the regression coefficients β are plotted in Fig. 10.4 for different values of λ, on a log scale. Less restricted models are on the left side and more restrictive on the right. Similarly, the estimated β become attenuated, moving left to right in this figure. Two of the most outstanding regression coefficients are identified: fractal dimension and concave points. Fractal dimension and concave points measure the complexity of the cell's surfaces and are associated with abnormal cell reproduction. The cross-validated estimated minimum deviance is identified with a vertical line in this figure.

We notice in a neighborhood of the cross-validated estimate of λ the parameter estimates are bunched close together so there is no clear indication of which parameters should be included in our model. One way to proceed is to plot those estimates of β in a narrower range of values near the estimate for λ. We can do this by providing specified values of λ to the glmnet function and plotting the corresponding estimated β's of the fitted models. The resulting plot appears as Fig. 10.5.

In the narrow range of values near the cross-validated λ, we can see the fractal dimension remains the single most important covariate in the restricted logistic

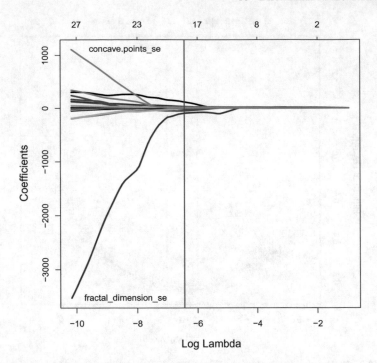

Figure 10.4 Restricted lasso estimates of β in logistic regression for breast cancer data. The cross-validated optimal value of λ is identified by a vertical line

Figure 10.5 Restricted lasso estimation of β in logistic regression for breast cancer data. Values are plotted in a narrower range than in Fig. 10.4, closer to the cross-validated optimal value of λ, identified by a vertical line

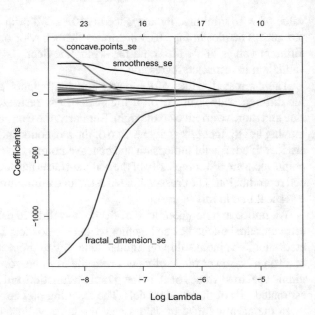

Figure 10.6 Observed
diagnosis and fitted logistic
model for the probability of
malignant diagnosis. Fractal
dimension and smoothness
are on a log scale

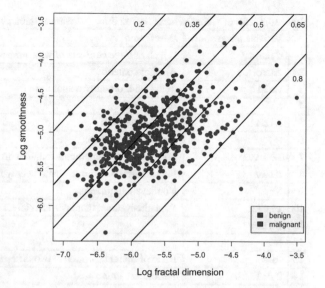

regression model. There is also a trade-off for second place: Concave points appear
as the second most important in Fig. 10.4. But on closer examination, in Fig. 10.5,
we see smoothness takes over concave points in the lasso restriction.

The final fitted logistic regression model is given in Fig. 10.6. The contour lines of
the model are plotted in this figure. The values of smoothness and fractal dimension
are both very skewed and a better presentation is given when these are plotted on a
log scale.

There are some final lessons to be learned from this section. The first of these is
restricted regression is useful but the conclusions can be sensitive to small changes
in the restriction λ. Specifically, Fig. 10.4 identifies the set of useful covariates but
upon closer examination, in Fig. 10.5, our conclusion changes.

Another, more subtle, point can be made when we examine the fitted model in
Fig. 10.6. The lasso restriction helps us in identifying important covariates to put in
our model and which ones can be omitted. Lasso does not suggest the inclusion of
these covariates might be better expressed on a different scale, the log in this case.
Perhaps we should include all of the covariates *and their logarithms* in an even larger
restricted logistic regression model to identify a better model.

10.3 Several Categorical Groups

Let us begin by introducing an example and then carry it through the remainder of
this chapter. Data on three varieties of wine cultivars are given in the data set `wines`
(Forina et al. 1988). The entire data set is also available online along with additional
information on the variables and a list of references to other, published analyses of

Table 10.3 List of variables measured on three cultivars of Italian wine grapes

	Variable name	Description
1	Class	Which of three cultivars of wine grapes
2	Alcohol	Alcohol content
3	Malic	Malic acid: provides a sour taste
4	Ash	Ash content
5	Alcal	Alkalinity of ash
6	Mg	Magnesium content
7	Phenol	Total phenols: compounds found in drugs and plastics
8	Flav	Flavanoids: compounds found widely in plants
9	Nonf	Nonflavanoid phenols
10	Proan	Proanthocyanins: tannins which affect color and aging
11	Color	
12	Hue	
13	Abs	Ratio of light absorption at two different frequencies
14	Proline	Proline, an amino acid

these data. There are 178 different wines examined. A list of the 14 variables in this data set is listed in Table 10.3.

We can read these data directly from the website using

```
wines <-
read.table(
  "http://archive.ics.uci.edu/ml/machine-learning-databases/wine/wine.data",
  sep = ",")
```

The pairs() matrix scatterplot is given in Fig. 10.7. The **R** code to produce this figure is

```
colors <- c("green", "red" ,"blue")[wines[ , 1]]
newwine <-   cbind(     # new dataframe with jittered Class variable
        jitter(as.integer(wines[ , 1])),
        wines[ , -1])
names(newwine)[1] <- names(wines)[1]  # old name to new variable
pairs(newwine, pch = 16, cex = .3, gap = 0, col = colors,
   xaxt = "n", yaxt = "n")
```

The Class variable is jittered to make it easier to view. The pairs() command uses options to remove the axes and spaces ween individual panels. These instructions create a new data frame called newwine in which the integer values of Class variable have been jittered.

Discriminant analysis helps us identify the distinguishing characteristics of the different groups. One approach is to examine each of the individual measurements separately in a univariate, marginal analysis. In the top row and left column in Fig. 10.7, we can identify individual variables demonstrating how individual variables differ

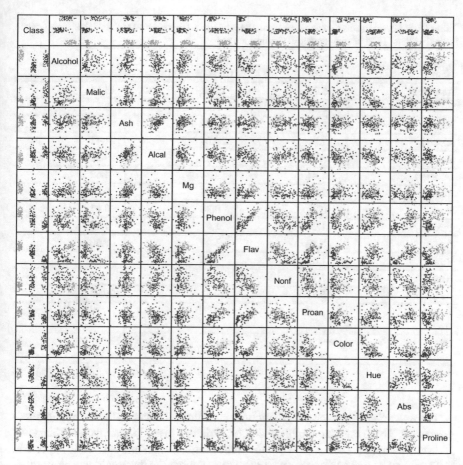

Figure 10.7 Matrix scatterplot for wine data. The colors correspond to the three cultivars

across the three groups of wines. We can quantify these individual relationships in terms of a separate one-way analysis of variance for each. Specifically, we can perform a hypothesis test the means of each of the variables are the same across the three groups. If we do this, we find the one-way analysis of variance demonstrates an extreme level of statistical significance for every variable in the data set. The individual group means are given in Table 10.4 for each variable in the data set.

This marginal approach is intuitive for identifying group means, but it fails to identify discriminatory characteristics for individuals. One individual cultivar may have a high or low value for a specified measurement, but the histograms of the three groups may exhibit considerable overlap, making the assessment of group membership difficult. This overlap is readily apparent in the parallel coordinate plot given in Fig. 10.8. Not all variables are included in this figure. The choice of axes in this figure was subjective and performed with a little trial and error. Parallel coordinates were introduced in Sect. 3.5.

Table 10.4 Group means for each variable in the wine data. In every row, the statistical significance is smaller than 10^{-4} testing equality of group means

Name	Means Class=1	Class=2	Class=3
Alcohol	13.74	12.28	13.15
Malic	2.01	1.93	3.33
Ash	2.46	2.24	2.44
Alcal	17.04	20.24	21.42
Mg	106.34	94.55	99.31
Phenol	2.84	2.26	1.68
Flav	2.98	2.08	0.78
Nonf	0.29	0.36	0.45
Proan	1.90	1.63	1.15
Color	5.53	3.09	7.40
Hue	1.06	1.06	0.68
Abs	3.16	2.79	1.68
Proline	1115.71	519.51	629.90
Sample sizes	59	71	48
Color codes	green	red	blue

The univariate approach fails to include correlations between the individual measurements. There may be combinations of variables providing a much higher level of discriminatory precision between the three cultivars than this univariate approach.

Figure 10.7 suggests another way of distinguishing the three cultivars. A number of plotted pairs are useful in identifying and discriminating between the three cultivars in Fig. 10.7. These include (Abs, Proline), (Alcohol, Hue), and (Color, Flav) as examples. The object of discriminant analysis is to identify distinguishing characteristics between the different groups. Even though there are many small plots in the figure, the use of color helps us identify those pairs of variables having high value in discriminating between the three cultivars.

The following two sections describe discriminatory methods based on linear combinations of all variables in this data set. The support vector approach, described in Sect. 10.6, identifies specific observations helping to define regions of high discriminatory value and does not necessarily seek linear combinations to achieve these goals.

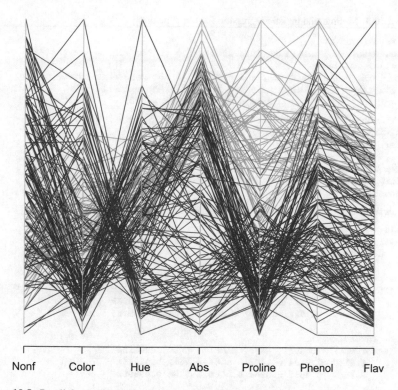

Figure 10.8 Parallel coordinate plot for wine data. The colors correspond to those in Fig. 10.7

10.4 Multinomial Logistic Regression

We next describe the generalization of logistic regression when there are more than two groups we want to discriminate between. The most commonly used approach selects one category as a reference or baseline and compares all other categories to it. This approach performs a pairwise comparison between each of the categories to the single baseline, reference category. This approach has a useful interpretation when there is an obvious baseline standard, and it makes sense all categories should be compared to it. In the case of the wine cultivar data, there is no obvious comparison group, and we will arbitrarily set Class=2 as the reference.

The generalization of (10.1) to model the three categories for the wine data is the pair of simultaneous equations

$$\log\left(\frac{\Pr[\,\text{Class}=1\mid x\,]}{\Pr[\,\text{Class}=2\mid x\,]}\right) = \beta_1' x$$
$$\log\left(\frac{\Pr[\,\text{Class}=3\mid x\,]}{\Pr[\,\text{Class}=2\mid x\,]}\right) = \beta_3' x \ .$$

Output 10.3 Multinomial logistic regression for the wine data

```
> require(nnet)
> wines$Class <- as.factor(wines$Class) # create factor categories
> wines$rClass <-
+       relevel(wines$Class, ref = 2)      # set reference category
> winelogit <- multinom(rClass ~ Alcohol + Ash + Alcal + Abs  + Proline,
+                         data = wines, maxit = 200)

# weights:  21 (12 variable)
initial  value 195.552987
iter   10 value 38.789908
  ...        ...
iter 170 value 13.330023
final  value 13.325689
converged

> print(ws <- summary(winelogit), digits = 4)

Call:
multinom(formula = rClass ~ Alcohol + Ash + Alcal + Abs + Proline,
    data = wines, maxit = 200)


Coefficients:
   (Intercept) Alcohol    Ash    Alcal      Abs Proline
1      -124.00   6.213 22.849 -3.3478 10.354 0.029383
3       -46.46   2.927  6.192  0.3032 -7.483 0.005955

Std. Errors:
   (Intercept) Alcohol    Ash   Alcal      Abs Proline
1       0.1139  1.6304 0.1403 1.0161 0.2612 0.032351
3       0.3588  0.4539 2.8564 0.2566 1.8766 0.003968

Residual Deviance: 26.65138
AIC: 50.65138

> tratio <- ws$coefficients / ws$standard.errors
> # two tailed p values from the t with $edf = effective df
> print( 2 * (1 - pt(abs(tratio), df = ws$edf)), digits = 4)

   (Intercept)    Alcohol     Ash    Alcal      Abs Proline
1            0  2.482e-03 0.00000 0.006404 4.308e-14  0.3816
3            0  3.169e-05 0.05101 0.260270 1.802e-03  0.1592
```

In this pair of equations, probabilities Pr[Class = 1] and Pr[Class = 3] are separately compared to the reference category Pr[Class = 2] with respective regression coefficients β_1 and β_2.

We next see how to estimate the regression coefficients β_1 and β_3 in **R**. The program and output appear in Output 10.3. This code begins by defining the new variable rClass as type factor and then sets the reference category.

These regression coefficients are the pairwise comparisons between Class=1 and =3 with the reference category. The fitted coefficients represent log-odds ratios of the change in classification probabilities when the independent variable changes by one unit. This is the same interpretation as with binary response logistic regression.

The models are specified by

```
rClass ~ Alcohol + Ash + Alcal + Abs  + Proline
```

in the `multinom` routine, using the notation also used to specify linear models in the previous chapter.

Following some trial and error, we found this choice of covariates provided a good fit. Output 10.3 ends by showing how to test the statistical significance of these regression coefficients and computes two-tailed p-values using a t distribution with *effective df* determined by `edf`.

The fitted multinomial distribution for each observation is obtained as follows:

```
ws$fitted.values

                2            1            3
1    6.405531e-18 1.000000e+00 2.109756e-21
2    3.942623e-16 1.000000e+00 1.247350e-20
3    3.273230e-11 1.000000e+00 2.887328e-12
        . . .                      . . .
176  3.195637e-03 2.996409e-10 9.968044e-01
177  3.295305e-03 4.418253e-09 9.967047e-01
178  2.347762e-05 3.582232e-15 9.999765e-01
```

Every row of these fitted values sums to one (or within a rounding error of one). Each row is the estimated probability of class membership for this wine.

Let us introduce some graphical diagnostics for this model. Figure 10.9 plots the fitted model and standardized residuals using `wine$Class=2` as the reference category. Fitted values only appear below the diagonal because $Pr[Y = 1]$ and $Pr[Y = 3]$ must sum to less than one. A perfect fit would have all of these values in each of the corners of the triangle: green (for Class=1) in the lower right, red (Class=2, the reference category) at the origin in the lower left, and blue (Class=3) at the upper left.

Let us define standardized residuals for this model:

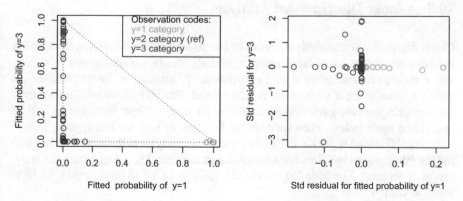

Figure 10.9 Fitted and standardized residuals in multivariate logistic model wine data using `Class=2` as the reference category. These plots use the same color codes as in Figs. 10.7 and 10.8

$$(obs - \widehat{p})\Big/\sqrt{\widehat{p}(1 - \widehat{p})}. \tag{10.4}$$

There are three residuals for each observation in the wine data. The three $\widehat{p}$ values are obtained from `ws$fitted.values`, above. The *obs* is the indicator of observed group membership for each category. In the wine data, with three categories, an observation in Class=3 will have *obs* = (0, 0, 1).

The residuals are standardized to have zero means and unit variances. We should not expect these to look normally distributed, because *obs* is binary-valued so residual values close to zero are not possible. Every observation will yield one residual for every category so every cultivar will have three residuals. Figure 10.9 shows the scatterplot of residuals for the Class=1 and =3 categories. The residuals of observed values all fall into different orthants, again because the obs values are either zero or one. Specifically, when one of the three residuals is positive-valued, then the other two must be negative. There is one extreme residual with an absolute value of five and only a few with values greater than three, so we conclude the model contains few outliers.

Let us conclude this section with a brief discussion of this generalization of logistic regression to more than two categories. Multinomial logistic regression does not have a large collection of diagnostics unlike logistic regression for binary-valued responses. We described a set of residuals in this section.

An advantage to the approach of comparing all categories to a reference is it supports the *independence of irrelevant alternatives*. Specifically, if observations from a new category are added then the results remain unchanged. Similarly, if observations from a non-reference category are deleted, then, again, the results remain unchanged. The independence of irrelevant alternatives follows from the approach of performing a series of pairwise comparisons with a baseline category. See Exercise 10.9 for another approach to generalizing logistic regression to multinomial data.

10.5 Linear Discriminant Analysis

Linear discrimination analysis allows us to identify a linear combination of variables used to estimate the group membership of all individuals. Unlike logistic regression which makes no assumption about the explanatory variables x, linear discriminant analysis assumes the x's have multivariate normal distributions with different means for each group but the same covariance across all groups. These assumptions will be made clear again below, when we develop the methodology for this approach.

In Fig. 10.10, we apply the linear discrimination analysis to the wine data and plot the resulting groups in colors and identify Class number. The `lda()` function is the program we need. The code to perform the analysis in **R** and produce Fig. 10.10 is given in Output 10.4.

The first and second discriminators are linear combinations of variables best discriminating between the three cultivars of wines. The linear weights are listed as LD1

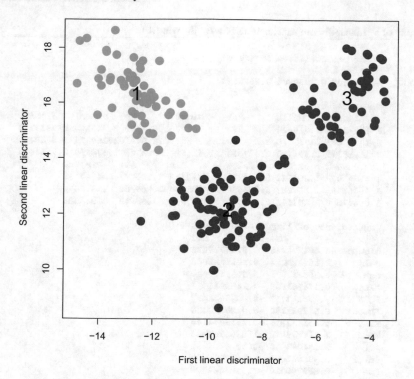

Figure 10.10 Linear discrimination for wine data using the same color codes as in Figs. 10.7 and 10.8

Output 10.4 Code to produce Fig. 10.10

```
library(MASS)
ld <- lda(Class ~ ., data = wines)
loading <- as.matrix(wines[ , 2 : 14])   %*%   ld$scaling

plot(loading, col = c(6, 2, 4)[ wines[ , 1] ],
   pch = 16, cex = 1.25,
   xlab = "First linear discriminator",
   ylab = "Second linear discriminator")
for (i in 1 : 3)                    # add class number to each centroid
{
   centx <- mean(loading[wines[,1] == i, ] [ , 1] )
   centy <- mean(loading[wines[,1] == i, ] [ , 2] )
   text(centx, centy, i, cex = 2)
}
```

and LD2 in Output 10.5. The loadings are the linear combinations of the explanatory variables, calculated in the code and plotted in Fig. 10.10. This figure illustrates a clear distinction between the three cultivars.

Output 10.5   Linear discriminant analysis lda for the wine data

```
Prior probabilities of groups:
      1         2         3
0.3314607 0.3988764 0.2696629

Group means:
    Alcohol     Malic      Ash    Alcal       Mg   Phenol      Flav
1 13.74475 2.010678 2.455593 17.03729 106.3390 2.840169 2.9823729
2 12.27873 1.932676 2.244789 20.23803  94.5493 2.258873 2.0808451
3 13.15375 3.333750 2.437083 21.41667  99.3125 1.678750 0.7814583
      Nonf    Proan    Color      Hue      Abs   Proline
1 0.290000 1.899322 5.528305 1.0620339 3.157797 1115.7119
2 0.363662 1.630282 3.086620 1.0563380 2.785352  519.5070
3 0.447500 1.153542 7.396250 0.6827083 1.683542  629.8958

Coefficients of linear discriminants:
                 LD1             LD2
Alcohol  -0.403274956   0.8718833272
Malic     0.165185223   0.3051811048
Ash      -0.368792093   2.3459219420
Alcal     0.154783909  -0.1463931519
Mg       -0.002162757  -0.0004611477
Phenol    0.617931702  -0.0324979420
Flav     -1.661172871  -0.4916834144
Nonf     -1.495756932  -1.6303752589
Proan     0.134093115  -0.3070371492
Color     0.355006846   0.2530559406
Hue      -0.819785218  -1.5182643908
Abs      -1.157612096   0.0512054337
Proline  -0.002690475   0.0028540202

Proportion of trace:
   LD1    LD2
0.6875 0.3125
```

The fitted (posterior) estimated probabilities of group membership can be obtained as predict(ld)$posterior. The plot of these appears in Fig. 10.11. This plot is much better than the corresponding Fig. 10.9 for the multinomial logistic regression.

The remainder of this section introduces some methodology and shows how the mechanics of linear discrimination work. As we work out the theory, we will refer to an idealized example of discriminating between a mixture of two normal distributions depicted in Fig. 10.12. Then we will return to the example of the three wine cultivars.

Suppose we have K different populations (for some $K = 2, 3, \ldots$) and each population is expressible as a p-dimensional normal population with respective means μ_j ($j = 1, \ldots, K$) and all with the same covariance matrix Σ. (It will be useful to review the functional form of the multivariate normal distribution (7.2) at this point.) We also have mixing probabilities π_j representing the probability a randomly selected observation is sampled from Population j.

The parameters π_j are called *prior probabilities* because they represent characteristics of the population known to us before any data is observed. Of course, these

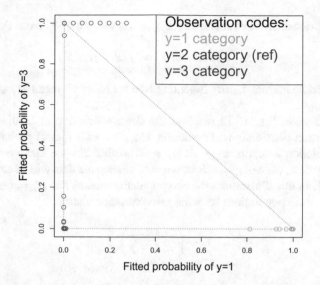

Figure 10.11 Fitted linear discrimination posterior probabilities for wine data using the same color codes as in Figs. 10.7 and 10.8

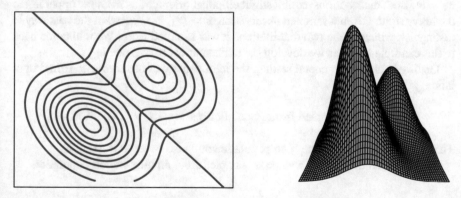

Figure 10.12 A mixture of two bivariate normal density functions plotted as contours and perspective. The red line is the boundary of the linear discriminator, given at (10.8)

can be estimated from the data, as is frequently the case in practice. In Output 10.5, for example, these prior probabilities are the observed sample proportions of the three wine cultivars. The means μ_j and the covariance Σ common to all populations will be assumed to be known, but in practice, these will also be estimated from the data.

Given a p-dimensional observation x, we can express the prior probabilities

$$\Pr[\text{Population } j] = \pi_j$$

a randomly selected observation is sampled from Population j.

The conditional density function of x given it was sampled from Population j is

$$f(x \mid \text{Population } j) = f(x \mid \mu_j, \Sigma)$$

for a multivariate normal density function given at (7.2) with mean μ_j and variance Σ.

As an example, Fig. 10.12 displays the density function of a mixture of two bivariate normal distributions. Population 1 occurs with (prior) probability $\pi_1 = .6$ and Population 2 occurs $\pi_2 = .4$. By *prior probability* we mean before having observed any data, we will guess there is a 60% chance the data will be sampled from Population 1. In this illustration, the two population means are $\mu_1' = (-1, -1)$ and $\mu_2' = (1, 1)$. Both populations have the same variance matrix

$$\Sigma = \begin{pmatrix} 1 & -.4 \\ -.4 & 1.2 \end{pmatrix}.$$

This example is illustrated in Fig. 10.12, both as a perspective and as contour plots. The front/left normal (with $\pi_1 = .6$) is a little taller than the second population with $\pi_2 = .4$. Both distributions exhibit slight elliptical orientations from the upper left to the lower right. Given a sampled observation $x = (x_1, x_2)$, we want the best way to distinguish which of the two distributions it was sampled from. We will come back to this example again as we develop the mathematical background.

Getting back to the general setting, the joint density of observing x from Population j is

$$f(x \text{ was sampled from Population } j) = \pi_j f(x \mid \mu_j, \Sigma).$$

That is, we have to select the j-th population and also observe x from it.

The marginal density for a value x sampled from an unspecified population

$$f(x) = \sum_{j}^{K} \pi_j f(x \mid \mu_i, \Sigma)$$

is the sum over all possible population values of $j = 1, \ldots, K$.

The *posterior probability density* of sampling from Population k for a given observation x is

$$f(\text{Population } k \mid x) = \pi_k f(x \mid \mu_k, \Sigma) \Big/ \sum_{j}^{K} \pi_j f(x \mid \mu_j, \Sigma). \qquad (10.5)$$

This is the basic formula needed to estimate the population observation x was sampled from. The *maximum a posteriori* (MAP) estimator $\widehat{k}$ directs us to choose the value of k making the probability in (10.5) as large as possible. Intuitively this makes sense. We want to identify the most likely population. The *mode* is one way to estimate this. The `lda()` routine in **R** calculates the K different values of (10.5) for us. The remainder of the mathematical development provides the detail of the computation when the data x is sampled from one of K different multivariate normal populations.

Notice the denominator of (10.5) is the same for every value of k so the MAP estimator of k

$$\widehat{k} = \text{Value of } k \text{ maximizing } \pi_k f(x \mid \mu_k, \Sigma)$$

is the value maximizing the numerator of (10.5).

The value of k maximizing $\pi_k f(x \mid \mu_k, \Sigma)$ will also maximize the logarithm of this quantity.

We next need to use the mathematical form of the multivariate normal density f. Recall from (7.2) the p-dimensional multivariate normal distribution with mean μ_k and variance Σ has density function

$$f(x) = \frac{1}{2\pi^{p/2}\text{Det}(\Sigma)^{1/2}} \exp\left\{-1/2(x - \mu_k)'\Sigma^{-1}(x - \mu_k)\right\}.$$

Then we can write

$$\log\left\{\pi_k f(x \mid \mu_k, \Sigma)\right\} = \log(\pi_k) - \log\left\{(2\pi)^{p/2}\text{Det}(\Sigma)^{1/2}\right\} - 1/2\,(x - \mu_k)'\Sigma^{-1}(x - \mu_k).$$

The second term involving $(2\pi)^{p/2}$ and $\text{Det}(\Sigma)$ does not depend on either k or the data x, so this term can be ignored and will be omitted from further discussion.

We next want to find the value of k to maximize

$$\log(\pi_k) - 1/2\,(x - \mu_k)'\Sigma^{-1}(x - \mu_k)$$
$$= \log(\pi_k) + x'\Sigma^{-1}\mu_k - 1/2\,\mu_k'\Sigma^{-1}\mu_k - 1/2\,x'\Sigma^{-1}x$$

after we expand the quadratic form in x.

The last term in $x'\Sigma^{-1}x$ does not depend on the choice of k and can also be ignored.

Finally, the discriminant function defined by

$$\delta_k(x) = x'\Sigma^{-1}\mu_k - 1/2\,\mu_k'\Sigma^{-1}\mu_k + \log(\pi_k)$$

is the function we need to evaluate in order to choose the appropriate population x was sampled from. Our MAP estimate of k is the value which maximizes $\delta_k(x)$. We only have to evaluate these K functions $\delta_k(x)$ and pick the largest.

Only the first term in $\delta_k(x)$ depends on the data x. This is a linear function of x, leading us to use the name, *linear discrimination*. In practice, the parameters (μ_k, Σ) are replaced by their usual estimators. The `lda()` function in **R** calculates the $\delta_k(x)$ and evaluates the posterior probability (10.5) for every observation in the data.

Let us be specific and ask how the linear discrimination process distinguishes between two different populations denoted by j and k. The *boundary* of this process occurs for values of x for which

$$\delta_j(x) = \delta_k(x).$$

In other words, the solution to this equation is a set of hypothetical data values x providing equal amounts of evidence for both of these different populations.

The solutions of the equation $\delta_j(x) = \delta_k(x)$ occur for values of x in which

$$\log(\pi_k/\pi_j) - 1/2\,(\mu_k + \mu_j)'\Sigma^{-1}(\mu_k - \mu_j) + x'\Sigma^{-1}(\mu_k - \mu_j) = 0 \quad (10.6)$$

or more simply,
$$\text{Constant} + x'\Sigma^{-1}(\mu_k - \mu_j) = 0 \quad (10.7)$$

where the Constant depends on j and k but not on x.

If we return to the parameter values in the example of normal mixtures, (10.6) becomes

$$0.40546 + (x_1,\ x_2)'(-3.08, -2.69) = 0$$

or

$$x_2 = .1506 - 1.1428x_1. \quad (10.8)$$

This last equation is plotted as the red line in Fig. 10.12 and clearly provides a good dividing line to discriminate between the two mixed populations.

We can generalize this example by examining the linear function of x in (10.7). Specifically, the *Fisher linear discriminant function* between populations j and k is

$$L_{jk}(x) = x'S^{-1}(\widehat{\mu}_k - \widehat{\mu}_j). \quad (10.9)$$

Parameter values in (10.7) have been replaced by their usual estimates in (10.9) and the constant term has been ignored. Specifically, Population means μ_k are replaced by the sampled within-group means. The covariance matrix Σ is replaced by the sample covariance matrix S assuming the covariance is the same in all groups. The discriminator in (10.9) is a scalar-valued, linear function of a vector of data values, x. More generally, when discriminating between K groups, there will be (at most) $K-1$ linear discrimination functions. Two linear discriminant functions are plotted in Fig. 10.10 for the three wine cultivars.

We next describe a method allowing the computer to identify a more general classification rule between groups of individuals. This rule does not begin with any pre-specified functional form.

10.6 Support Vector Machine

The support vector machine (SVM) is a group of classification algorithms including a variety of parametric and nonparametric models. Parametric models include straight lines and similar regression methods. The nonparametric methods contain a variety of kernel smoothing techniques. The programs in **R** include features to estimate the classification probabilities using cross-validation as well as training samples in machine learning.

Two examples are presented in Fig. 10.13. The left panel illustrates a linear SVM classifier. Line A does not completely classify the red and blue groups of samples. Line B classifies correctly but has small margins for misclassification. Line C, the product of a SVM, provides the largest possible margins. These margins are given with dotted lines.

Clearly, those observations closest to the margins are most important to the determination of the classification regions. Such observations are referred to as *support vectors*. The support vectors in this figure are plotted with black circles. Observations defining and lying on the periphery of the regions of different colored points are support vectors, as well. Support vectors will be discussed again below.

The right panel of Fig. 10.13 is the result of a SVM with a kernel smoothing classifier. Kernel smoothing is closely related to the *loess* fits in Fig. 3.16 and in the kriging map of altitudes of US cities in Fig. 3.14. Unlike the linear classification regions assumed in the previous two sections of this chapter and in the left panel of Fig. 10.13, kernel smoothing on the right panel of this figure makes no assumption on the shape of the regions.

The kernel smooth produced by SVM classifies future observations with confidence based on the intensity of the plotted color. The lighter-colored regions have

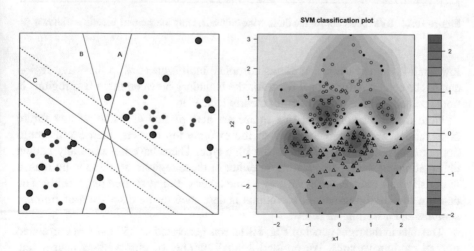

Figure 10.13 Examples of support vector methods: linear and kernel classifiers

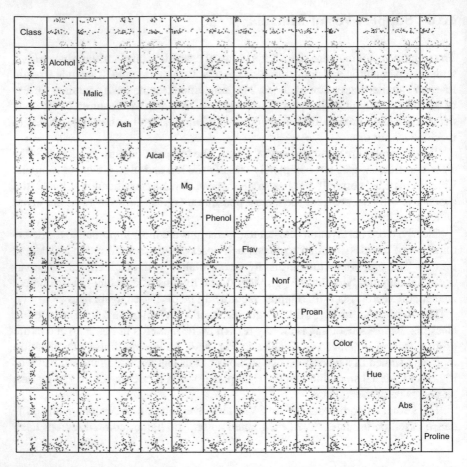

Figure 10.14 SVM classifier for the three wine cultivars. Only the support vectors are shown

low confidence and white represents complete indifference, as in the wavy region across the center. A functional form for the boundary between these two regions is not specified, but the SVM program clearly locates it.

Note the upper corners of this figure are also plotted as white. If any future observations were to fall in either of the extreme top corners, then SVM would not automatically classify these as the blue type. There have not been any known observations of the type appearing in either of these regions, so there is no reason to classify new observations one way or the other with any degree of certainty. The concept of classifying new observations is described in the discussion of *training samples* and *test samples* below.

The data in the right panel of Fig. 10.13 was generated as 250 pairs of correlated normal random variates. We omitted a small number of observations near a sine wave region running through the data. The groups above and below this sine wave are plotted as circles and triangles, respectively. Those observations are identified

Output 10.6 Create a non-linear classification and identify the support vectors in Fig. 10.13

```
library(kernlab, mvtnorm)              # for ksvm and rmvnorm
x <- rmvnorm(n = 250, mean = c(0, 0),
    sigma = matrix(c(1, .1, .1, 1), 2, 2))
wavy <- sin(pi * x[,1]) / 2            # wavy boundary
include <- (abs( wavy - x[,2]) > .25 )# 2x width of boundary
x <- x[include, ]                      # include those inside
wavy <- wavy[include]                  #    the wavy boundary
group <- 1 + (x[,2] > wavy)            # above or below boundary?
all <- data.frame(x = x[,c(2, 1)],
    group = group)                     # build a data.frame
colnames(all) <- c("x2", "x1", "group")

sv <-ksvm(group ~., data = all, type = "C-svc")
plot(sv, data=all)
```

as support vectors. These are critical to estimating the boundaries plotted in solid. The search for support vectors is similar to observations located on the convex hull, except the classification regions are not necessarily convex. (An example of a plotted convex hull appears in Fig. 3.11.) The SVM algorithm, then, includes a search for classification regions as well as those observations bounding and determining the regions.

The right panel of Fig. 10.13 was produced by the **R** code in Output 10.6. In this code, we begin by generating 250 pairs of bivariate normals. The sine wave-shaped classification region is called `wavy`. The code removes all observations close to this region. A `data.frame` is created, and only `group` membership is identified to the `ksvm` program. The first and second indexes are reversed in the `data.frame`. By default, plotted SVM output puts the axis for the second variable on the bottom and the axis for the first variable on the left. This is contrary to the usual way this is done in **R**.

The index of the support vectors is obtained and the support vector in the original data is available in **R** using

```
svi <- alphaindex(sv)[[1]]
all[svi, ]
```

This code was used to identify and highlight the support vectors in the left panel of Fig. 10.13.

The SVM works well for these two artificial examples. Before we apply the SVM to the wine data, let us introduce a method of testing the accuracy of a classification model called *cross-validation*.

As with any classification method, we are deluding ourselves if, after fitting the model to some data, we then claim how well the model appears to predict all of the observations in the data. The model was built around the data so such a claim is hollow. A much stronger claim would be to see how well the model correctly classifies some future observations not part of the model-building process. We rarely have access to additional data so the idea of cross-validation is to fit the model and then test it with different parts of the existing data.

Cross-validation, then, is a method for allowing us to fit and then test on different portions of the data set. Specifically, an *n*-fold cross-validation randomly partitions a data set into *n* nearly equally sized sets. (Typically, *n* is an integer in the range between 5 and 10.) One set, called the *testing data set*, is omitted. Then the model is fitted using the remaining *n* − 1 sets. These are referred to as the *training data set*.

One training data set is fitted and then cross-validation examines how well the resulting model classifies the observations in the omitted, testing data set. The cross-validation process then systematically replaces the omitted data and removes a different set. This process is repeated, separately fitting and testing *n* different models. Cross-validation produces a more reliable estimate of the fitting accuracy. We can also compare the *n* different fitted models to examine the consistency of the model-building process.

The process of cross-validation produces an estimate of the accuracy of the model but also has a hidden benefit, referred to as *machine learning*. In the process of producing an *n*-fold estimate of the classification error, the SVM also had to fit *n* different models. Some of these models may have better properties than the original model fitted from the entire data. In this manner, the SVM appears to learn about better models.

Some useful **R** code for the wine example includes

```
> (svw <- ksvm(Class ~ . , data = wines,
+      type = "C-svc", cross = 5))

        .    .    .

Cross validation error : 0.01127
```

which illustrates how we obtain an estimate of the five-fold cross-validation error. See Exercise 10.8 for more on the fold parameter when performing a cross-validation.

The `alphaindex()` command produces three separate lists of support vectors: one for each of the three cultivars. There may be some duplication when support vectors are on the boundary for more than one of the three groups. We can combine these lists and remove duplicates as follows:

```
> svi <- ( c(alphaindex(svw)[[1]], alphaindex(svw)[[2]],
+          alphaindex(svw)[[3]]]))   # master list of support vectors
> svi <- svi[!duplicated(svi)]      # remove duplicates
```

using the `duplicated()` function in **R**.

We can use this code to identify and plot the support vectors in the wine data. The original data has 178 observations on three cultivars. In Fig. 10.14, only the support vectors are plotted, using the same colors as before. There are 69 support vectors plotted in this figure, a considerable simplification over the corresponding plot in

Fig. 10.7. This approach would also be beneficial with a much larger sample size and each panel would be overwhelmed with data.

The SVM will also produce estimated multinomial prediction probabilities of individual observations belonging to each of the different groups. In the case of the wine cultivar data, we have

```
> svw <- ksvm(Class ~ . , data = wines, type = "C-svc", prob.model = T)
> print(predict(svw, wines[,-1], type="probabilities"), digits=2)

             1        2       3
  [1,]  0.99129  0.00280  0.0059
  [2,]  0.98174  0.00977  0.0085
       .    .    .

 [177,]  0.00826  0.00470  0.9870
 [178,]  0.00690  0.00451  0.9886
```

where each row sums to one and estimates the probability this observation belongs to the three different cultivars.

From these estimated multinomial probabilities, we can plot the fitted and residual values, with an analogy to Fig. 10.9. Again, we use the second category as a reference and continue to use the same color codes for the three classes in this example.

The SVM fit in Fig. 10.15 is clearly accurate: The fitted probabilities for the three cultivars place them squarely in the three corners of the triangle-shaped figure, just as we would expect of a well-fitting model. There is no overlapping of fitted categories as visible in Fig. 10.9 showing SVM produces a much better fit. However, the residual plot is not useful and exhibits a distorted horizontal scale, owing to the small probabilities involved.

Much more can be said about SVM including the many options and different kernel smoothing functions available, but this is a good place to stop and review.

What are the good and bad features of the different discrimination methods described so far in this chapter? Figure 10.15 illustrates an excellent discrimination of the three wine cultivars. This figure illustrates a much better fit to the data

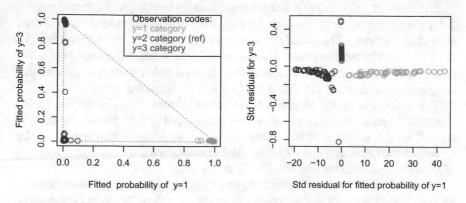

Figure 10.15 SVM fitted probabilities and residuals for the wine cultivars

than the corresponding plot multinomial logistic regression provides us in Fig. 10.9. Unfortunately, SVM produces estimates but no model can be expressed as a mathematical formula. Conversely, SVM is extremely flexible and able to detect the wavy boundary in Fig. 10.13 without any additional specifications on our part.

Linear discrimination provides both a mathematical form as well as a useful diagram in Fig. 10.10. The two axes of this figure are made of linear-weighted composite measures lacking a simple explanation. Similarly, multinomial logistic regression also expresses discrimination functions on the basis of linear combinations of the data values.

We next describe a classification method combining the regression models of the previous chapter with a classification tree.

10.7 Regression Trees

We can also build classification rules based on hierarchical trees. These methods will work well for classifying groups based on a continuous outcome (see Exercise 10.16), but we will concentrate on discrete group membership in this section. The methods of this section are also referred to as *recursive partitioning* and as *computer-aided regression trees (CART)*.

Let us look at a regression tree for the wine data. The regression tree appearing in Fig. 10.16 was built using the **R** code:

```
winetree <- mvpart(Class ~ . , data = wines, method = "class",
        size = 4)
```

The **R** program mvtree (in the library of the same name) was used to draw this picture. At the tips of the leaves, this program draws a small histogram of the three different categories of wines. The **R** program rtree (also in a library of the same name) has a similar function.

The mvpart program has a syntax identical to the regression program specifying the dependent variable (Class) and a list of the explanatory variables to be considered in the model. The period in the notation Class ~ . is shorthand for a list of all variables in the data frame. The size variable specifies the number of leaves on the tree. The program will choose a value for you if this number is not included. Diagnostics for choosing the size of the tree will be discussed below.

The printed tree in Fig. 10.16 can be described in words. The first split on Proline separates the mode of the Class=1 wines. The second split on Flavonoids removes a small number of the other two classes from this initial split. The branch on Abs segregates the Class=2 and =3 wines. At the bottom of the tree, there is a summary of several diagnostics we will describe next in a larger example.

Let us introduce another data set to explain CART in more detail. The crabs data set in the MASS library lists five dimensions made on each of 200 crabs *Leptograpsus variegatus*, 50 each of the combinations of two sexes and two color variants (blue

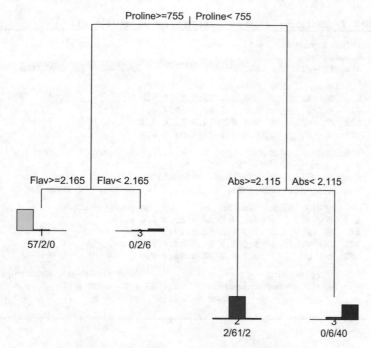

Proline>=755 | Proline< 755

Flav>=2.165 | Flav< 2.165

Abs>=2.115 | Abs< 2.115

57/2/0

0/2/6

2/61/2

0/6/40

Error : 0.131   CV Error : 0.252   SE : 0.0447
Missclass rates : Null = 0.601 : Model = 0.0787 : CV = 0.152

Figure 10.16 Regression tree of wines

or orange). The five measurements (in mm) and symbols are frontal lobe size (FL), rear width (RW), carapace length (CL), carapace width (CW), and body depth (BD). We will use the regression tree approach to classify the four categories of sex and color on the basis of these five measurements.

The program in Output 10.7 creates four group categories and appends these to the original crab data, producing a new data frame called cp. The groups of sex/color combinations are coded as 1–4 and also using character symbols indicating color (B and O) and upper/lower case for M/F. This code prints out one observation from each of the four groups before and after this transformation. Printing out some data allows us to see if this is being done correctly. This is a good programming habit to develop.

The regression tree for the crab data appears in Fig. 10.17. Sometimes, the regression tree can grow to unmanageable complexity so the maximum number of branches is specified by the size = option in the mvpart statement in Output 10.7. Every branch ends with a set of the frequencies of the four categories of crabs and plots a small histogram. The symbol of the modal category is also printed for us. The first split, for example, is made on large values (≥13.95mm) of rear width RW and this branch segregates a majority (35) of the orange female crabs from all others.

Output 10.7 Program to create four groups of crabs and produce Fig. 10.17

```
> library(MASS)
> data(crabs)
> crabs[c(1, 51, 101, 151),]              # look at some raw data
     sp sex index    FL  RW   CL   CW  BD
1     B   M     1   8.1 6.7 16.1 19.0 7.0
51    B   F     1   7.2 6.5 14.7 17.1 6.1
101   O   M     1   9.1 6.9 16.7 18.6 7.4
151   O   F     1  10.7 9.7 21.4 24.0 9.8
> group <- 1 + 2 * (crabs[,1] == "O") + (crabs[,2] == "F")
> groupch = c( "B", "b", "O", "o")[group]
> cg <- cbind(crabs, group, groupch)
> cg[c(1, 51, 101, 151), ]               # look at the appended data
     sp sex index    FL  RW   CL   CW  BD group groupch
1     B   M     1   8.1 6.7 16.1 19.0 7.0     1       B
51    B   F     1   7.2 6.5 14.7 17.1 6.1     2       b
101   O   M     1   9.1 6.9 16.7 18.6 7.4     3       O
151   O   F     1  10.7 9.7 21.4 24.0 9.8     4       o
> library(mvpart)                        # draw the regression tree
> crabtree <- mvpart(groupch ~ FL + RW + CL + CW + BD, data = cg,
+                    method = "class", size = 7)
```

There are a number of useful diagnostics available helping guide us to identify an optimal tree size and to estimate the predictive value of the tree. As with many statistical models, there is a trade-off between complexity and precision. A tree with more branches will fit the data better but suffers from the additional burden of its complexity. Similarly, a tree built from a data set will appear to classify those values well. Ideally, we would like to make a statement about how a given tree predicts some new set of additional data.

A useful way to approach the competing goals of prediction and complexity is to consider cross-validation, a topic introduced in Sect. 10.6. Specifically, a number of the observations are omitted and a new regression tree is built based on the remaining observations. Then we measure how well the resulting tree classifies the omitted values.

We can perform a cross-validation simulation of the regression model method by fitting a large tree with many splits and then computing statistics on each of the smaller-sized trees. In **R**, we do this for the crab data as follows:

```
crabtree <- mvpart(groupch ~ FL + RW + CL + CW + BD, data = cg,
                   method = "class", size = 20)
crabcp <- printcp(crabtree)
```

The printcp() program produces cross-validated errors on models up to the size specified by the size parameter in mvpart(). This program also calculates a complexity parameter (CP) taking into account the size of the tree in addition to its predictive value. These values are plotted in Fig. 10.18 for the crab data.

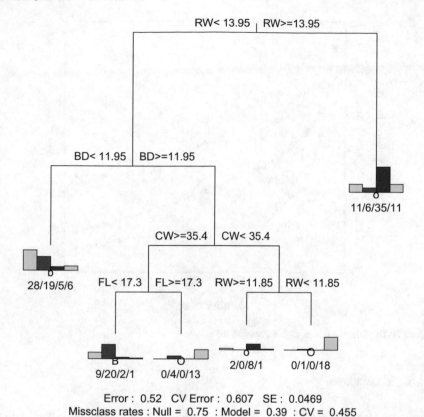

Error : 0.52   CV Error : 0.607   SE : 0.0469
Missclass rates : Null = 0.75 : Model = 0.39 : CV = 0.455

Figure 10.17   Regression tree classification of 200 crabs

The cross-validation errors (left scale) and CP statistic (right scale) decrease with model size. The largest gains appear among the smallest models. There is a much slower improvement in models with more than five splits. This figure was used to choose the model size in Fig. 10.17.

Finally, it is possible to completely automate the model-building process. For example, we can specify the regression tree continues branching until no additional splits result in a specified improvement in the CP statistic.

Some colorful language has also been developed among those who study this methodology. Reducing the complexity of an existing tree is called, appropriately enough, *pruning* and the many random trees resulting from cross-validation studies are often referred to as a *forest*.

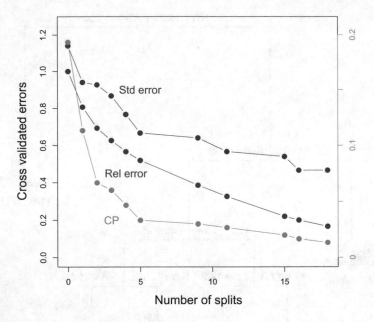

Figure 10.18   Diagnostics of crab regression tree

10.8   Exercises

Exercises 10.5 through 10.8 refer to the analysis of large data sets. The data is available in the `kernlab` library in **R** and also in the University of California at Irvine Machine Learning Repository. This repository is located at

                        http://archive.ics.uci.edu/ml/index.html

and is an excellent resource for other data sets.

10.1   In times of stress, the body undergoes a process called vasoconstriction in which blood vessels at the extremities are closed, forcing blood to the central organs. Vasoconstriction can also occur after taking a deep breath. The data set `vaso` in the `robustbase` library summarizes the vasoconstriction (or not) of subjects' fingers along with their breathing volumes and rates.

   a. Plot the breath rates and volumes using different colors for those with and without vasoconstriction. Perform any of the discrimination methods and see how well these distinguish between the two groups.
   b. Repeat your analysis of part a. but first take logs of the explanatory variables. Which analysis do you prefer?

10.2   The human leukocyte antigen system (HLA) is a group of genes on chromosome 6 linked to the immune system. The data set `hla` in the `gap` library contains HLA data on six markers for 177 schizophrenia patients and 94 matched healthy controls. How can we use these six markers to distinguish between the patients and their controls?

10.3 The data set `skulls` in the HSAUR2 library lists four-dimensional measurements made on ancient Egyptian skulls from five different epochs, hundreds of years apart. Differences are attributed to interbreeding with different immigrant populations. Even though the epochs are ordered in times, do you see a break in the ordering, equivalent to a major change in the genetic mix?

10.4 The data set `iris` has four measurements on three different species of 150 irises. Figure 3.23 shows the parallel coordinate plot of these data. Describe the factor loadings from a discriminant analysis and try to reconcile these with what you see in this figure.

10.5 The `musk` data set in the `kernlab` is an example of a discrimination problem on a large data set. In this data set, there are 476 molecules: 207 are classified as a musk and the remaining 269 are not. The goal is to identify a classification of the musks from non-musks using any combination of the 166 explanatory variables. These explanatory variables measure molecular distances in different directions. The original data appears at

https://archive.ics.uci.edu/ml/datasets/Musk+(Version+1)

with additional information including a complete description of the explanatory variables. The UCI website contains a list of other methods having been tried on these data.

10.6 The `promotergene` data set in the `kernlab` is another example of a discrimination problem in a large data set. This data set contains 106 gene sequences, half of which are classified as being either promoters or not. The explanatory variables are the lists of DNA base values preceding the gene of interest. The base values take the values a, c, g, or t corresponding to adenine, cytosine, guanine, and thymine, respectively. Use the base values to find a rule for discriminating between promoters and non-promoters. Additional information on these data can be found on the UCI website.

10.7 The `spam` data set in the `kernlab` library was gathered in an attempt to distinguish advertisement emails (spam) from non-spam. There are 4601 email messages collected by Hewlett-Packard and of these, 1813 are classified as spam and 2788 are non-spam. There are 57 explanatory variables measuring the frequency of various words such as "free" or "credit". Other explanatory variables count the frequency of different punctuation symbols or the length of strings of all capital letters. See the help file for a detailed explanation of the variables in this data set. Can you find a good rule to distinguish spam from non-spam?

10.8 The UCI data set at

> https://archive.ics.uci.edu/ml/datasets/Post-Operative+Patient

lists outcomes of 90 post-operative patients and several attributes such as blood pressure, body core temperature, and oxygen saturation. The object is to classify where patients should be sent from the post-operative recovery area. There are three choices: intensive care, regular hospital floor, or discharge. Use any of the methods discussed in this chapter to build a suitable model classifying patients.

10.9 Another approach to generalizing logistic regression to multinomial data has been developed by McFadden (1974). This method compares each category to all others, combined. McFadden, an economist, was concerned with modeling consumer choices, made to the exclusion of all other options. This explanation motivates models of the form

$$\log \left(\frac{\Pr[\, y = i \mid x \,]}{\Pr[\, y \neq i \mid x \,]} \right) = \beta_i' x$$

for each choice i.

a. Solve for $\Pr[\, y = i \,]$ and show this model is over-parameterized. (What happens when you add the same vector to all β's?) One solution to this problem is to restrict $\beta_1 = \mathbf{0}$.

b. Compare this restricted model to the approach taken in Sect. 10.4 where the reference category corresponds to $y = 1$. Are these two approaches the same? How are they different?

c. Does this approach support independence of irrelevant alternatives?

10.10 How large should n be in an n-fold cross-validation? Try different values of n to see how much these error estimates vary. Useful code may include

```
(sv <- ksvm(group ~., data = mydata, type = "C-svc", cross = 5))
cross(sv)
```

using the `cross()` function to capture the cross-validation error estimate. Plot these estimates for different values of n and comment on the effect of changing the sample size.

10.11 The `GlaucomaM` data frame in the `TH.data` library contains 62 measurements on 196 eyes in two classes: normal and glaucomatous. The subjects in the two groups were matched by age and sex to provide balance. This represents a large number of measurements on each eye. Use the methods described in this chapter to identify a much smaller set of measurements used to characterize the two groups.

10.12 The data frame `stagec` in the `rpart` library summarizes observations made on 146 men treated for Stage C prostate cancer. There are eight measurements made on each patient including whether or not the cancer has progressed. Use regression tree methods to indicate important prognostic measures on whether the cancer will progress from these data.

10.13 Kyphosis is a severe curvature of the spine. The `kyphosis` data frame in the `rpart` library presents the history of 81 children who had corrective spinal surgery and whether this resulted in kyphosis. The data frame includes three additional variables indicating the extent of the surgery and the child's age in months.

    a. Use regression trees to identify risk factors for kyphosis.
    b. Similarly, use logistic regression to build a linear model of the log-odds risk of kyphosis.
    c. Discuss these two different approaches to modeling kyphosis. Which model is more intuitive? Which is easier to explain and use?

10.14 The data set `mammoexp` in the `TH.data` library describes a survey of 412 women's attitudes to and experiences with mammography. Among the data are the respondent's perceived benefits of mammography and whether a close female relative had been diagnosed with breast cancer. A suitable response to these measurements is the variable ME measuring the time since the woman had her last mammography. The categorical responses to this variable are never, within a year, and over a year ago. Use a regression tree approach to model the time since the last mammography. If you were a public health official in charge of educating the public about the importance of periodic mammography examinations, what is the most effective message you can give?

10.15 A *haplotype* is a strand of genetic material on one chromosome inherited as an intact gene from one parent. Lander et al. (2011) collected and examined the lengths of haplotypes at 27 loci on 1915 beech trees (*Fagus sylvatica*) in France. The authors of this study examined historical data to verify these stands of trees existed at least 200 years ago. The trees were growing in three geographically separated areas, referred to as East, South, and West in the data. The data is available for download at

    `http://dx.doi.org/10.5061/dryad.q98202jk.`

Use linear discriminant analysis to show the East and South populations can be clearly distinguished but the West population overlaps both of these.

10.16 Regression trees are not limited to classifying individuals into discrete groups. These methods will also estimate cut points in continuous measurements and thereby create groups of data. Build a regression tree to model the mpg values in the car data introduced in Table 9.1. Show the most important classification is the number of cylinders and, to a smaller degree, the displacement.

10.17 Repeat the analysis of the breast cancer data examined in Sect. 10.2 using other restrictions in logistic regression.

    a. Set `alpha = 0` in the code in Output 10.2. Does this ridge restriction draw you to a different model?

    b. Examine the methods of Sect. 9.4 for restricted linear regression and identify an optimal value for α.

Chapter 11
Clustering Methods

C LUSTERING is a nonparametric method of arranging similar observations together, often in a graphical display used to detect patterns of grouping and outliers. The approach is usually considered nonparametric because there is no specified underlying distribution or model we need to assume. **R** offers great flexibility in graphical capability making these methods possible. The largest difference between these methods and those considered in the previous chapter is in this chapter we do not know group membership a priori, or whether in fact there are different groups at all. Similarly, part of the methods discussed here includes estimates of the number of dissimilar groups present in the data.

11.1 Hierarchical Clustering

Consider the statistics on the number of health care workers in Canada given in Table 11.1. This table lists the number and type of health care workers per 100,000 population in each Canadian province or territory.

Figure 11.1 depicts a hierarchical cluster representation of these data. This figure is interpreted as a tree or *dendrogram*. The root is at the top and the observations are represented as leaves toward the bottom. The vertical scale of the branches indicates how far individual observations and groups of observations are from each other using a distance metric we will discuss later in this section.

This representation is different from a regression tree or CART, as in Fig. 10.17. In regression trees, there is a single variable of greatest interest. In Fig. 10.17, for example, we model the species and/or sex of the crabs. In contrast, in Fig. 11.1, the variables are of equal importance; our goal is to identify provinces with similar characteristics overall.

Yukon is identified as very different from all others because of the huge number of doctors (331) per unit population. (In 2001, this figure was only 70, so something has clearly changed during this five-year period.) Manitoba and Saskatchewan are

© Springer Nature Switzerland AG 2022
D. Zelterman, *Applied Multivariate Statistics with R*, Statistics for Biology and Health,
https://doi.org/10.1007/978-3-031-13005-2_11

Table 11.1 Number of Canadian health care workers per 100,000 residents in 2006, listed by province or territory

Province or Territory	Doctors	Nurses	Psychologists	Social workers	Other
Newfoundland and Labrador	137	1149	45	179	1843
Prince Edward Island	97	1203	22	101	2153
Nova Scotia	153	1066	47	141	2268
New Brunswick	115	1121	53	172	2215
Quebec	142	825	95	150	2259
Ontario	127	825	45	166	1874
Manitoba	121	1061	36	197	2421
Saskatchewan	114	992	42	179	2354
Alberta	131	989	54	149	2096
British Columbia	134	584	45	134	1956
Yukon	331	1110	50	348	1722
Northwest Territories	97	1047	61	207	1595
Nunavut	85	648	34	222	801
Canada, overall	132	881	58	157	2052

Source Statistics Canada

similar in many ways and form the tightest cluster between any pair. The maritime provinces (Newfoundland, Nova Scotia, New Brunswick, and Prince Edward Island) also appear close together in this figure.

The **R** code producing Fig. 11.1 is as follows:

```
Cmed <- read.table(file = "Canmed.txt",
    header = TRUE, row.names = 1)
Cmed <- Cmed[-14, ]      # omit  "Canada total" row
d <- dist(scale(Cmed))   # distances between provinces
clust <- hclust(d)       # build hierarchical cluster
plot(clust, xlab = "", sub = "", main = "", ylab = "", yaxt = "n")
```

Another example of clustering appears in Fig. 11.2. The statistics on the three species of iris flowers are summarized in terms of their Euclidean distances from each other. These data also appear in Fig. 3.23 using another clustering method.

The branches of the dendrogram summarize the distances between each flower's observations. The leaves at the end of each branch are color-coded according to the three different species. The resulting dendrogram shows the relative distances of the various clusters. These distances determine how far back from the leaves we have

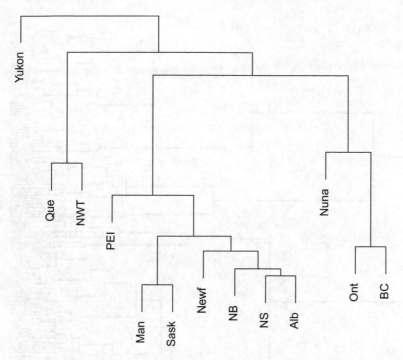

Figure 11.1 Clustering dendrogram of Canadian provinces and territories of data in Table 11.1

to go to obtain the junction with a different branch. Branches are joined with other branches, farther apart, until the tree is joined at a single root. The method is called *hierarchical* because each branch depends on all previous branches leading to it. See also Exercise 11.9 for other methods to cluster these data.

In Fig. 11.2, we see the algorithm does a reasonable job of grouping together the individual species into three separate regions of the tree. There is some overlap of the species seen in this figure, of course. However, we made no assumptions and specifications. The Euclidean distances between every pair of irises were the only criteria used to construct the tree. Unlike CART, the algorithm does not have the species information when constructing the tree. At the completion of the clustering, these values were used to draw the final figure.

The program creating this figure is as follows:

```
id <- dist(scale(iris[ , 1 : 4]))  # find euclidean distances
fit <- hclust(id)                  # build the tree
library(ape)                       # graphics for trees
plot(as.phylo(fit), type="phylogram", cex = .5, label.offset = .1,
    tip.col = c(rep("red", 50), rep("blue", 50), rep("green", 50)))
```

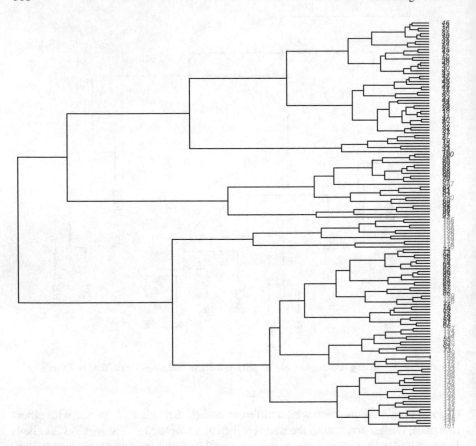

Figure 11.2 Clustering dendrogram of iris data

When we begin, the data columns are usually scaled to have the zero means and unit variances. This is done so no one variable dominates the others simply by nature of having greater variability. See Exercise 11.1 for details.

The `dist()` program calculates the Euclidean distance between every pair of observed flowers. That is, the whole data set was reduced to a set of pairwise comparisons specifying the distance between observations. Euclidean distances are the default, but there are other options, and these are discussed at the end of this section. The clustering tree is built by **R** in `hclust` from the matrix of distances. The `ape` library offers a number of options to present these trees.

Let us consider a more detailed example and use it to illustrate some of the many additional graphical options available to us. The data in Table 11.2 summarizes the records of all major league baseball teams in 1986, attendance totals, and average 1987 salaries. There are two leagues (American and National) and two divisions (East and West). Teams are ranked within each of the four combinations of leagues and divisions. The number of wins has a strong negative correlation with the number

Table 11.2 Baseball team records for 1986 and total attendance in 1,000s. The 1987 average salary data is in $1,000's

Name	League	Division	Rank	Wins	Losses	Attendance		Average
						At home	Away	salary
NYMets	N	E	1	108	54	2768	2178	$527
Phi	N	E	2	86	75	1933	1721	541
StL	N	E	3	79	82	2472	1696	445
⋮	⋮	⋮	⋮	⋮	⋮	⋮	⋮	⋮
Min	A	W	6	71	91	1255	1707	432
Sea	A	W	7	67	95	1029	1559	186

Source http://lib.stat.cmu.edu/datasets/baseball.data

of losses, but this correlation is not perfect because not all teams played the same number of games.

The top four panels in Fig. 11.3 are produced using

```
d <- dist(scale(baseball[,c(-1,-2)])) # scale numerical values
library(ape)                           # offers plotting options
fit <- hclust(d)
plot(fit, main = "Plain dendrogram", hang = -1, cex = .8,
    xlab = "", ylab = "", sub = "", axes = FALSE)
plot(as.dendrogram(fit), type = "triangle",
    main = "Triangle branches", cex = .8, axes = FALSE)
plot(as.phylo(fit), type = "unrooted", cex = .8,
    main = "Unrooted tree")
plot(as.phylo(fit), type = "fan", cex = .8,
    main = "Leaves spread in a circle")
```

In the iris data, this method appears to confirm our understanding of the data. Identical species of flowers have much in common. However, in the case of the baseball data, it is not obvious why some teams appear to cluster. For example, the two New York teams and Boston always appear in the same tight cluster, but except for their geographic proximity, it is not clear why these teams belong together. (This, despite the long-standing rivalry between Red Sox and Yankees fans.) Clearly, **R** can demonstrate the clusters, but it remains for us to interpret the resulting figure.

As a final example in this section, let us point out some data sets lend themselves to the tree-like structure and are stored in **R** as such. The chiroptera data set in the ape library is a *supertree*, a composite tree constructed from many different sources, describing the complete phylogeny of 916 species of bats (Mammals of the order *Chiroptera*). This data is best displayed as a tree, and two versions appear in Fig. 11.4. The **R** code producing this pair of figures is

```
library(ape)
data(chiroptera)
plot(chiroptera, type = "r", cex = .1)
plot(chiroptera, type = "u", cex = .1)
```

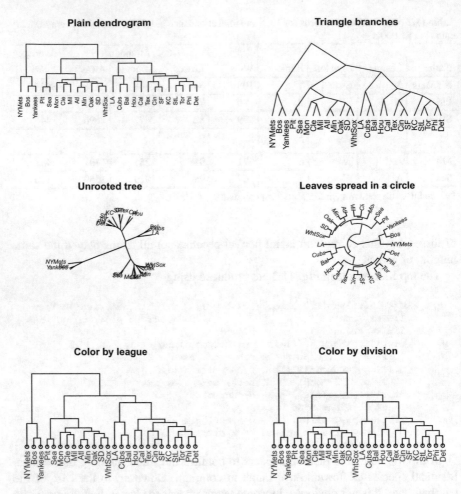

Figure 11.3 Hierarchical clustering of baseball teams using a variety of displays

Similar tree structures for birds are available as `bird.orders` and `bird.families`, both in the `ape` library.

Let us end this section with a discussion of options for the distance between two observations. In a `data.frame`, it usually makes sense to start by scaling or normalizing the columns (different variables) to have the same variances. Otherwise, a column (variable) with a large variance will dominate any reasonable distance, and a column with a small variance will tend to be ignored. That is, we should usually employ the template

```
d <- dist(scale(mydata))
```

when using `dist`.

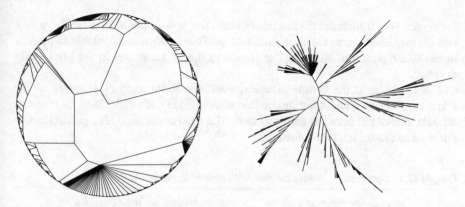

Figure 11.4 Two displays of the `chiroptera` data

The `dist` function will calculate the distance between every pair of observations (rows) in a data.frame. Consider, then, two observations (rows in a `data.frame`) denoted by the vectors $x' = (x_1, \ldots, x_n)$ and $y' = (y_1, \ldots, y_n)$. There are several useful options available, depending on how we define distance.

The most popular distance is the Euclidean distance.

$$\text{Euclidean distance}(x, y) = \sqrt{\sum (x_i - y_i)^2}$$

is the default distance for the `dist` function.

The Euclidean length of a vector was introduced at (4.4). It corresponds to the length of the shortest, straight line connecting x and y.

The *maximum* or *supremum norm*

$$\text{Maximum norm}(x, y) = \max_i |x_i - y_i|$$

is the largest component-wise difference.

The *Manhattan norm* is

$$\text{Manhattan distance}(x, y) = \sum_i |x_i - y_i|$$

which is calculated as though we had to walk along rectangular, city blocks.

The *Minkowski norm*[1] which is

$$\text{Minkowski distance}(x, y) = \left\{ \sum |x_i - y_i|^p \right\}^{1/p}$$

---

[1] Hermann Minkowski (1864–1909). Mathematician and mathematical physicist, lived in Germany.

for power $p > 0$ includes the Euclidean norm for $p = 2$; the Manhattan for $p = 1$ and the maximum norm for large values of p. These norms are available as options in the `dist` program, including the choice of the p parameter in the Minkowski distance.

Finally, there is the *Gower distance*, available in the `daisy` program of the `cluster` library. The Gower metric first standardizes each variable by its range so all data values fall between zero and one. The Gower distance also generalizes to allow us to cluster interval-valued data.

Output 11.1   **R** program to produce the plots with colored leaves in Fig. 11.3.

```
colLab <- function(n)            # function on dendrograms
{                                # to get colored labels
    if (is.leaf(n))              # when we find a leaf...
    {
        a <- attributes(n)       # capture its attributes
                                 # which team number is it?
        teamn <- match(a$label, row.names(baseball))
                                 # color for league or division
        leafcolor <- c("red", "blue") [teamtype[teamn]]
                                 # assign new attributes to leaf
        attr(n, "nodePar") <- c(a$nodePar, lab.col = leafcolor)
    }
    return(n)                    # return the dendrogram
}

league <- baseball[ , 1]
division <- baseball[ , 2]
d <- dist(scale(baseball[ ,c(-1, -2)])# scale numerical values
library(ape)                     # offers plotting options
fit <- hclust(d)
teamtype <- league               # leaf color by league
colfit = dendrapply(fit, colLab)        # dendrapply to tree
plot(colfit, main = "Color by league",
    cex = .8, axes = FALSE)

teamtype <- division                   # leaf color by division
colfit = dendrapply(fit, colLab)
plot(colfit, main = "Color by division",
    cex = .8, axes = FALSE)
```

Sourced, in part from: www.http://gastonsanchez.com.

11.2   *K*-Means Clustering

The *K-means* clustering algorithm is based on the principal there are a specified number, K, multivariate normal populations present in the data and these differ only in terms of their means. The cluster members and their mean are estimated in such a way as to minimize the within-cluster variability. The algorithm uses an analysis of variance (ANOVA) approach to estimate the K different multivariate means as well as estimate the group membership of each observation. The ANOVA approach also suggests the clustering algorithm proposed by Hartigan and Wong (1979). The algorithm determines the group membership of each observation so the program minimizes the sums of squares within each group.

Let us begin with a small example. Table 11.3 gives the characteristics of 11 male Japanese cigarette smokers who participated in a larger study of the health effects of smoking. The data in this table includes demographic variables (age, weight, height), characteristics of their cigarette brands (nicotine, tar), and smoking history (age at start, cigarettes per day, and pack-years).

The K-means program is in the `stats` library. The program fitting $K = 4$ clusters and produces Fig. 11.5 as follows:

```
require(graphics, stats)
(cl <- kmeans(smokers, centers = 4))
plot(smokers[ ,c(3, 9)], xlab = "Weight in kg",
    ylab = "Pack  years", pch = 16, col = cl$clust, cex = 2.5)
text(smokers[ ,3], smokers[ ,9], labels = row.names(smokers),
    pos = 2)
```

Figure 11.5 plots the four different clusters by color by their pack-years and weights. This figure identifies two unusual individuals: a low-smoking, obese man (#5) in the lower, right-hand corner of this plot and a heavy smoker (#4) at the top of the figure. The remaining nine individuals are either classified as five light smokers (red) or four heavy smokers (black).

Let us begin with the choice of axes in this plot. These were chosen with a combination of interpretation and visual appeal. The visual appeal works because

Table 11.3 Characteristics of 11 Japanese smokers

	Age	Height in cm	Weight in kg	Nicotine	Tar	Age start	Cigarettes per day	Years smoking	Pack years
1	36	168	50	0.7	8	20	15	16	12
2	41	170	64	0.7	8	20	20	21	21
3	35	169	65	0.8	10	20	30	15	23
4	55	177	68	1.0	12	20	20	35	35
5	21	172	80	0.7	10	16	15	5	4
6	46	165	53	1.4	17	20	20	26	26
7	38	167	57	0.1	1	20	10	18	9
8	37	165	58	0.1	1	20	20	17	17
9	40	156	53	0.4	5	18	20	22	22
10	36	172	55	0.5	6	20	20	16	16
11	39	168	65	0.7	8	16	10	23	12

Source Takahashi et al. (2013)

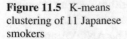

Figure 11.5 K-means
clustering of 11 Japanese
smokers

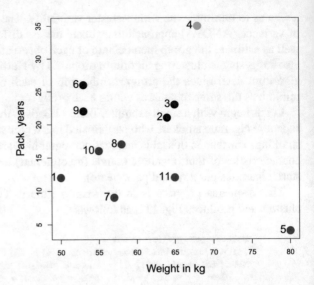

the clusters separate nicely and do not overlap in this display. The interpretation also
aligns with our sense of the overall health effects of smoking. Unfortunately, useful
axis choices in this figure are found by trial and error, so the user will have to do
some experimenting in order to produce an appealing display.

A graphical display can help us choose an appropriate value of K. The analysis of
variance has an interpretation we can use here and is introduced at (9.2). The simple
idea of the ANOVA is that the total sum of squares can be decomposed as

$$\text{Total sum of squares} = \text{Between cluster sum of squares}$$
$$+\text{Within cluster sum of squares}$$

or, more simply, the total sum of squares is the sum of *explained sum of squares* plus
the *unexplained sum of squares*.

The total sum of squares is the same for every choice of K. We can examine the
within-cluster variability which will decrease as K increases. Another reasonable
summary of how well we are doing is to examine the percent of explained variability.
That is,

$$\text{Percent variability explained} = \frac{\text{Between group sum of squares}}{\text{Total sum of squares}}$$

and this will decrease as K is increased.

These two summary measures represent a trade-off and can be compared to each
other. Figure 11.6 plots these two summaries for different values of K.

This figure confirms our intuition the percentage of explained variability increases
with the number of clusters, K. Similarly, the within-cluster variability decreases

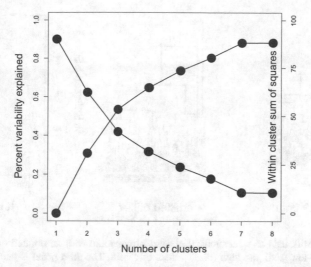

Figure 11.6 Percentage of variability explained (blue) and within-cluster sum of squares (red) in K-means clustering of 11 Japanese smokers

Table 11.4 Variable names and their definitions in the `milk` data

dens	density
fat	fat content
prot	protein content
casein	casein content
Fdry	cheese dry substance measured in the factory
Ldry	cheese dry substance measured in the laboratory
drysub	milk dry substance
cheese	cheese product

with the number of clusters. At $K = 1$, the data is estimated to have originated from one population, and nothing is explained. At the other extreme, if K is equal to the sample size, then 100% of the variability is explained by having each observation in its own cluster, but nothing is learned. We look at Fig. 11.6 to see if we can identify a compromise. The percent variability explained increases steeply up to $K = 4$ and then starts to level off for larger values of K. This choice of K is somewhat arbitrary and $K = 3$ might also have done a good job.

Let us compare K-means with hierarchical clustering. We begin by introducing the `milk` data set in the `robustbase` library. This data set consists of eight measurements on each of the 86 separate containers of milk. The variables are labeled `X1` through `X8` in the original. Table 11.4 renames these and gives their definitions.

In the first panel of Fig. 11.7, a clear outlier (observation #70) appears in the hierarchical clustering method. In the second, middle panel, this observation has been removed and the `hclust` has been repeated, indicating two distinct clusters of observations. These two clusters are largely determined by the values of casein,

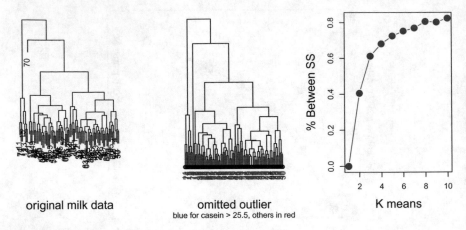

Figure 11.7 Milk data as a hierarchical cluster: original and with an omitted outlier. Color is determined by low (red) and high (blue) values of casein. The third panel is percent variability explained in K-means

although other variables could provide similar discrimination. In the middle panel, values of casein over 25.5 are in blue, others in red.

The third panel in this figure plots the percent variability explained in terms of the number of K-means clusters. This third panel illustrates a big change for $K = 2$ and $K = 3$ but larger values of K yield only small improvements.

Figure 11.8 is the `pairs()` plot of the K-means clusters for milk data with values of $K = 2$ in the lower panels and $K = 3$ in the upper panels. In this figure, we see a strong linear relationship between each of the pairs of variables `prot`, `cassein`, `Fdry`, and `Ldry`. Both K-means clustering indicates evidence clusters appear along the lengths of these lines.

Figure 11.8 was produced using the **R** code in Output 11.2. In this code, we begin by omitting the outlier, renaming the variables, and identifying the color schemes for 2 and 3 K-means. The `panel.up` function tells the `pairs()` program how to process separate scatterplots. In this case, we use it to provide separate, colored plots in the panels above and below the diagonal. Specifically, the `upper.panel=` is an option on `pairs` to be assigned the value of this function. There are other analyses we can do with these data. See Exercise 11.6 for some suggestions.

The K-means clustering, then, is a simple and intuitive method for clustering data and is dependent only on the user's choice of K. To complete our illustration of the method, let us try a small simulation to show the effect of mis-specification of K.

Consider a simulation in which we generate 100 samples from each of three different multivariate normal populations with different means and a slight negative correlation. These samples are plotted at the top of Fig. 11.9 with different colors for each of the three populations. The plot of percent variance explained seems to indicate $K = 3$ clusters should be appropriate and little is to be gained using larger values.

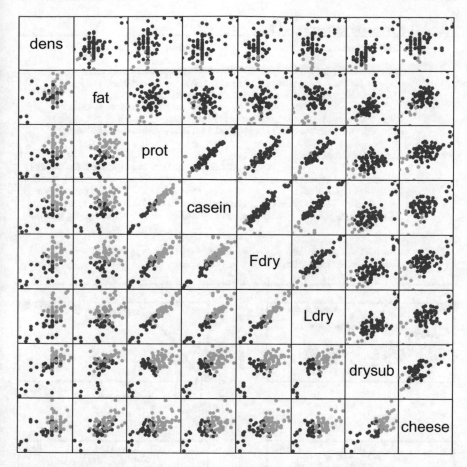

Figure 11.8 K-means for milk data with $K = 2$ (below) and $K = 3$ (above)

The next four graphs in Fig. 11.9 summarize the results of using different values of K. The plot with $K = 2$ clearly misses one group by combining the two dissimilar groups at the bottom. The $K = 3$ plot closely reproduces the original figure, albeit with different colors. Plots with larger values of $K = 4$ and 5 tend to pull apart clusters seeming adequate to our eyes. Exercise 11.4 asks the reader to further explore what can go wrong if the specified value of K is not appropriate.

In summary, what can we say about the K-means clustering algorithm? The approach is not limited to small data sets. The choice of K can be estimated from graphics such as Fig 11.6. The interpretation of the K clusters is up to us. A useful plot such as Fig. 11.5 requires us to identify appropriate choices for the axes and, again, requires we are able to interpret the resulting figure. In the following section, we describe methods for assessing the quality of the clusters identified by these algorithms.

Output 11.2 R code to produce Fig. 11.8

```
library(robustbase)                    # library with the milk dataset

milk2 <- milk[-70, ]                   # omit outlier
colnames(milk2) <- c("dens", "fat", "prot", "casein", "Fdry",
  "Ldry", "drysub", "cheese")          # supply new names
                                       # color schemes for K-means
 colorlow <- rainbow(3)[kmeans(scale(milk2), centers=2)$cluster]
 colorup  <- rainbow(3)[kmeans(scale(milk2), centers=3)$cluster]


panel.up <- function(x, y, ...)
   {                                   # function to produce scatterplot in pairs()
    usr <- par("usr")                            # save par() values
    on.exit(par(usr))                            # set par() at end
    par(usr = c(max(y), min(y), max(x), min(x))) # set bounds
    points(y, x, col = colorup, pch = 16)        # plot data points
   }

pairs(milk2, pch = 16, gap = 0, xaxt = "n", yaxt = "n",
   col = colorlow, upper.panel = panel.up)
```

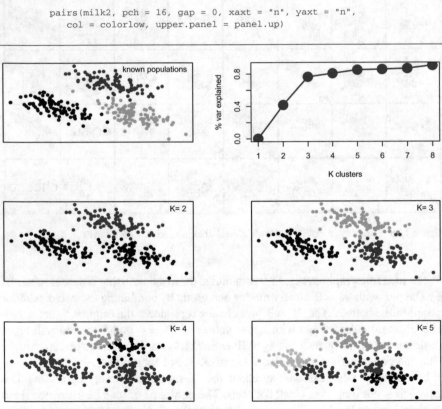

Figure 11.9 Simulation of K-means clustering

11.3 Diagnostics and Validation

Clustering algorithms provide a data diagnostic to help our exploration. Figure 11.6 has shown us this illustration can be an aid in identifying the number of clusters in a K-means procedure. How many clusters are appropriate? It is reasonable to see a clustering figure and then ask whether such a diagram could have occurred by chance alone. Will a set of randomly generated data values naturally appear to cluster into two or more groups? The clustering procedures are nonparametric, so it is reasonable to retain this model-free approach in any study of validation.

Three popular methods to assess the quality of a clustering procedure are jittering, bootstrap resampling, and the cluster silhouette. We will go over these methods and illustrate them in this section.

Jittering adds a small amount of random noise to the data and then repeats the clustering procedure. The bootstrap randomly samples from the observed data before repeating the clustering procedure. Both methods are repeated several times. The goal is to check the stability of the outcomes. (Jittering also appears as a graphical tool in Fig. 3.6.)

Clustering, most generally, breaks the sample into subsets of the total. We will then need a way to compare the results of two different clustering processes. There are three popular measures of agreement in the clustering of sets. These are attributed to Jaccard, Dunn, and Rand.

Let us introduce a measure of similarity between two sets. Let S and T be finite-sized sets. The *Jaccard Index*[2] is defined as

$$J(S, T) = \frac{\text{\# of elements in } (S \cap T)}{\text{\# of elements in } (S \cup T)}.$$

If S and T are both empty, then $J = 0$.

Clearly, $0 \leq J \leq 1$ with larger values indicating a greater percentage of agreement. The relevance here is to compare a set S identified by a clustering algorithm based on the observed data with a set T obtained from simulated data. The simulated measure J will then have a distribution. We will need to look at a summary of the randomly generated values such as their histogram or mean value. We don't assign a statistical significance to the value of the Jaccard index, but it is possible to do so. See Exercise 11.7 for details.

A commonly used measure of cluster quality is the Dunn Index (Dunn 1973). The Dunn Index is the ratio of the smallest distance between clusters divided by the diameter of the largest cluster. Ideally, we want small clusters located far apart, so larger values of the Dunn Index are better. Of course, there are many possible definitions of distance, as we pointed out in Sect. 11.1, so there are many variations on how the Dunn Index may be defined. The general idea of this measure is similar to other metrics frequently encountered in applied statistics. See Exercise 11.7 for details.

---

[2] Paul Jaccard (1868–1944). Swiss professor of botany and plant physiology.

Another general measure of agreement is the Rand Index (Rand 1971). Suppose we have two sets of sets $X = \{x_1, \ldots x_n\}$ and $Y = \{y_1 \ldots, y_m\}$ both making up partitions of the sampled observations. Imagine taking all possible observations, two at a time. The Rand Index counts the proportion of times these observations occur in the same x_i and same y_j or else in different x's and different y's. See Exercise 11.7 for more on this.

The *cluster silhouette* is a method for assessing cluster quality and is often used as a quantitative determination of the appropriate number of clusters when we perform a K-means. Roughly speaking, the silhouette $s(i)$ of the i-th data point compares the difference of the average distance to all other points in the same cluster to the average distance to all other points in the nearest cluster. By "distance" we mean any choice of metrics described in Sect. 11.1.

Specifically, let $a(i)$ be the average distance between the i-th data point and every other point in the same cluster. Let $d(i, C)$ be the average distance between this data point and every data point in the cluster C. Then let $b(i)$ denote the smallest value of d taken over all clusters C this data point does not belong to. The silhouette of the i-th data point is then

$$s(i) = \frac{b(i) - a(i)}{\max(a(i), \ b(i))}$$

Intuitively, if $s(i)$ is large (close to one) then this point is well clustered, meaning it is close to members in the same cluster and still far away from the nearest cluster. Similarly, if $s(i)$ is close to zero then this point is probably on the boundary between two clusters: about as far from its own cluster as the nearest neighboring cluster. A negative silhouette is not rare and is indicative of a data point not fitting well into any of the existing clusters. A detailed explanation and method for nearest neighbor clustering appear in Exercise 11.21.

Finally, there is a nonparametric method for assessing the quality of the clustering. The **R** program `prediction.strength()` in the fpc library provides a cross-validated measure of the quality of a cluster. This program randomly divides the data into two equal-sized number of observations, called A and B. The set A is used to estimate the k clusters and then records the percent of times observations in B are clustered into the same clusters as in the original, full data. The procedure is then reversed, fitting B and predicting A. The simulation is repeated for different partitions of A and B and then for different values of k. The prediction strength will generally decrease with k, and the authors of this method recommend we choose values of k resulting in a prediction strength over .8 or .9. An example of this simulation appears in Fig. 11.10, below.

Now let us examine a data set involving genetic markers measured using an Affymetrix DNA microarray. These data will be used in **R** to illustrate the methods described in this section. In this example, three sets of mouse mesenchymal cells from each of two anatomic strictures (mesodermal and neural crest) were examined. Mesenchymal cells can develop into a variety of different tissues including bone, cartilage, as well as parts of circulatory and lymphatic systems. Many genetic markers

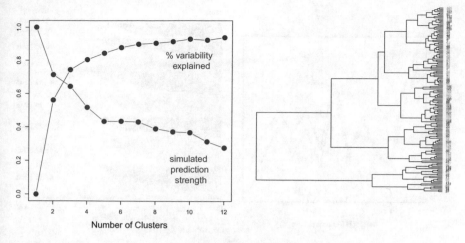

Figure 11.10 Clustering of genetic markers in mouse masenchymal cells

were measured in the original data, but only those 147 exhibited a large difference between the mesodermal and neural crest cells which are included here.

A portion of these data are obtained and displayed

```
> library(clValid)
> data(mouse)
> print(mouse, digits = 4)

        ID      M1    M2    M3    NC1   NC2   NC3                   FC
1   1448995_at 4.707 4.528 4.326 5.568 6.915 7.353 Growth/Differentiation
2  1436392_s_at 3.868 4.052 3.475 4.996 5.056 5.184    Transcription factor
3  1437434_a_at 2.875 3.380 3.240 3.877 4.460 4.851              Miscellaneous

          ...                     ...                         ...

145 1417129_a_at 6.694 6.019 7.037 5.770 5.149 4.541    Transcription factor
146 1425779_a_at 6.109 5.960 5.999 4.537 4.068 4.251    Transcription factor
147   1450723_at 5.948 5.753 6.001 5.027 4.187 3.111    Transcription factor
```

The six cells are listed as `M1`, `M2`, `M3` for the mesodermal and `NC1`, `NC2`, `NC3` for the neural crest. The `ID` is the specific genetic address and `FC` refers to the gene's functional class. There are nine different functional classes of genes in these data.

Notice these data are presented transposed from our usual manner of displaying data: observations as rows and variables as columns. In our applications of clustering so far in this chapter, the object has been to cluster individuals. In this case, the data is *wide* in the sense there are many more variables than observations. Similarly, the object of the clustering analysis in these data is to group similar genes together, rather than different cell samples.

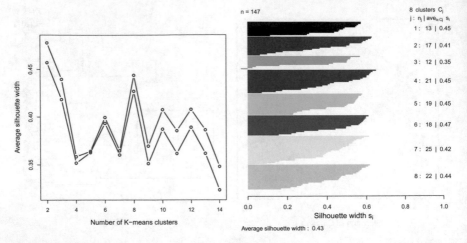

Figure 11.11   Average silhouette width by cluster size (Manhattan metric in *blue*; Euclidean in *red*.) On the right is the silhouette plot for all data points, $k = 8$ clusters using the Manhattan metric

Figure 11.10 includes a plot of the percent variability explained by cluster size and a dendrogram. The simulated prediction probability decreases with a larger number of clusters. The dendrogram plots the functional class of each marker in a separate color but does not demonstrate a clear indication of the homogeneity of these clusters. Together, the two panels in Fig. 11.10 suggest there should be three cluster centers, maybe four at most.

We can also examine the silhouette of the clustering in these data. Figure 11.11 presents the mean silhouette width (left panel) using the Manhattan and Euclidean metrics. These figures are very similar indicating either $k = 2$ or $k = 8$ k-mean clusters would be appropriate. The right panel of Fig. 11.11 plots all individual silhouette values, by cluster. The right panelof Fig. 11.11 is produced using the code:

```
short <- mouse[ , 2 : 7]        #   remove text columns
dman <- daisy(short, metric = "manhattan")  # Manhattan distance matrix
kmm <- kmeans(short, 8)
plot(silhouette(kmm$cluster, dman), col = 1:8, main = "", cex.lab = 1.25)
```

The `clusterboot` program in the `fpc` library simulates cluster stability by simulating K-means clustering using a variety of methods including jittering or bootstrap methods. The mean Jaccard Index for $K = 3$ clusters in the `mouse` data using jittering yields

```
cbj <- clusterboot(short, bootmethod = "jitter",
    krange = 3, clustermethod = kmeansCBI)
cbj$jittermean

[1] 0.9960000 0.9957377 1.0000000
```

The same simulation using a bootstrap gives

```
cbb <- clusterboot(short, bootmethod = "boot",
   krange = 3, clustermethod = kmeansCBI)
cbb$bootmean

[1]  0.9170135 0.9179769 0.9026569
```

The authors of these programs suggest average Jaccard Index values above 0.75 indicate stable clusters. Clearly, these simulations indicate $K = 3$ clusters is a reasonable number.

A simulation with $K = 4$ on these data gives

```
> cbb$bootmean

[1]  0.5059524 0.8515681 0.6708926 0.4336492

> cbj$jittermean

[1]  0.8069331 0.9293281 0.8260002 0.8801505
```

These second sets of simulations yield somewhat ambiguous results. The bootstrap simulation provides much lower mean Jaccard values for $K = 4$ than we saw for $K = 3$, above. The jittered simulation provides lower mean values but these are considerable higher than those of the bootstrap and much closer to the values for $K = 4$. From these simulations, we may conclude $K = 3$ clusters is a reasonable conclusion, and there is weaker evidence $K = 4$ is appropriate.

The Dunn Index for $K = 3$ clusters is 0.087, but we have no context to understand this value. We can perform a bootstrap simulation to examine the distribution of the statistic. The **R** code to perform this simulation is given in Output 11.3.

Output 11.3 **R** code to perform bootstrap for K-means clustering

```
short <- mouse[ , 2 : 7]                # remove text columns
d <- dist(short)
cl <- kmeans(short, centers = 3)
dunn <-                                 # Dunn Index of original data
   cluster.stats(d, cl$cluster)$dunn

n <- dim(short)[1]
for (i in 1 : 100)                      # number of bootstrap samples
   {
   booti <-  as.integer(1 + n * runif(n)) # bootstrap indices
   bd <- dist( short[booti, ])        # distances of bootstrap sample
   clb <- kmeans(bd, centers = 3)     # cluster bootstrap sample
   dunn <- c(dunn,                    # bootstrapped Dunn values
      cluster.stats(bd, clb$cluster)$dunn )
   }
```

Figure 11.12 Bootstrap simulation of Dunn Index in mouse data. The value for the observed data is highlighted

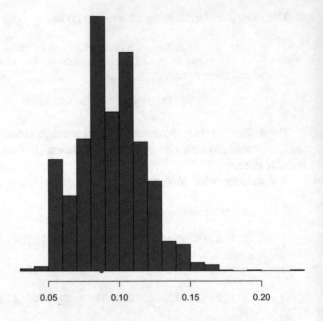

0.05	0.10	0.15	0.20

   This simulation produces values presented in Fig. 11.12. The Dunn Index for the observed data is highlighted and appears near the center of a right-skewed distribution which may also have a bimodal distribution. It is also possible to perform a bootstrap simulation to describe the behavior of the Dunn Index assuming a model in which there are no clusters, with the data sampled from a single population. See Exercise 11.10 for details on this simulation.

   A generalization of the single-linkage clustering is a simultaneous clustering of both rows and columns of a data matrix, also known as a *heatmap*. We used a heatmap in Fig. 9.6 to summarize the statistical significance of a large number of regression coefficients. Figure 11.13 displays clusters of mouse mesenchymal markers (by rows) and cells (by columns) in a way blocks of high and low data values are grouped together. The data values are displayed by color, as hotter (larger) or colder (smaller) values. The blocks of colors are clear in this figure because the data only includes markers exhibiting large differences between the two cell types. The margins of this figure include separate dendrograms. The colors along the left edge are the same as those used in Fig. 11.10.

   This figure can be produced with the **R** code

```
library(ape)
library(clValid)
library(stats)
data(mouse)
iclass <- as.integer(mouse$FC)   # integer categories
heatmap( as.matrix( mouse[, 2 : 7] ),
    RowSideColors = rainbow(max(iclass))[iclass] )
```

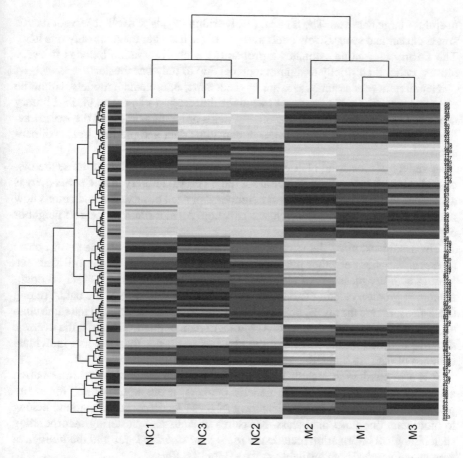

Figure 11.13 Heatmap for genetic markers in mouse mesenchymal cells

This code begins by loading the three necessary libraries. The FC column of the mouse data contains the functional class as factor levels and the as.integer function recodes these as integer values. Columns 2 through 7 contain the numerical values of the gene expression data. The heatmap program operates on a matrix of numerical values so the data.frame also needs to be reformatted. The RowSideColors option adds colors corresponding to the functional class of the genetic markers. There are many more options and enhancements available in the heatmap.2 program in the gplots library.

Let us end this section by pointing the reader toward a number of other clustering methods available in **R**. The cluster package contains a number of useful programs including pam() which performs K-means using a variety of metrics more robust than the within-group sums of squares. The agnes() program implements the popular unweighted pair group method with arithmetic mean algorithm. The clara() algorithm (also in cluster) uses a faster algorithm than pam() and is useful for large data sets. The `diana()` algorithm begins with all observations in a single cluster and successively peels away until each cluster contains only one item. The `fanny()` routine estimates a probability each observation belongs to every cluster, rather than strictly assigning membership to only one cluster.

Neural networks assume there are unobservable, intermediate models within the observed data. The self-organizing tree algorithm `sota()` in the `clValid` library uses neural networks. The self-organizing maps program `som()`, in the `kohonen` library, is useful for visualizing high-dimensional data and plotting in two dimensions.

A variety of clustering metrics have also been proposed. Many of these are discussed at length in the documentation for the `clValid` library in **R**. *Connectivity* is a measure of the number of "nearest neighbors" of each observation and counts how many of these occur in the same cluster partition. An algorithm for nearest neighbor clustering is given in Exercise 11.21.

The usual jackknife deletes individual observations (or rows of a `data.frame`) to assess variances or other properties of statistics measured on the full data set. Various stability measures of clustering that are discussed in the `clValid` documentation propose deleting variables (`data.frame` columns) of the data. Among these measures are the *average distance* between observations fitted in the same cluster with the full data and then, with a column of data omitted. Similarly, the *average distance between means* measures the changes in cluster means when individual columns of data are omitted.

It is also possible to include biological information about clusters. Information about the functional class of the genetic markers in the `mouse` data, for example, should be included in any clustering of these markers. Some markers belong to more than one functional class. Measures of statistical clustering incorporating such biological information include the *biological stability index* and the *biological homogeneity index*, both available in the `clValid` library.

11.4   Clustering Application: Image Processing

This is an example of a data analysis where we wouldn't normally anticipate seeing data. When you take a digital photo with a camera or cell phone, the image is converted into millions of tiny pixels, each with its own unique color. These pixels are displayed together and we see the resultant picture. There are popular software packages making it possible to enhance the colors, delete unwanted features, and change the background. As a natural extension of clustering, in this section, we show how a photographic image containing millions of data points can be greatly reduced in size and complexity yet still retain much of the original fidelity.

The code in Output 11.4 uses the `OpenImageR` library to read a `.jpg` file and display it in **R**. In this case, we will use a photo the author took with his cell phone. The image is stored as a three-dimensional $2376 \times 2393 \times 3$ matrix, or over 17 million double precision numbers in **R**. The call to the `resizeImage` program

Output 11.4 Code to read an image, display it, and change the resolution to fewer pixels. The two images produced by this code appear in Fig. 11.14

```
library(OpenImageR)                      #  image processing package
original <- readImage("Dog.jpg")         #  original cell phone image
imageShow(original)                       #  display it in R
dim(original)                             #  it is a large 3-dim matrix

[1] 2376 2393    3

fewer <- resizeImage(original, 200, 200, method = 'bilinear')
dim(fewer)                                #  expressed in fewer pixels

[1] 200 200    3

imageShow(fewer)                          #  lower resolution display
fewer[1 : 5, 1, ]                         #  look at color in pixels

           [,1]         [,2]          [,3]
[1,]  0.6891035  0.61067216  0.17144000
[2,]  0.5721075  0.48489176  0.27579373
[3,]  0.1397757  0.09216784  0.03740314
[4,]  0.2146855  0.15949490  0.08461176
[5,]  0.6457137  0.54283137  0.25699608
```

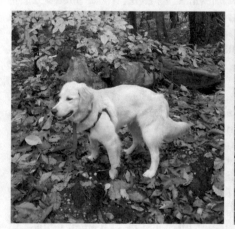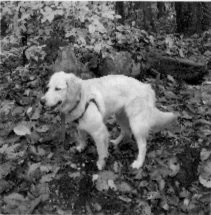

Figure 11.14 Original photo on the *left* and reduced resolution image with the number of pixels reduced to about 0.7%, produced by the **R** code in Output 11.4

reduces this image to a $200 \times 200 \times 3$ matrix with 120,000 entries, a reduction to about 0.7% of the original size. This size reduction makes our clustering experiment much more manageable.

The original photo and the reduced resolution image are displayed in Fig. 11.14. The image with a reduced number of pixels is slightly grainy but otherwise little has been lost in this large reduction in the amount of information needed to store and display the photo. In order to apply clustering methods and further reduce the size of the image, we next need to describe how this image is stored.

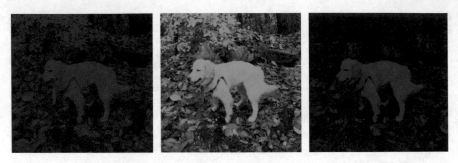

Figure 11.15 Photo separated into its RGB component colors

If we look again at Output 11.4, we see the image is stored as a three-dimensional array. The first two indexes refer to the (x, y) address of each individual pixel, with addressing starting from the upper-left corner of the image. The third index of the image matrix describes the color of the pixel, represented in three columns of values.

Every color is expressed as three continuous values. These specify how much red, green, and blue go into this color, often abbreviated as RGB. These three separate components of color are sometimes called *channels*. The three columns of values in Output 11.4 can be treated as any other numerical values and studied or altered to change the image. As an example, we can marginally examine each of these three columns of values individually by zeroing out the other two. This results in the three separate images appearing in Fig. 11.15.

Think of the individual color channels in Fig. 11.15 as three marginal distributions. We can also draw histograms of the overall distributions of red, green, and blue in the pixels of the photos. These are given in Fig. 11.16.

Overall, there is an even distribution of red (earth-tones) across the photo. The green also gives us browns and yellow for the leaves. Most of the pixels have very low levels of blue and this is reflected in its strongly biased distribution.

Consider the three-dimensional values for colors as sampled from a small number of discrete categories or clusters. We can now apply K-means to cluster these different colors in the original photo. Every pixel then belongs to one of a small number of color clusters.

The eight colors and their relative frequencies are expressed in Fig. 11.17. The four most common clusters are rather similar earth-tones. Their similarity made the K-means clustering difficult and produced warnings (not given here) indicating the failure of the algorithm to converge. This necessitated the use of several random starting values to obtain convergence. Different starting values were performed using the `nstart = 10` option in Output 11.5. This difficulty to converge indicates a smaller number of colors (clusters) may be appropriate.

The resulting photo with fewer pixels and color palette appears in Fig. 11.17. Compared to the original `.jpg` image, this is reminiscent of an early, inexpensive cell phone image. The dog's orange collar is now yellow, like the leaves, for example. Even so, this new image represents a huge reduction in the amount of data needed to represent the photo.

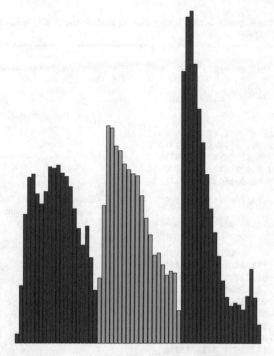

Figure 11.16 Histograms of the RGB components in the pixels of the photo

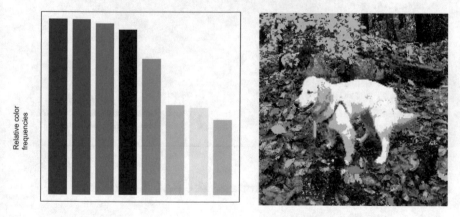

Figure 11.17 K-means clustering into eight colors and the frequencies of each color

Output 11.5 Perform K-means on the image colors, replace the colors with cluster centers, and print the image in K colors

```
fewer.vect <- apply(fewer, 3,as.vector)  #  express image as a matrix
dim(fewer.vect)                          #  how big is it?

[1] 40000      3

fewer.vect[1:4, ]                                 #  see how the image is stored

          [,1]         [,2]          [,3]
[1,] 0.6891035 0.61067216 0.17144000
[2,] 0.5721075 0.48489176 0.27579373
[3,] 0.1397757 0.09216784 0.03740314
[4,] 0.2146855 0.15949490 0.08461176

dog.df <- as.data.frame(fewer.vect)      #  data frame for K-means
K <- 8                                   #  K-means: how many colors?
dog.k <- kmeans(dog.df, centers = K, nstart = 10)
dog.k$centers                            #  the K colors

          V1          V2          V3
1 0.7569583 0.71328493 0.65519253
2 0.6407123 0.55007712 0.45153567
3 0.2850400 0.19915888 0.12463532
4 0.5531898 0.43202167 0.29309464
5 0.9070588 0.89874709 0.87380404
6 0.7992250 0.69439013 0.17196018
7 0.1509825 0.09570056 0.05445707
8 0.4306363 0.31083674 0.19331394

reduced <- dog.k$centers[dog.k$cluster, ] #  replace colors with centroids
reduced[1:6, ]                            #  look at a few

          V1          V2          V3
6 0.7992250 0.69439013 0.17196018
4 0.5531898 0.43202167 0.29309464
7 0.1509825 0.09570056 0.05445707
3 0.2850400 0.19915888 0.12463532
4 0.5531898 0.43202167 0.29309464
6 0.7992250 0.69439013 0.17196018

dim(reduced) <- c(200, 200, 3)           #  back to 3-dimensional matrix
imageShow(reduced)                       #  draw image in K colors
```

11.5   Gaussian Mixture Model and the EM Algorithm

In   the Gaussian mixture model (GMM), every cluster is expressed as a multivariate normal population with different means and variance matrices. As with K-means clustering, we need to specify the number of clusters, but we will illustrate tools to help in making this choice. A big difference between GMM and K-means is the use of the EM algorithm, used to estimate the multivariate parameters.

Every individual has a probability of belonging to each of the multivariate normal distributions. The membership probability allows us to express our uncertainty of the clustering output. In GMM, the EM algorithm estimates the percent of the member-

Output 11.6 Obtain AIC and BIC for burger data in order to judge the number of GMM clusters

```
library(ClusterR)
burger <- read.table("burger.txt", header =TRUE, row.names = 1)
burger

    CalFat  Cal Fat SatFat Sodium Carbs Protein
  1    612 1050  68     21   1750    53      55
  2   1197 2120 133     38   4200   139      65


         .   .   .   .   .   .

 38    440 1010  49     19   2190    91      52
 39    690 1120  76     28   1670    66      45
cbur <- center_scale(burger, mean_center = TRUE,
                     sd_scale = TRUE)  # centered and scaled burgers
burgerAIC <- Optimal_Clusters_GMM(cbur, max_clusters = 10, criterion = "AIC",
                                  dist_mode = "maha_dist")
burgerBIC <- Optimal_Clusters_GMM(cbur, max_clusters = 10, criterion = "BIC",
                                  dist_mode = "maha_dist")
```

ship in each cluster as well as the multivariate normal parameters for each cluster. We will see that the membership probabilities usually indicate observations belonging to a single cluster with very little uncertainty. Instead, these probabilities aid in the estimation process using the EM algorithm. In this section, we give a simple use of GMM and then delve into the details of the EM method.

Let us begin with an examination of the nutritional data on hamburgers, given in Table 1.6. There are seven nutritional values for each of 39 different hamburgers. Output 11.6 reads the data, normalizes the values to mean zero and variance one in each column, and then fits GMM models with up to 10 clusters using two different criteria.

As with any program, always print out the data and make sure it was correctly read into **R**. The `center_scale` program creates standardized values with zero means and unit variances. The `Optimal_Clusters_GMM` program fits up to 10 clusters using Mahalanobis distance between observations and their estimated multivariate normal means. We could also use Euclidean distance, which would be appropriate if the different nutritional measures were uncorrelated.

The available metrics for measuring the quality of clustering are either the Akaike information criterion (AIC) and the Bayesian information criterion (BIC). These two measures are the log-likelihood with a different penalty for every parameter added to the model. Specifically,

$$\text{AIC} = -2 \, \text{Log Likelihood} + 2p$$

and

$$\text{BIC} = -2 \, \text{Log Likelihood} + p \, \log(N)$$

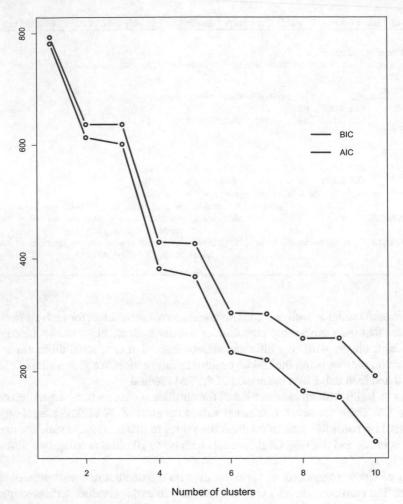

Figure 11.18   AIC and BIC for different cluster sizes using GMM clustering

where p is the number of parameters and N is the sample size.

The values of AIC and BIC are plotted in Fig. 11.18. This graphical diagnostic serves the same role as the screeplot, used in Chap. 8 to decide on the number of principal components.

The AIC and BIC statistics are different in value but tell a similar story in Fig. 11.18. There is a large benefit going from one cluster to two. Little is gained between two and three clusters. Similarly, four clusters are much better than three but five has little improvement over four.

A basic **R** code to fit the GMM model and plot the clusters is given in Output 11.7. The GMM program fits the model with a specified number of multivariate

Output 11.7   Fit and plot GMM with two clusters

```
gmm <- GMM(cbur, gaussian_comps = 2, dist_mode = "maha_dist")
pr <- predict_GMM(cbur, gmm$centroids, gmm$covariance_matrices, gmm$weights)
plot(burger, gap = 0, col = pr$cluster_labels)
```

components. The `predict_GMM` program provides cluster membership labels in `$cluster_labels`.

Figure 11.19 plots the results of two and four clusters obtained using GMM. The standout (in *green*) with four clusters is the group with a single member corresponding to the one burger with extreme levels of several nutritional values. Output 11.2 is an illustration in **R** of how to plot different matrix scatter plots values in the same `pairs` figure.

This covers the basic fitting of GMM in **R**. Let us next explain how the model is fitted with an explanation of the EM algorithm. The expectation–maximization (EM) algorithm was popularized by Dempster et al. (1977) as a method for imputation of missing or unobservable values in data analysis. Briefly, the method specifically

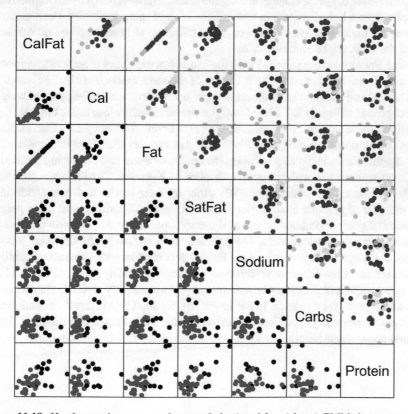

Figure 11.19   Hamburger data expressed as two (below) and four (above) GMM clusters

applied to clustering alternates between estimating the probability of group membership and then estimating the multivariate normal parameters of those groups. In this section, we used the `ClusteR` package in **R** to illustrate GMM. We next work out an example in detail to explain the details of EM.

Let us return to the US state cancer rate data in Table 11.8. Exercise 11.14 used K-means to demonstrate there were probably two cluster groups in these data. Let us continue to assume there are two groups and apply the EM clustering method to fit GMM.

We begin by assigning probability weights w_i and $1 - w_i$ each state belonging to one of the two clusters. These should not all be initialized to exactly 1/2 but values close to 1/2 are necessary to make this algorithm work correctly. See Exercise 11.17 for details.

Given weights, we use maximum likelihood to estimate the means and variances of the separate normal populations. This is the "M" or maximum likelihood step.

Given these estimates for the parameters of the normal populations, we replace the weights for each state's membership with the respective likelihoods of belonging to each population. This is the "E" or expectation step.

The program in **R** is not long and given in Output 11.8. Output 11.8 begins with a K-means to identify two clusters among the states. The weights (`wt`) are initialized as samples from a beta distribution with means 1/2 and small variances. For a given set of weights, the M-step uses these weights to calculate weighted means and variances using the `cov.wt()` function in **R**.

Next, the weights are replaced with the respective multivariate normal likelihoods, calculated with `dmvnorm` in the **R** library of the same name. This is the E-step.

These E and M-steps are alternated eight times and the resulting sets of weights w_i are plotted in Fig. 11.20. The 51 weights are all initially close to 1/2 but after eight iterations, these have all converged to either zero or one. The weights in Fig. 11.20 are color-coded, corresponding to the two different clusters identified using K-means. Clearly, there is little overlap between the results of these two clustering methods.

Let us contrast this with the approach taken by K-means. The K-means clustering method of Sect. 11.2 assumes clusters differ by their means and every individual is a member of just one cluster. The GMM clustering method is both more general in terms of group membership and at the same time restrictive because clusters are expressed in parametric models. The populations identified by the Gaussian mixture model will generally overlap because the clusters have larger estimated variability.

The results of the different clustering approaches are readily apparent in Fig. 11.21. The upper-right half illustrates how K-means seeks to identify separate clusters in the top row of plots, for example. In the lower left, we see GMM identifies overlapping multivariate normal populations, each with different means and variances. These normal populations identified by GMM overlap as do the members in each.

Output 11.8 R code to perform EM Gaussian mixture clustering for two groups of states' cancer rates. Results are compared with K-means in Fig. 11.21

```
cc <- kmeans(cancer, centers = 2)        # K-means cluster with 2 groups
cc$cluster                               # initially, every state
                                         # membership

AL AK AZ AR CA CO CT DE DC FL GA HI ID IL IN IA KS KY LA ME MD MA MI MN MS MO MT
 1  1  2  1  2  2  1  1  2  2  1  2  1  2  1  1  1  1  1  1  1  1  2  1  1  1  1
NE NV NH NJ NM NY NC ND OH OK OR PA RI SC SD TN TX UT VT VA WA WV WI WY
 1  2  1  1  2  1  1  1  1  1  1  2  1  1  1  1  1  2  2  1  2  1  1  1  2

library(mvtnorm)                         # for multivariate normal
                                         # functions
wt <- rbeta(dim(cancer)[1], 1e5, 1e5)    # initialize weights
estep <- t(wt)                           # initialize list of E-step
                                         # weights
reps <- 8                                # number of iterations
for(i in 1 : reps) {
  M1 <- cov.wt(cancer, wt, center = TRUE)    # M-step: Weighted means and
                                             # vars
  M2 <- cov.wt(cancer, 1 - wt, center = TRUE)
                                         # two likelihoods
  L1 <- dmvnorm(cancer, mean = M1$center, sigma = M1$cov)
  L2 <- dmvnorm(cancer, mean = M2$center, sigma = M2$cov)
  wt <- wt * L1 / (wt * L1 + (1 - wt) * L2) # E-step: update weights
  estep <- rbind(estep, wt)                  # save the weights at each E-step
}                                        # end of E-M loop
                                         # plot the weights: Fig. 12.3
plot((0 : reps), xlim = c(0, reps), ylim = c(0, 1), type = "n",
    xlab = "Iteration number", ylab = "Estimated weights", cex.lab = 1.25)
for(i in 1: dim(estep)[2]) {
  lines( 0 : reps, estep[, i], type = "l", lwd = 2,
        col = c("red", "blue")[cc$cluster[i]]) }
                                         # draw the clusters: Fig. 12.4
up <- function(x,y){points(x, y, col = c("tomato", "peachpuff")[cc$cluster],
        pch = 19, cex = 1.5) }
down <- function(x,y) { points(x, y, pch = 19, cex = 1.5,
                col = c("seagreen", "steelblue2")[1 + round(estep[reps, ]) ])}
pairs(cancer[,c(1:3, 9:12)], gap = 0, upper.panel = up, lower.panel = down)
```

11.6 DBscan

Unlike K-means or Gaussian mixture models, DBscan does not require us to specify the number of clusters to be generated. Instead, we must specify the minimum number of members of each cluster along with a maximum relative size for each cluster. The name DBscan is shorthand for *density-based clustering of applications with noise*. Similarly, the output of DBscan is the identification of clusters and their members. Data points not falling into any of these clusters are classified as outliers. DBscan can find any shape of clusters: these do not have to be convex shapes. The clusters are identified by nearest neighbor clustering. Objects within the same cluster must

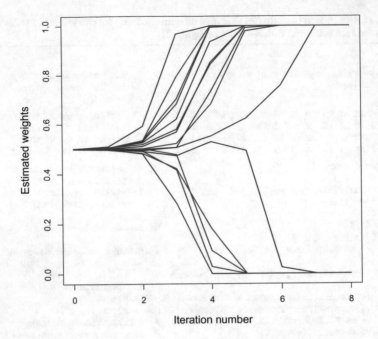

Figure 11.20   Estimated weights w_i for each iteration of the EM clustering of the US states' cancer rates. The colors correspond to the two groups identified using K-means clustering

be density-accessible, explained later in this section. A good reference for DBscan is Hahsler et al. (2019).

We will illustrate DBscan using the baseball team data given in Table 11.2. The attendance numbers and salaries are very large so we replaced these values with their logarithms. In Output 11.9, we examine three different cluster sizes. The *dbscan* program (in the **R** library of the same name) prints a summary of the clusters found and the number of observations in each. The number of outliers is aggregated in the "0" category.

The eps parameter sets the size of the clustering window. Output 11.9 demonstrates dbscan using the eps parameter values of 2, 5, and 7 with the baseball team data. These values were chosen using trial and error until we obtained a reasonable clustering summary. The output of dbscan for the value of eps = 2 is summarized as two small clusters and many outliers. The value of eps = 5 yields two clusters with fewer outliers. Finally, eps = 7 gives us one large cluster with a single outlier. We will continue to work with the middle of these three choices (eps = 5) in this example.

In every trial value of eps, we also specified a minimum cluster size minPts = 3. Similarly, different values of minPts will change the outcome. See Exercise 11.18 for more details.

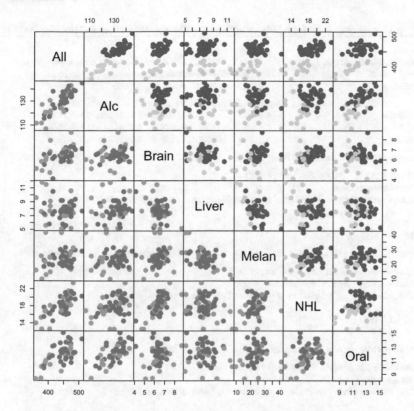

Figure 11.21 US states fitted into two cancer rate clusters. The upper half used K-means and the lower are Gaussian mixture model clusters fitted using EM

The league and division values are omitted in Fig. 11.22 because these are binary-valued and did not present much use in clustering. Similarly, losses and rank are determined by the number of games won and are omitted as well. The two clusters appear in *red*: high number of games won and *green*: high lost games. In this figure, we see the teams' number of wins is related to both at-home and away attendance as well, but not their salary figures. The points in *black* are considered as outliers by DBscan. These outliers are five teams with either the very best or the very worst records.

In the *dbscan* package, there is an implementation of other clustering algorithms and diagnostics. One of these is the HDBscan, a DBscan algorithm with simplified usage. Specifically, HDBscan estimates the value of the eps parameter for us. The downside, of course, is we lose some of the control of the process, as we saw by varying the cluster sizes in Output 11.9.

A useful diagnostic is called the *local outlier factor,* (or *lof*) which is a measure of how far each observation is located from the center of the cluster. A similar diagnostic is referred to as optics or its reachability. These are different concepts and will be explained below. Briefly, two objects may be physically located close together but are also separated by a region of low density.

Output 11.9 **R** code to perform DBscan clustering of baseball team data and produce Fig. 11.22

```
library(dbscan)
bb <- read.table(file = "baseball_teams.txt", header = T, row.names = 1)
bb[ ,6:8] <- log(bb[ , 6:8])  # scale attendance and salary values
bb[1:3, ]                     #  examine some of these

         league division rank wins losses  HomeAtt  AwayAtt   salary
NYMets        1        1    1  108     54 14.83349 14.59328 13.17476
Phi           1        1    2   86     75 14.47476 14.35850 13.20105
StL           1        1    3   79     82 14.72053 14.34363 13.00594

dbscan(bb, eps = 2, minPts = 3) #  Two small clusters, mostly outliers

DBSCAN clustering for 26 objects.
Parameters: eps = 2, minPts = 3
The clustering contains 2 cluster(s) and 16 noise points.

 0  1  2
16  5  5

(db <- dbscan(bb, eps = 5, minPts = 3)) #  two clusters, some outliers

DBSCAN clustering for 26 objects.
Parameters: eps = 5, minPts = 3
The clustering contains 2 cluster(s) and 5 noise points.

 0  1  2
 5  9 12

dbscan(bb, eps = 7, minPts = 3) #  one large cluster

DBSCAN clustering for 26 objects.
Parameters: eps = 7, minPts = 3
The clustering contains 1 cluster(s) and 1 noise points.

 0  1
 1 25

pairs(bb[, -1:-2], col = db$cluster + 1, gap = 0, xaxt = "n", yaxt = "n",
      pch = 19, cex = 2)              #  Produce Fig. 12.5
```

In Fig. 11.23, we plot the HDBscan clustering of the baseball teams where the size of the figures represents *lof* and the density of color is its reachability. The **R** code to produce this figure is given in Output 11.10.

In order to describe the DBscan algorithm and the concept of reachability, consider the clustering of simulated data given in Fig. 11.24. In this simulated example, DBscan identifies two clusters. The observations within both clusters are closely located to other members of their cluster but the two clusters are also separated by a region of low density. In contrast, the K-means run on the same data is unable to identify these types of clusters. This figure will help illustrate the concept of reachability, described next.

To describe the DBscan algorithm and how it is able to identify clusters, let us recall the parameters we need to specify to the dbscan program, as in Output 11.9. Specifically, there is a eps parameter to determine the maximum core size and the minPts parameter to restrict the minimum number of observations in each cluster.

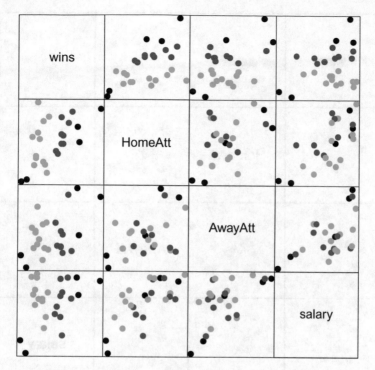

Figure 11.22 DBScan for baseball teams

Output 11.10 R code to perform HDBscan clustering of baseball team data and produce Fig. 11.23

```
hdb <- hdbscan(bb, minPts = 3)          #  hierarchical DBscan
lof <- lof(bb, minPts = 3)              #  local outlier factor
opt <- optics(bb, eps = 5, minPts = 3) #  reachability
opt <- extractDBSCAN(opt, eps_cl = 5)
colors <- mapply(function(col, i) adjustcolor(col,
           alpha.f = hdb$membership_prob[i]),
           palette()[hdb$cluster + 1], seq_along(hdb$cluster))
plot(bb[, -c(1:3, 5)], col=colors, pch=20, gap = 0, cex = 2*lof^2.5,
     xaxt = "n", yaxt = "n" )
```

Observations are classified as being of one of three types: core, border, or outlier. These are classified in terms of the number of neighboring points within eps distance. Specifically,

- A *core point* is a point with at least minPts neighbors within a distance of less than eps.
- A *border point* is located within eps of a core point but has fewer than minPts neighbors at a distance of eps.
- An *outlier* is neither a core or border point.

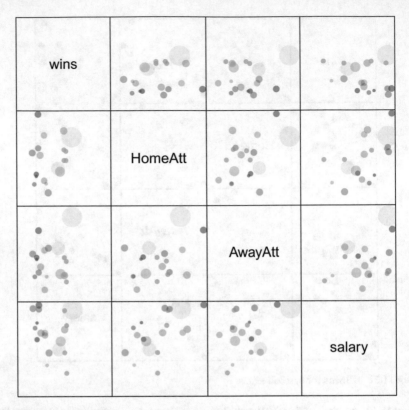

Figure 11.23 DBScan diagnostics for baseball data: each figure size is *lof* and color density is reachability. The outliers have been omitted

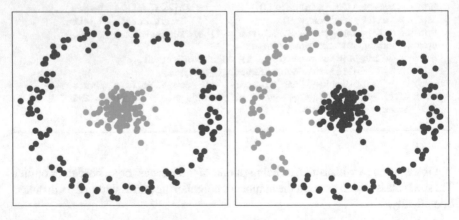

Figure 11.24 DBScan on simulated data (*left*) and K-Means clustering on the same data (*right*)

Briefly, a core point is in a data-dense region, with many neighbors, in the interior of a cluster. An outlier is located in a sparse region with few neighbors and none of these are core points. Border points have few neighbors but at least one of these is a core point.

The BDscan algorithm builds clusters by connecting contiguous, dense regions containing core points. Specifically, a pair of core points are said to be density-accessible or reachable if there is a sequence of core points within eps of each other connecting these. Border points are accessible only if they are at the end of one such sequence, but not the middle. Such reachable sequences of eps sized regions define the DCscan clusters.

In the example of Fig. 11.24, we see two clusters defined by data-dense regions separated by low-density, sparse regions which are not reachable. This ability to create non-convex cluster regions is a clear advantage of DBscan over other methods such as K-means. In contrast, for massive data sets, DBscan will run much slower than K-means. A disadvantage to DBscan is the specification of the eps and minPts parameters. In Exercise 11.18, we examine how their mis-specification can lead to strikingly different conclusions.

11.7 Exercises

11.1 How critical are the use of scaling and choice of distance metric in hierarchical clustering? (See Exercise 11.14 for the effect of scaling on K-means.)

   a. Try different distance metrics on the iris data. Do these do better or worse than the plot in Fig. 11.2?
   b. Redraw Fig. 11.1 without using scale to transform the data columns to the same variances. Has the scaled figure changed? Which figure is easier to interpret: scaled or unscaled? Explain your reasoning. Try different distance metrics. Do these yield very different appearing dendrograms?

11.2 Look at the swiss data examined in Chap. 6 using clustering methods. Is there evidence some cantons were making the demographic transition sooner than others?

11.3 Table 11.5 lists the annual returns to investors (as of Sept., 2010) of government bonds, listed by duration and issuer. These returns are influenced by the respective rates of inflation and strengths of the various currencies as well as market perceptions for these rates into the future. Perform a hierarchical cluster of these returns to identify countries with similar financial situations. Comment on how the dendrogram clusters countries in similar geographic regions, as well.

11.4 Repeat the example summarized in Fig. 11.9. What happens when the sample means are much further apart?

Table 11.5 Government bond returns by issuer and duration

Issuer	1mo	3mo	6mo	8mo	1yr	3yr	5yr
USGovt	1.88	4.45	6.37	8.39	7.97	7.68	5.94
AustAsia	−0.19	9.47	4.94	5.52	13.93	10.46	9.13
Canada	2.22	3.98	5.48	7.30	7.07	7.27	5.20
Eurozone	2.42	2.73	4.30	5.92	6.55	6.92	4.11
Japan	0.66	2.20	3.08	3.14	3.94	3.01	2.04
Switzerland	2.18	2.89	5.06	6.64	8.59	7.00	3.61
UK	4.70	6.12	10.35	10.69	8.69	9.01	5.99

Source © 2010 Morningstar, Inc., Morningstar Bond Market
Commentary, September, 2010. All Rights Reserved
Used with permission

11.5 The `coleman` data set in the `robustbase` library lists summary statistics for 20 different schools in the northeast US. The six variables measured on each school include demographic information (such as percent of white-collar fathers) and characteristics of each school (such as staff salaries per pupil). Read the help file of `coleman` for the complete list of demographics and references to others' analyses of these data.

    a. A suggested analysis is a regression model explaining the mean verbal score of all sixth graders.

    b. Perform a hierarchical cluster of these data using all explanatory variables. Is there evidence of different types of schools?

    c. Similarly, does a K-means clustering provide evidence of different types of schools?

    d. Which of these four types of statistical analyses seems most appropriate for the data? Is there strong evidence there are no clusters? What might such data look like?

11.6 Try some other examinations of the `milk` data. First omit the suspected outlier (observation #70) and `scale` the data.

    a. Perform the K-means clustering and plot the first two principal components by color of cluster membership.

    b. Read about the `pam()` program in `cluster` library. The syntax is similar to that of `kmeans`, but `pam()` is more robust against outliers and has a useful display of the clusters. Describe the influence the outlier (observation #70) has on this algorithm when it is re-introduced to the data.

11.7   a. Show how we can assign statistical significance to the Jaccard Index. Suppose we have a finite-sized population containing n items. One sampling method identifies m of these items and a different, independent method identifies m' items. Let X denote the random variable counting the number of items common to both samples. Identify the distribution of X.

b. Suppose the set S is completely contained in the set T. What are the largest and smallest possible values of $J(S, T)$? Comment on the suitability of J as a measure of agreement.

c. Suppose the set Σ contains $2n$ items and the partitions $X = \{x_1, x_2\}$ and $Y = \{y_1, y_2\}$ are both composed of two sets of sets, each containing n items. When n is large, what are the largest and smallest values of $\text{Rand}(X, Y)$?

d. Suppose x_1 and y_1 of the previous question both contain only one item, then what is the range of $\text{Rand}(X, Y)$?

e. Compare the Dunn Index with the F-ratio used to assess statistical significance in a one-way analysis of variance.

11.8 Examine the `lung` data set in the `pvclust` library. This data has gene expression on 916 genes for 72 human lung tissues, including 67 lung tumors. See how much of the analysis of Sect. 11.3 you can repeat on this much larger data set. How many clusters of genes do you estimate? What evidence do you use to support this claim?

11.9 The Older Americans Act (OAA) is a federal program begun in 1965 to provide social services and nutritional assistance to senior citizens. Table 11.6 lists the percent composition of people served in each state. Examine these data using hierarchical clustering methods. Are there unusual groups of states? Do geographically similar states cluster together?

11.10 Simulate the Dunn Index in the `mouse` data under a model of no clustering.

a. Specifically, generate bootstrap samples by separately generating random columns of genetic marker values. Calculate the Dunn Index on each sample, draw a histogram of these values, and compare these to the index on

Table 11.6 Composition of seniors served by the OAA, Title III in 2011

State	Percentage			
	Poverty	Minority	Poverty and Minority	Rural
AL	9	28	3	26
AK	39	34	21	80
AZ	26	42	16	48
⋮	⋮	⋮	⋮	⋮
WI	22	6	3	70
WY	18	3	1	73
US Total	30	25	11	37

Source US Department of Health & Human Services, Administration on Aging

the original value. Comment on this figure. What evidence does the Dunn Index provide of the validity of $K = 3$ clusters in the original data?

b. Can you give a possible explanation for the bimodal distribution of the simulated Dunn Index appearing in Fig. 11.12?

11.11 The `car90` data frame in the `rpart` library cites an article from 1990 *Consumer Reports* on 34 measurements on 111 different car models. There are many *NA*'s in these data, so you might want to use the `complete.cases` command to eliminate those cars with incomplete data.

a. Use K-means clustering to identify groups of similar cars. What is an appropriate value of K? What are the defining characteristics of these car groups?

b. Consider recursive partitioning methods to classify the reliability measurement. Reliability is coded using the ordered categories:

much worse < worse < average < better < much better

Use a regression tree approach to identify those variables associated with the most and least reliable cars. Briefly, which types of cars appear to have the most and least problems?

11.12 The data frame `wpbc` in the `TH.data` library contains 34 measurements on the tumors of 198 women with breast cancer treated in a clinic in Wisconsin.

a. Examine these data using K-means and estimate how many different tumor types there are in these data.

b. The `help` file for this data frame contains a list of suggested regressions. These can be fitted to model different response variables. Examine one of these models using a regression tree approach. How well does the regression tree coincide with the K-means approach you found in part a.?

11.13 Table 11.7 lists the largest oil companies and their production statistics for 2006 and the change from 2005.

a. Use hierarchical clustering to show Gazprom, the world's largest producer of natural gas, is very different from the other companies in this table. Without GASPROM, the oil companies cluster into three distinct groups.

b. Apply K-means or other methods to demonstrate the clustering pattern of these companies. Figure 11.25 is an example.

11.14 Table 11.8 lists cancer cases and deaths in 2016 for each of the 50 US states and DC. (U.S. Cancer Statistics working Group, 2019). The "Alcohol" heading is a risk factor for six combined categories of cancer-related diseases: mouth and throat, voice box (larynx), esophagus, colon and rectum, liver, and breast (in women). Similarly, there is some overlap and correlation in this table.

a. Use K-means and try to identify different types of states. Build a figure, similar to Fig. 11.10 to see how many different groups of states there are.

Table 11.7 Reserves and production of global oil companies

Company	Reserves (MM boe)	Current Years of Production	2006 Oil & Gas Production	
			Amount	% Change
BP	17,368	10.4	3,926	−1.9
ChevronTexaco	11,020	10.9	2,667	6.1
ExxonMobil	21,518	11.3	4,238	3.8
Royal Dutch Shell	11,108	6.7	3,474	−1.0
Hess	1,243	7.9	358	7.0
BG Group	2,149	6.2	601	19.0
ConocoPhillips	6,676	8.7	2,359	29.7
ENI	6,406	11.2	1,770	5.8
Marathon	1,262	7.1	377	9.0
Norsk-Hydro	1,916	9.3	573	2.0
Petro-Canada	1,301	8.4	345	−3.1
Repsol YPF	2,600	5.2	1,128	−3.0
Petrobras	11,458	14.2	2,287	4.5
CNOOC	503	3.0	455	11.7
Gazprom	144,668	39.7	9,965	6.0
LUKOIL	18,144	27.2	1,838	4.5
PetroChina	16,260	15.6	2,907	5.0

Figure 11.25 Clustering of oil-producing companies

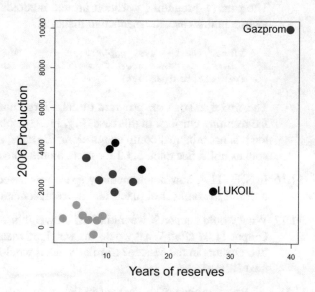

Table 11.8 Cancer incidence in US states

State	All	Alcohol	Brain	⋯	Thyroid	Bladder
AL	457.8	138.9	6.3	⋯	10.1	17.5
AK	405.8	121.9	7.9	⋯	12.4	19.3
⋮	⋮	⋮	⋮		⋮	⋮
WI	458.6	129.2	6.8	⋯	14.0	21.8
WY	402.3	117.1	6.6	⋯	15.7	18.5

Source https://gis.cdc.gov/Cancer/USCS/DataViz.html

    b. Show part (a.) identifies two types of states. Plot these clusters using `pairs()` to illustrate K-means has identified those states with high and low overall cancer rates.

    c. Repeat part (a.) after using `scale()` to normalize all cancer types to have the same variances across the various states. Show the percent variability measure in K-means is highly dependent on the different variances.

11.15 K-means minimizes the sum of squares within each of the clusters. There are generalizations to any of the other distances described in Sect. 11.1. Specifically, K-medoids are similar to K-means but minimize the sum of distances within each cluster.

The `pam()` program ("partition around medoids") allows you to choose a metric, in this case, the manhattan distance:

```
library(factoextra, ggplot2, fpc)
pam.out <- pam(cancer, 2, metric = "manhattan", stand = FALSE)
fviz_cluster(pam.out)
```

The `fviz_cluster` program offers a large number of options to display the resulting clusters. In this case, Fig. 11.26 displays K=2 state clusters plotted against principal components along the axes, enclosed in their respective convex hulls. See Sect. 3.3.2 for more on the convex hull.

11.16 In Sect. 11.4, how much memory space was saved by reducing the image in terms of the number of pixels and the representation of colors?

11.17 What would happen if we initialized all weights $w_i = 1/2$ in the program in Output 11.8? *Hint:* What would the weighted means and variances be for the two clusters in the M-step? Similarly, what would the new weights be at the next E-step?

11.18   a. Examine the `milk` data set in the `robustbase` library using DBscan. Other clustering results of these data are also given in Fig. 11.7 where we

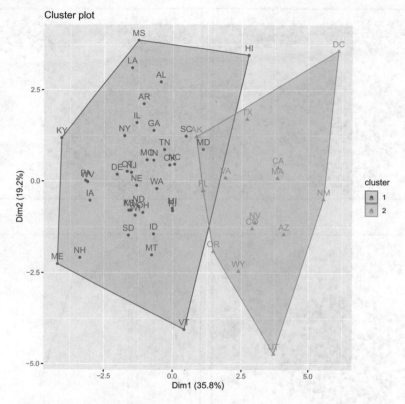

Figure 11.26 K-Medoid clusters of state cancer rates

noted an unusual outlier. Try different values of the eps and minPts
parameters. Are there combinations of these parameters producing a small
number of reasonable-sized clusters with not too many outliers? Is DBscan
a suitable tool for these data? Comment.

b. As in part a., examine the mouse genetic marker data in the clValid
library. Use DBscan and identify suitable cluster sizes and minimum
members. Look at a pairs plot in **R** to plot the clusters identified by
DBscan. Notice how all of the markers are highly correlated. Is clustering
an appropriate approach to summarize these data?

11.19 Use DBscan to cluster the iris data in the data sets library. This data is
often chosen to illustrate clustering methods because there are three identified
species. See if you can identify the values of the eps and minPts parameters
yielding three clusters. How well do these clusters correspond to the known
species? Compare your results with those in Fig. 11.2.

11.20 Another clustering algorithm is called the self-updating process or *SUP*. This
method has the advantage over DBscan because it is designed to detect clusters

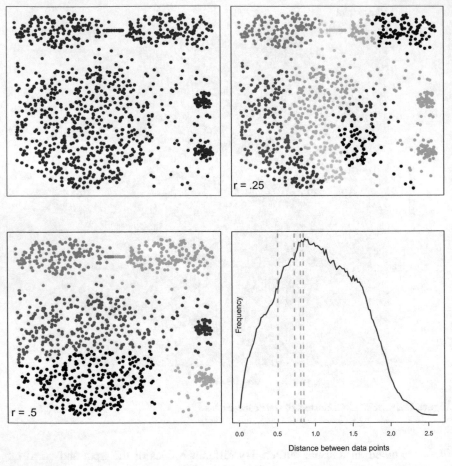

Figure 11.27 Raw data and SUP clustering for $r = .25$ and $r = .5$. The histogram of distances between data points identifies valleys

of different densities. It is similar to the clustering using representatives or *CURE* algorithm. Both of these methods are suitable for the analysis of large data sets.

As an example, the authors of the CURE algorithm proposed the artificial data given in the *upper left* of Fig. 11.27. There are five clusters in this figure: a large diffuse group in the lower left; two dense clusters on the right; and two oblong clusters joined by a small, dense set of points at the top. There are also many outliers not clearly belonging to any of these clusters.

a. The **R** code to produce Fig. 11.27 is given in Output 11.11. Specifically, the **R**code needed is

```
supcl(trial, r = .25)
```

Output 11.11 R code to perform SUP clustering and produce Fig. 11.27

```
library(supc)
trial <- as.matrix(shape)
trial[1:3,]                               #  look at the data


             V1          V2
[1,]  0.3799643 -0.4223201
[2,] -0.3986451 -0.4131589
[3,] -0.4028908  0.2429166

plot(shape)                               #  plot raw data
supc.out <- supc1(trial, r = .25)         #  sup cluster
plot(trial, col= supc.out$cluster)

dshape <- dist(trial)         # Euclidean distances between points
shape.freq <- hist(dshape, breaks = 125, plot = F)
plot(shape.freq$mids, shape.freq$density, type = "l")  # draw histogram
dist.freq <- cbind(dist = shape.freq$mids[-1],
                   freq = shape.freq$count[-1],
                   diff = diff(shape.freq$count))
(valleys <- dist.freq[dist.freq[,3] < 0,]  [1:4, ])

      dist freq diff
[1,] 0.51 6229  -56
[2,] 0.73 7695  -69
[3,] 0.81 8531  -30
[4,] 0.85 8565  -83

abline(v = valleys)                    #  identify valleys in histogram
```

which requires us to specify the r parameter, determining the size of the cluster, similar to the eps parameter we used in DBscan.

Try to identify a suitable value for r in this example. A value of r=.25 breaks apart the single large, diffuse cluster in Fig. 11.27. A larger value of .5 also breaks this cluster but into just two parts. Find a useful value of r in this data example.

b. The authors of the CURE algorithm suggest we look at the histogram of the distances between all possible pairwise pairs of observations. The *valleys* are those distances whose frequencies are lower than those of the next smaller distance. These are computed in Output 11.11 and identified in the histogram in Fig. 11.27. Perhaps, these valleys occur when the outer reaches of dense clusters give rise to sparse regions with lower frequencies. Try the values of the valleys in identifying suitable values of the r parameter. Are these resulting clusters better than the trial-and-error value you identified in part a.?

11.21 Jarvis–Patrick clustering (Jarvis and Patrick 1973) is a simple idea based on nearest neighbor clustering. There are two parameters we need to specify for this method. Initially, for every data point, we need to identify the k other data points closest to it. After identifying the k nearest neighbors of every data

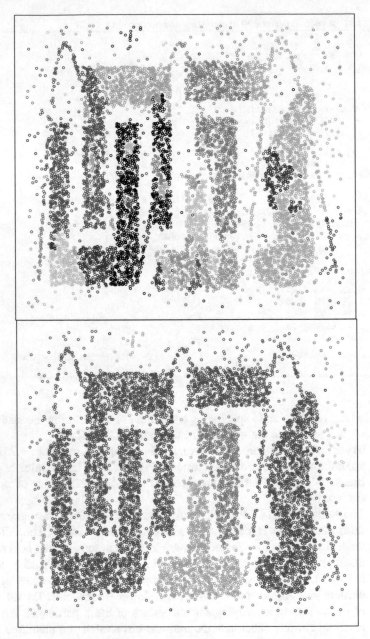

Figure 11.28 Jarvis–Patrick (nearest neighbor) clustering with parameter values k = 15, kt = 10, above, and k = 20, kt = 12, below

Output 11.12 R code to perform nearest neighbor clustering and produce Fig. 11.28

```
library(dbscan)
data(DS3)
cl <- jpclust(DS3, k = 15, kt = 10)
plot(DS3, col = cl$cluster + 1, cex = .5)
```

point, we say two data points share the same cluster if they share at least kt neighbors.

The artificial data DS3 is the dbscan library and is useful for illustrating clustering algorithms. These data consist of several dense clusters, separated by sparse regions. There are also many outliers and a sinusoidal wave crossing over all. An example of nearest neighbor clustering of these data is given in Fig. 11.28. The program to generate this figure is given in Output 11.12.

Run this program with different parameter values of k and kt. The values given in Output 11.12 result in several dense areas being separated from other nearby dense areas. The authors of the software recommend using k = 20 and kt = 12. The resulting clustering using these parameters appears in the lower plot of Fig. 11.28. This later set of parameter values does not identify some of the clusters we see.

Chapter 12
Basic Models for Longitudinal Data

Longitudinal studies is a common form of studies including clinical trials where the treatment effect is visible only after several measurements are made on the same individual over a period of time. This chapter begins with an example of a randomized trial of an experimental medication.

Stanish et al. (1978) summarized a clinical trial of a treatment for a skin condition. Patients with the condition were randomized to either active treatment (88 subjects) or a placebo (84 subjects). Table 12.1 summarizes the frequencies of the follow-up patterns for each of the 172 patients in the trial. Every patient was scheduled to be observed three times after the initial randomization to active or placebo treatment. At each of the three scheduled visits, every patient's skin condition was categorized as:

1: Rapidly improving from previous visit
2: Improving
3: No change
4: Worsening
0: Missed visit

Missed visits are coded as zero (0) in Table 12.1, and we will discuss these again later. The original report also gave a separate category of rapidly worsening (5) we reclassify as worsening (4).

As an example of how to read Table 12.1, the last column shows there were two active treatment patients whose disease condition continually worsened at each of the three visits (the 4–4–4 pattern) and there were 14 placebo subjects with this response pattern. The categorical data in Table 12.1 uses the summary given by Landis et al. (1988). The original article by Stanish et al. gives additional information on the initial severity of the skin condition and at which of six clinics each of the patients was enrolled. We will ignore these additional covariates in our description of this data.

Given the longitudinal, categorical data in Table 12.1, the statistician will be asked if there is a treatment difference. If so, is the active therapy better than the

© Springer Nature Switzerland AG 2022
D. Zelterman, *Applied Multivariate Statistics with R*, Statistics for Biology and Health,
https://doi.org/10.1007/978-3-031-13005-2_12

Table 12.1 Frequency of follow-up patterns in change of skin condition by treatment at each of three follow-up visits. Codes: 0 = missing; 1 = rapidly improving; 2 = improving; 3 = no change; 4 = worsening or rapidly worsening. Source: Stanish et al. (1978)

Visit																	
1	0	0	0	1	1	1	1	2	2	2	2	2	2	2	2	2	3
2	1	3	4	0	1	1	1	0	1	1	1	2	2	2	2	3	0
3	0	2	4	1	0	1	2	1	0	1	3	0	1	2	3	3	0
Frequency:																	
Active	1	1	1	1	2	19	0	1	1	10	1	0	11	10	0	0	3
Placebo	0	0	0	1	1	1	2	0	0	0	0	2	3	5	2	2	0
Visit																	
1	3	3	3	3	3	3	3	3	3	3	4	4	4	4	4	4	4
2	0	0	1	2	2	3	3	3	3	4	0	2	3	3	4	4	4
3	3	4	1	1	2	0	2	3	4	4	0	4	3	4	0	3	4
Frequency:																	
Active	1	0	3	3	6	0	1	4	1	2	2	0	1	0	0	0	2
Placebo	0	1	0	0	0	1	0	9	3	2	6	1	13	2	11	2	14

placebo—and, importantly, what do we mean by "better"? How can we demonstrate a treatment effect and make it apparent to someone without a sophisticated statistical background? More generally, what is an appropriate statistical analysis for longitudinal data such as this?

This all depends on the questions we want to answer. There are two major approaches: marginal and transitional. Unfortunately, each of these approaches do not easily address the questions addressed by the other.

12.1 Marginal Models

The answers to these broad questions are not easy to give but by carefully posing less general, more specific questions, several different summaries of this data will suggest themselves. These analyses fall into two general categories: marginal models and transitional models. We will describe both with regard to the data in Table 12.1. Each of these two types of analyses answers specific questions about the data that, unfortunately, are not easily answered by the other type. We will begin with the marginal model.

A marginal analysis of longitudinal data examines the data separately at each time point. Table 12.2 is a marginal summary of the skin condition data. This table displays the number of individuals categorized by treatment type and clinical evaluation for each of their three scheduled visits. This table can be found using the **R** program in Output 12.1.

Table 12.2 The marginal frequencies of visits categorized by skin condition and each of three scheduled visits. These tables are obtained using the program in Output 12.1

| | Active treatment | | | | Placebo | | | |
| | Visit number | | | | Visit number | | | |
Condition	1	2	3	Total	1	2	3	Total
1	22	37	48	107	5	4	5	14
2	34	30	18	82	14	13	7	34
3	24	8	7	39	16	30	28	74
4	5	5	6	16	49	29	23	101
Missed visit	3	8	9	20	0	8	21	29
Total	88	88	88		84	84	84	

The marginal summary in Table 12.2 can be used to answer questions such as Do active treatment patients experience more improving visits (categories 1 and 2) than the placebo group? Does the proportion of 1's and 2's increase with subsequent visits? Are there more 3's and 4's (no change or worsening) in the placebo patients? Which of the two treatment groups misses more visits? Do missed visits become more common as the study progresses? In other words, without regard to the results of an individual patient's previous history or subsequent visits, a marginal summary of this longitudinal data describes the frequency of classifications of visits for each of the five clinical outcome categories. The units counted in Table 12.2 are visits, not patients.

Answers to the questions posed in the previous paragraph can be obtained from the marginal summary of the data given in Table 12.2. Under the "Total" columns in this table we see most of the active treatment patients' visits were given improving scores (1 or 2) and most of the placebo subjects' visits were classified as no change (3) or worsening (4). The number of rapidly improving (1) visits doubled from 22 to 48 for the active treatment group between the first and third visits but the number of 1's remained small and steady for the placebo group. The number of no change (3) visits decreased from 24 to 7 for the active treatment group and increased from 16 to 28 for the placebo patients. The declining number of worsening (4) visits among placebo patients may be evidence that, when left untreated, the skin condition has a natural tendency to reverse itself.

Mosaic plots such as in Fig. 12.1 are a natural way to display marginal summaries of longitudinal data. The column for each visit is a familiar pie chart except the marginal probabilities are displayed as colored tiles rather than pie slices. The ordered outcomes are listed from best, on top, to worst, ending with missing visits on bottom.

From this figure, we see the patients with the active treatment are observed with a greater fraction of rapidly increasing (1) visits in red. Those patients on the placebo have few of these visits. Instead, the placebo patients have many more no change or worsening visits (2, or 3, in green and blue) and missing visits (lavender, at the

Output 12.1 Program to read skin trial data and create marginal tables

```
> skin <- read.table(file = "skin.txt", header = TRUE)
> skin                              # print it to check
   visit1 visit2 visit3 active placebo
1       0      1      0      1       0
2       0      3      2      1       0
 ...          ...          ...
33      4      4      3      0       2
34      4      4      4      2      14
 af <- data.frame(matrix(0, 5, 3))    # active treatment, marginal table
 pf <- data.frame(matrix(0, 5, 3))    # placebo,marginal table
 row.names(af) <- row.names(pf) <- c("1", "2", "3", "4", "Missing")
 colnames(af) <- colnames(pf) <- c("visit1", "visit2", "visit3")
 for(visit in 1:3)
 {
     for (outcome in c(1 : 5))
     {
       screen <- (skin[, visit] == (outcome %% 5))   #  outcomes = 1,2,3,4,0
       af[outcome, visit] <- sum(skin$active[screen])
       pf[outcome, visit] <- sum(skin$placebo[screen])
 } }
 afm <- rbind(cbind(af, rowSums(af)), c(colSums(af), sum(af)))
 colnames(afm)[4] <- row.names(afm)[6] <- "Sums"
 afm                               # active treatment, marginal frequencies
          visit1 visit2 visit3 Sums
1             22     37     48  107
2             34     30     18   82
3             24      8      7   39
4              5      5      6   16
Missing        3      8      9   20
Sums          88     88     88  264
 pfm <- rbind(cbind(pf, rowSums(pf)), c(colSums(pf), sum(pf)))
 colnames(pfm)[4] <- row.names(pfm)[6] <- "Sums"
 pfm                               #  placebo, marginal frequencies
          visit1 visit2 visit3 Sums
1              5      4      5   14
2             14     13      7   34
3             16     30     28   74
4             49     29     23  101
Missing        0      8     21   29
Sums          84     84     84  252
```

bottom). The mosaic plot (also known as a Marimekko diagram or Mekko chart) has been popularized in a number of applications by Friendly (1999, 2002).

The mosaic plot in Fig. 12.1 was produced using **R** code given in Output 12.2. This code begins with the marginal frequencies af and pf obtained in Output 12.1 and converts these to proportions of outcomes for each of the visits. The code uses the rect() function to draw colored rectangles in the plot area.

To end this section, a summary based on the marginal frequencies such as in Table 12.2, describes the distribution of categories at each visit. Each visit's summary is described by summing over all patients' experiences for each visit.

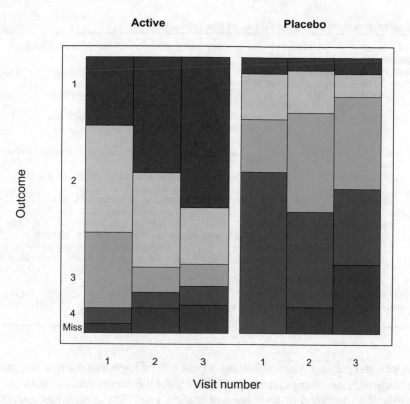

Fig. 12.1 Mosaic plot of marginal rates for skin clinical trial. Outcomes are listed as best (top) to worst and missing on bottom

12.2 Transitional Models

We cannot use Table 12.2, for example, to tell if a rapidly improving patient continues to do so on a subsequent visit. Such a question is addressed by transition models. Transitional models answer questions about the future status given past history. Typical questions answered by transitional models might be Does a deteriorating condition lead to the increased likelihood of a missed visit? Will an improving patient continue to improve? What are the chances a worsening patient on the active treatment will turn around and show an improvement in the next visit? Exercise 12.2 shows how to estimate the distribution of diagnoses at a hypothetical fourth visit based on the outcome of the (observed) third visit.

There were fewer placebo subjects than active treatment patients yet Table 12.2 shows that more visits were missed by the placebo group than the treated group (29 vs. 20). In subsequent visits, the rate of missed visits is increasing steadily for both groups, but this increase is at a much greater rate in the placebo group. Is there any information we can extract from the missed visits or should these be ignored? Could

Output 12.2 R code to produce the mosaic plot in Fig. 12.1

```
amp <- af / colSums(af)[1]      # convert marginal counts to column fractions
pmp <- pf / colSums(pf)[1]
colors <- rainbow(5)            # choose colors
plot(xlim = c(0, 6.5), ylim = c(0, 1), x=0, y=0, xaxt = "n",
     main = "Active                             Placebo",
     xlab = "Visit number", cex.lab = 1.25,
     yaxt = "n", ylab = "Outcome", type = "n")      # draw empty box
for(visit in 1 : 3)             # for each of the three visits . . .
{
   ybota <- 0                   # initialize bottoms of active, placebo boxes
   ybotp <- 0
   for (outcome in 5 : 1)       # for each of the outcomes, worst to best, . . .
   {
     rect(visit - .75, ybota, visit + .25, ybota + amp[outcome, visit],
          col = colors[outcome])              # colored rectangle for active
     ybota <- ybota + amp[outcome, visit]  # move up the bottom of the next box
     rect(visit + 2.5, ybotp, visit + 3.5, ybotp + pmp[outcome, visit],
          col = colors[outcome])              # colored rectangle for placebo
     ybotp <- ybotp + pmp[outcome, visit]  # move up the bottom of the next box
   }
}
axis(side = 1, at = c((1 : 3)-.25, 4 : 6), labels = c(1 : 3, 1 : 3), tick = F)
text(labels = c(1 : 4, "Miss"), x = rep(0, 5), y = c(.9, .55, .2, .07, .02))
```

it be placebo patients are experiencing a poor rate of improvement and drop out of the study after becoming discouraged? Does a deteriorating condition (category 4) increase the likelihood of a subsequent missed visit? These questions cannot be answered by the marginal description of the data given in Table 12.2. Instead, we need to introduce transitional models. We will return to a discussion of missed visits after that.

Table 12.3 gives the transition frequencies for the treated and placebo patient groups respectively. This table summarizes the original data in Table 12.1 in terms of a succession of outcomes from patient visits. Every patient generates two observations in this summary characterized by their change in conditions between the first and second visits, and then again between their second and third visits. In the second row of Table 12.3, for example, we see there were 26 visits of treated patients whose status went from improving (2) to rapidly improving (1) on the subsequent visit. This table does not show how many of the patients made this change between visits 1 and 2 or between visits 2 and 3.

Transitional models are concerned with making inference about the future status of a patient given their present condition. A sequence of categorical responses in which the distribution of each observation is dependent on the previously observed data is called a *Markov chain*. Every patient is categorized into one of five categorical "states" in each of a succession of visits. The Markov chain transitional model is a way of describing the probability distribution on the categories of the next visit as a function of current status.

Table 12.3 Transitional frequencies for the active and placebo treatment groups categorized by skin condition on the previous and following visits

		Active treatment					
		Skin condition on subsequent visit					
		1	2	3	4	Missing	Total
Condition	1	53	0	1	0	5	59
on	2	26	37	0	0	1	64
previous	3	3	11	11	3	4	32
visit	4	0	0	1	7	2	10
	Missing	3	0	2	1	5	11
	Total	85	48	15	11	17	176
		Placebo treatment					
		Skin condition on subsequent visit					
		1	2	3	4	Missing	Total
Condition	1	5	2	0	0	2	9
on	2	3	17	4	1	2	27
previous	3	0	0	37	7	2	46
visit	4	0	1	17	43	17	78
	Missing	1	0	0	1	6	8
	Total	9	20	58	52	29	168

For $i, j = 0, \ldots, 4$ define the transitional probabilities:

$$p_{ij} = \Pr[\text{ patient's next visit is } j \mid \text{ patient's current status is } i \,] \,.$$

These transitional probabilities p_{ij} describe the probability of making a change in status from condition i at the current visit to condition j at the next visit. Conditional on the patient's current status (i) we can describe the probability the next visit is classified as missing, no change, and so on. Markov chain transition probabilities p_{ij} not changing over time are said to be *stationary*. Stationary transition probabilities p_{ij} are the same for modeling the transitions between visits 1 and 2 as they are between visits 2 and 3.

Given the marginal frequency distribution at one visit from Table 12.2, we can estimate the frequencies of the subsequent visit using the transition frequencies of Table 12.3. At a given visit, let f_i $(i = 0, \ldots, 4)$ denote the marginal frequency of the ith skin condition, including a missed visit.

If the transition probabilities p_{ij} are stationary then the estimated marginal frequency of patients classified into category j at the next visit is

$$\sum_i p_{ij} f_i \,.$$

Exercise 12.2 uses this result to estimate the frequency distribution of treated patients at a hypothetical fourth visit.

A stationary Markov chain can also be extrapolated into the distant future. The long-term proportion π_i of patients in category i after a large number of transitions can be found by solving the Chapman–Kolmogorov equations:

$$\pi_i = \sum_j p_{ij}\pi_j \ .$$

The π_j might be used, for example, to estimate the proportion of patients who will never improve.

Another approach to the modeling of transitional effects in longitudinal data has been developed by Liang and Zeger (1986). These flexible generalized estimating equation (GEE) methods allow us to estimate the correlation structure of longitudinal observations within each individual. Even if the correlation structure is incorrectly specified, the GEE method allows iterative refinement to correct this misspecification.

This concludes the broad picture of the two main approaches to the analysis of longitudinal data. Marginal models give the "public health" view which describes the behavior of a group over time. In Table 12.2, for example, we see, as a whole, the treated patients do better than those on placebo. On the other hand, the transitional approach is more of a "medical" view which describes the paths of individual patients over time. The transitional approach views individual patients in terms of their past histories.

12.3 Missing Values

Finally, what can be said of the missed visits? Missing data is a common problem in longitudinal studies where subjects have to be observed on several different occasions. The reason for the missing values may be related to the response that would have been observed had this value been collected. This is referred to as *informative* missing data. In this skin condition study, some of the missing values contain useful information.

In Table 12.2, we see both groups experience an increasing rate of missed visits. This may be due to declining enthusiasm for the study on the part of the subjects or the investigators. The rate of missed visits among the placebo group increases faster than the active treatment group. From Table 12.3, a missed visit in the placebo group has probability 6/8 ($= 75\%$) of being followed by another missed visit. For the active treatment group, this rate is reduced to 5/11 ($= 45\%$). Table 12.3 also shows treated patients who miss a visit are as likely to have missed the previous visit as to have had a rapidly improving classification (1) on their previous visit. In contrast, in the placebo group 17/78 ($= 22\%$) of those who experience worsening conditions will miss their next visit.

To summarize the experience with missing visits, placebo patients seem to be discouraged by poor improvement and one missed visit is likely to be followed by another. The placebo subjects with the worst improvements are most likely to miss visits. On the other hand, missing visits in the active treatment group appear to be comparable to the non-missing visits. A missed visit among the active group is as likely to be followed by another missed visit as a return visit with a rapidly improving (1) report. The data on missing visits in the placebo group contains some information about the missed visit but a missed visit in the active treatment group does not tell us much about the patient's condition. That is, the missing data in the placebo group appears informative but missing values are not informative in the treated group.

12.4 Semiparametric Modeling with GEE

Generalized estimating equations or GEE and their applications to longitudinal data analysis are attributed to Liang and Zeger (1986). This publication noted the equations required to obtain maximum likelihood estimates are similar for a variety of different distributions of data including the normal and Poisson. The full generalization allows us to fit correlated observations without specifying the underlying distributions. The means are specified as in linear regression and the covariance structures can be specified and estimated. The overall approach is close to transitional methods given in Sect. 12.2 but describe the full set of observations for each individual. Two implementations in **R** of GEE are available: one for general, continuous measures and another specific to ordered categorical responses.

The lme4 library in **R** contains the sleepstudy data. This data summarizes a study of reaction times in 18 long-distance truck drivers who were restricted to three hours of sleep for each of 10 consecutive nights. Figure 12.2 is a spaghetti plot with of these data. See Exercises 12.5 for a more detailed examination of this example.

12.5 Exercises

12.1 In December, January, and again in February, we asked the same group of people whether or not they had flu symptoms or herpes simplex. Marginally, we found both of these illnesses had a constant rate of appearing across the three-month span. Is this an appropriate summary of the data?

12.2 (a) There are 176 observations in Table 12.3. What does this number represent?

(b) Convert the frequencies of Table 12.3 for the active treatment group into conditional transition probabilities by dividing the entries by the row sums.

(c) Given the frequency distribution of skin conditions of treated patients at their third visit from Table 12.2, estimate the distribution of conditions at a fourth hypothetical visit for the active treated group. Assume the transition probabilities derived in part (a) are stationary.

(d) Use part (c) and solve the Chapman-Kolmogorov equations to find the long-term proportion π_i of treated patients in each of the five outcome categories.

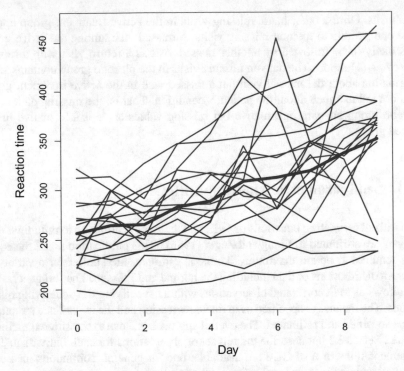

Fig. 12.2 Spaghetti plot of each subject's responses in the sleep study and mean line (in *red*)

12.3 The data in Table 12.4 was presented by Fitzmaurice and Lipsitz (1995). This data represents a summary of a randomized, double blind study comparing the drug Auranofin with placebo in arthritis patients. Patients reported their self-assessed response at baseline (week 0) as well as at weeks 1, 5, 9, and 13 of treatment.

(a) Is there evidence use of Auranofin is associated with a larger percentage of "good" responses than placebo? Do the frequency of the good responses on Auranofin increase over the course of the trial?

(b) Calculate the frequencies needed for a conditional analysis, separately for the two treatments. Is there evidence good responses are more likely to be followed by more of the same? Does there appear to be inertia of the form one type of response tends to be followed by more of the same?

(c) Secondary concerns were to identify any treatment differences by age or sex. Is there evidence of this? Fitzmaurice and Lipsitz (1995) reported a large treatment difference, a modest sex difference, and small effects due to age or change over the course of the study.

(d) Examine the missing values. Do these have value or do these appear at random? Argue once a patient has a missing observation then it is likely more will follow for the same subject.

Table 12.4 Self-assessed response in a clinical trial of an arthritis medication. Columns are: Patient number; Sex; Age; Treatment (A = Auranofin; P = placebo); and assessment at baseline, weeks 1, 5, 9, and 13 (Responses: 0 = good; 1 = poor; – = missing). Source: Fitzmaurice and Lipsitz (1995)

1	M	48	A	0	0	0	0	0		2	M	29	A	0	0	0	0	0
3	M	59	P	0	0	0	0	0		4	F	56	P	0	0	0	0	0
5	M	33	P	0	0	0	0	0		6	M	61	P	0	0	1	0	0
7	M	63	A	1	1	0	–	–		8	M	57	P	0	1	0	0	0
9	M	47	P	0	0	0	1	0		10	F	42	A	1	1	0	–	1
11	M	62	A	0	0	0	0	0		12	M	42	P	0	0	0	0	0
13	M	50	A	0	0	0	0	0		14	F	47	A	0	0	–	–	–
15	M	45	P	1	1	1	0	0		16	M	55	A	0	0	0	0	0
17	M	56	A	0	0	0	0	0		18	M	57	P	0	0	0	0	0
19	F	57	P	0	0	0	1	–		20	M	45	A	0	1	0	1	0
21	M	29	A	0	0	1	–	–		22	F	51	A	1	1	0	0	1
23	F	65	P	0	0	1	0	1		24	F	50	A	0	0	0	1	0
25	M	65	A	0	0	0	0	0		26	F	58	P	0	0	1	1	1
27	F	62	A	1	0	0	0	0		28	F	35	A	0	0	0	0	0
29	M	28	A	0	0	0	0	0		30	M	41	A	0	0	0	–	–
31	M	40	P	0	1	0	1	0		32	M	33	P	1	1	1	1	1
33	F	60	P	1	1	1	1	1		34	M	62	A	0	1	0	0	0
35	M	45	P	0	0	1	0	0		36	M	64	P	1	1	1	1	1
37	M	55	P	1	1	1	0	0		38	M	57	A	0	0	0	0	–
39	M	51	P	0	0	1	0	0		40	F	57	A	0	0	0	0	0
41	M	37	P	0	1	0	–	0		42	M	52	A	1	0	0	0	–
43	M	52	P	0	0	–	0	0		44	M	46	A	0	0	0	0	0
45	M	63	A	1	1	0	1	–		46	M	60	P	0	0	1	1	1
47	M	63	A	1	0	–	1	1		48	F	33	P	0	1	1	0	–
49	M	60	A	1	1	0	0	0		50	M	58	A	0	0	0	0	0
51	M	37	P	1	1	1	0	1										

12.4 The data in Table 12.5 came about from a longitudinal study of coronary risk factors in school children. Briefly, school children were surveyed in 1977, 1979, and 1981. At each of these three cross-sectional surveys, the children were classified as being either obese (O) or not obese (N) in relation to other same age/sex children. See Woolson and Clarke (1984) for more details. There was a wide variety in the patterns of participation and many observations are classified as missing (M). The data separately by sex and five age groups are given in Table 12.5.

(a) There are $3^3 = 27$ possible response patterns but only 26 are represented in this table. Why?

Table 12.5 Classification of children as obese (O) or not (N) at three different ages

Response pattern			Sex									
			Male					Female				
			Age in 1977									
			5–7	7–9	9–11	11–13	13–15	5–7	7–9	9–11	11–13	13–15
N	N	N	90	150	152	119	101	75	154	148	129	91
N	N	O	9	15	11	7	4	8	14	6	8	9
N	O	N	3	8	8	8	2	2	13	10	7	5
N	O	O	7	8	10	3	7	4	19	8	9	3
O	N	N	0	8	7	13	8	2	2	12	6	6
O	N	O	1	9	7	4	0	2	6	0	2	0
O	O	N	1	7	9	11	6	1	6	8	7	6
O	O	O	8	20	25	16	15	8	21	27	14	15
N	N	M	16	38	48	42	82	20	25	36	36	83
N	O	M	5	3	6	4	9	0	3	0	9	15
O	N	M	0	1	2	4	8	0	1	7	4	6
O	O	M	0	11	14	13	12	4	11	17	13	23
N	M	N	9	16	13	14	6	7	16	8	31	5
N	M	O	3	6	5	2	1	2	3	1	4	0
O	M	N	0	1	0	1	0	0	0	1	2	0
O	M	O	0	3	3	4	1	1	4	4	6	1
M	N	N	129	42	36	18	13	109	47	39	19	11
M	N	O	18	2	5	3	1	22	4	6	1	1
M	O	N	6	3	4	3	2	7	1	7	2	2
M	O	O	13	13	3	1	2	24	8	13	2	3
N	M	M	32	45	59	82	95	23	47	53	58	89
O	M	M	5	7	17	24	23	5	7	16	37	32
M	N	M	33	33	31	23	34	27	23	25	21	43
M	O	M	11	4	9	6	12	5	5	9	1	15
M	M	N	70	55	40	37	15	65	39	23	23	14
M	M	O	24	14	9	14	3	19	13	8	10	5

(b) Marginally, does the incidence of obesity increase or decrease with age? Is this change markedly different for boys and girls?

(c) Using a transitional approach, are obese children more or less likely to stay the same as they age?

(d) What can be said about the missing data in this table?

12.5 The data in Table 12.6 is presented by Lumley (1996) who reports on the results of a randomized surgical trial of abdominal suction to reduce shoulder pain

Table 12.6 Pain scores (1 = lowest, 5 = highest) on six times following surgery. Source: Lumley (1996)

Active treatment								Usual care							
		Visit number								Visit number					
Sex	Age	1	2	3	4	5	6	Sex	Age	1	2	3	4	5	6
f	64	1	1	1	1	1	1	f	20	5	2	3	5	5	4
m	41	3	2	1	1	1	1	f	50	1	5	3	4	5	3
f	77	3	2	2	2	1	1	f	40	4	4	4	4	1	1
f	54	1	1	1	1	1	1	m	54	4	4	4	4	4	3
f	66	1	1	1	1	1	1	m	34	2	3	4	3	3	2
m	56	1	2	1	1	1	1	f	34	3	4	3	3	3	2
m	81	1	3	2	1	1	1	f	56	3	3	4	4	4	3
f	24	2	2	1	1	1	1	f	82	1	1	1	1	1	1
f	56	1	1	1	1	1	1	m	56	1	1	1	1	1	1
f	29	3	1	1	1	1	1	m	52	1	5	5	5	4	3
m	65	1	1	1	1	1	1	f	65	1	3	2	2	1	1
f	68	2	1	1	1	1	2	f	53	2	2	3	4	2	2
m	77	1	2	2	2	2	2	f	40	2	2	1	3	3	2
m	35	3	1	1	1	3	3	f	58	1	1	1	1	1	1
m	66	2	1	1	1	1	1	m	63	1	1	1	1	1	1
f	70	1	1	1	1	1	1	f	41	5	5	5	4	3	3
m	79	1	1	1	1	1	1	m	72	3	3	3	3	1	1
f	65	2	1	1	1	1	1	f	60	5	4	4	4	2	2
f	61	4	4	2	4	2	2	m	61	1	3	3	3	2	1
f	67	4	4	4	2	1	1								
f	32	1	1	1	2	1	1								
f	33	1	1	1	2	1	2								

after laparoscopic surgery. It was thought removing any residual abdominal gas remaining after surgery would relieve the pressure felt in the shoulder. Patients were asked to rate their pain on a scale of 1 (low) to 5 (high) every three days after surgery.

(a) Comment on the randomization. Are nearly equal numbers of men and women, and old/young people assigned to the treated and untreated groups?

(b) Marginally, are pain scores increasing, decreasing, or holding constant for all patients taken together?

(c) Does the treated group differ substantially from the untreated group as far as this marginal progression?

(d) Does the abdominal suction help those in the highest levels (3 or higher) of pain? Do the treated patients get relief from their pain faster?

Table 12.7 Wheezing among children at four ages

Mother smokes			Age 10		Nonsmoking mother			Age 10	
Age 7	Age 8	Age 9	No	Yes	Age 7	Age 8	Age 9	No	Yes
No	No	No	118	6	No	No	No	237	10
		Yes	8	2			Yes	15	4
	Yes	No	11	1		Yes	No	16	2
		Yes	6	4			Yes	7	3
Yes	No	No	7	3	Yes	No	No	24	3
		Yes	3	1			Yes	3	2
	Yes	No	4	2		Yes	No	6	2
		Yes	4	7			Yes	5	11

(e) Is there evidence the greatest pain is not experienced immediately after surgery, but rather, after a few days' time?

12.6 The data in Table 12.7 is taken from Ware et al. (1984) as part of the Six Cities study of the health effects of pollution. Children in Steubenville, Ohio were examined for wheezing at each of ages 7 through 10 years of age. The mothers' smoking habits were recorded at the start of the study.

(a) Marginally, does wheezing increase or decrease with age? Is the pattern for children of mothers who smoke different from that of children of nonsmokers?

(b) Estimate the transition matrixes for pairs of adjacent ages, separately for children of smokers and nonsmokers. Is there a change in these transition matrixes at different ages? Stationary Markov chains are those whose transition matrixes do not change over time.

(c) Assume the process is stationary and estimate the incidence of wheezing at age 11 for those children whose mothers do and do not smoke.

(d) Is there a marked difference in the rates of wheezing in children of smokers and nonsmokers? How would you make a formal comparison of these rates?

12.7 The `sleepstudy` in the `lme4` library summarizes the reaction times of long-distance truck drivers who have been sleep deprived for 10 consecutive days.

(a) Figure 12.2 plots the raw data and adds the marginal means for each day to summarize these data. Does this marginal line provide a reasonable summary of these data? Comment on the variability. Does the variance increase with the mean? Is it useful to take logs of the reaction times?

(b) Examine the log reaction times in the linear model using

```
lm(log(Reaction) ~ Days + Subject + Days * Subject,
   data = sleepstudy)
```

where every subject has a different slope and intercept. Run this again but omit the interaction of days and subjects. Compare the log likelihood values to see if every subject has the same slope. Recall the change in the likelihood after omitting a term provides a test of the statistical significance of that term. See Sect. 7.4.

(c) Plot the residuals against the jittered day. Note there are several very large residuals both above and below the expected reaction times.

Chapter 13
Time Series Models

T HE MODELS for data described so far have been concerned with independent observations on multivariate values. The data examined in this chapter are for settings where successive observations are also correlated. The subject matter is not usually associated with multivariate methods but our choice of applications makes these methods more relevant.

This type of data appears in studies where a sequence of observations is taken over an evenly spaced time period. Historically, time series methods are associated with economic and financial applications and are much studied in the business community. In contrast, the applications in this chapter are all associated with health and the environment. Specifically, we examine cancer trends in this chapter. Another example identifies periodic, seasonal patterns in birth rates. Finally, any study of climate change would be incomplete without a data analysis using time series methods. Similarly, this chapter also examines several measures of the global environment recorded monthly for more than three decades.

Such *time series* take into account the serial correlations: Adjacent observations are positively correlated, and observations farther apart in time act more independently.

A full study of time series methods is beyond the scope of this book, but a number of elementary procedures for this type of data are introduced and computed in **R**. We will concentrate on two types of analyses. One of these, *autoregressive models* is useful when the correlation between observations is related to the difference in time between their measurements. A different example of these models is described in Sect. 7.5. This second method, *spectral decomposition*, re-expresses the observed data in terms of cyclical patterns, repeating periodically within the observed data. Let us begin by introducing some examples of the type of data we are likely to encounter and then go over simple analyses performed in **R**.

© Springer Nature Switzerland AG 2022
D. Zelterman, *Applied Multivariate Statistics with R*, Statistics for Biology and Health,
https://doi.org/10.1007/978-3-031-13005-2_13

13.1 Introductory Examples and Simple Analyses

Table 13.1 presents the annual combined US cancer rates (per 100,000 persons) by race (black, white) and sex. This data was reported by the Surveillance, Epidemiology, and End Results (SEER) Program of the National Cancer Institute. The SEER program began in 1973 as part of the "War on Cancer" initiated under then-President Nixon. Currently, in addition to national-level statistics, SEER collects detailed information on all cancer cases, by diagnosis, in eight states, several metropolitan and rural areas, as well as in selected native-American populations.

A portion of the data in Table 13.1 is plotted in Fig. 13.1 for the overall population as well as separately for white and black females. The cancer rates are somewhat higher at the end of this time period than at the beginning. There was a sharp peak in 1991 followed by a quick reversal in the overall population, but this did not much affect some sub-populations. The generally increasing rates covered in this data are partly explained by the facts of longer life expectancy and advances in treating the competing risks of heart disease and stroke. People who would have died from other causes in an earlier time are now living long enough to develop cancer.

A simple examination of these data would be to fit a model of cancer rates as a linear or possibly quadratic function of the year. The problem with this approach is the statistical significance of the regression coefficients will be distorted because of the lack of independence of the observations from one year to the next. A high rate in one year is more likely than not to be followed by another high rate the following year.

There are some other questions we may want to address in these data. Does the year-to-year correlation carry over two or more years later? That is, do each year's rates depend on the past few years? Perhaps there is a random noise component, as we saw in regression models in Chap. 9. Do these random errors in one year influence cancer rates several years later? How do we express the correlation between two different series? Do these also have temporal correlations? That is, does a high rate

Table 13.1 Annual combined cancer rates in the US by sex and race 1975–2007

Year	All Races Both			Whites Both			Blacks Both		
	Sexes	Male	Female	Sexes	Male	Female	Sexes	Male	Female
1975	400.39	466.78	365.84	402.12	468.58	369.56	426.23	525.13	356.46
1976	407.40	481.17	367.40	409.69	481.86	373.12	427.38	553.02	340.44
1977	407.74	486.49	363.71	409.26	487.08	367.86	442.62	577.65	352.01
⋮	⋮	⋮	⋮	⋮	⋮	⋮	⋮	⋮	⋮
2006	462.14	535.72	410.08	471.25	539.95	423.20	487.43	614.56	400.20
2007	461.08	536.61	407.18	468.47	539.49	418.31	482.04	609.17	394.46

Source SEER

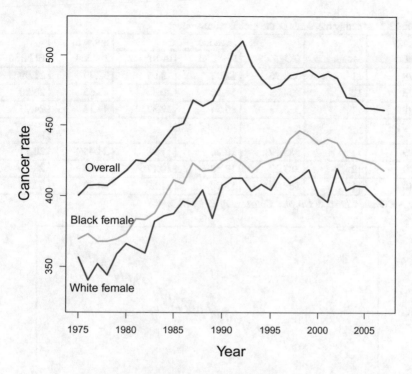

Figure 13.1 US cancer rates for selected populations, 1975–2007

or model error in one series influence another series a year later? We will describe models to answer these questions in Sect. 13.2.

Let us introduce another set of data to illustrate the methods of this chapter. The data in Table 13.2 summarizes a set of global environmental measures reported monthly from November 1978 through January 2010 for the northern hemisphere. The CO_2 values are atmospheric carbon dioxide, measured in parts per million. Sea ice is reported as both percentage of the extent and in millions of square km. Sea ice usually peaks in March/April and reaches its annual minimum in September or October. Snow cover is also reported in millions of square km. El Niño is a measure of the Pacific currents bringing rain and wind from the warm areas near the equator. A small number of missing values in this table have been linearly interpolated.

A plot of these data appears in Fig. 13.2. We see annual, cyclical patterns varying with the seasons in the northern hemisphere. There are trends, most clearly seen in CO_2 levels, but possibly in some of the other series, as well. The objective of the data analysis is to correct for the trends, if present, adjust for the annual cycle, and then examine the joint residuals in order to see if any additional information can be extracted from one data series to another. As with the cancer rate data, we are looking for correlations of temporally, closely spaced observations. These data will be modeled in Sect. 13.3.

Table 13.2 Monthly measures of the global environment

Year	Month	CO_2	Sea ice %extent	Sea ice in 10^6 km	Snow in 10^6 km	El Niño
1978	11	333.76	12.02	8.95	31.49	21.99
1978	12	334.83	14.12	10.85	43.65	23.30
1979	1	336.21	15.54	12.33	49.12	24.77
⋮	⋮	⋮	⋮	⋮	⋮	⋮
2009	11	385.99	10.26	7.98	34.44	22.11
2009	12	387.27	12.48	10.17	45.86	23.16
2010	1	388.45	13.78	11.59	48.27	24.82

Source Climate Charts & Graphs. Courtesy of Kelly O'Day

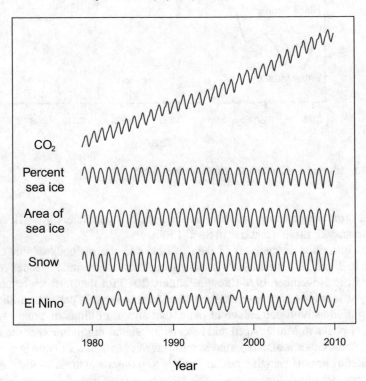

Figure 13.2 Plot of the five environmental time series appearing in Table 13.2

Let us end this section with a third data set and an illustration of some simple analyses we can perform in **R**. This data on the monthly birth rates in New York City can be read directly from the web, producing a data.frame as follows:

```
> NYCbirth <-
+    scan("http://robjhyndman.com/tsdldata/data/nybirths.dat")

Read 168 items

> print(NYCbirth, digits = 3)

 [1] 26.7 23.6 26.9 24.7 25.8 24.4 24.5 23.9 23.2 23.2 21.7 21.9 21.4 21.1
[15] 23.7 21.7 21.8 20.8 23.5 23.8 23.1 23.1 21.8 22.1 21.9 20.0 23.6 21.7
[29] 22.2 22.1 23.9 23.5 22.2 23.1 21.1 21.6 21.5 20.0 22.4 20.6 21.8 22.9
     . . .        . . .        . . .        . . .        . . .
```

In **R** there is a special data structure called ts acting as a data.frame but is better suited for some time series analyses. The ts() function creates a ts object, identifying the frequency period (months) and starting time. We create a ts object, adding these time coordinates:

```
> NYCts <- ts(NYCbirth, frequency = 12, start = c(1946, 1))
> print(NYCts, digits = 3)

       Jan  Feb  Mar  Apr  May  Jun  Jul  Aug  Sep  Oct  Nov  Dec
1946 26.7 23.6 26.9 24.7 25.8 24.4 24.5 23.9 23.2 23.2 21.7 21.9
1947 21.4 21.1 23.7 21.7 21.8 20.8 23.5 23.8 23.1 23.1 21.8 22.1
1948 21.9 20.0 23.6 21.7 22.2 22.1 23.9 23.5 22.2 23.1 21.1 21.6
     . . .        . . .        . . .              . . .
```

A simple time series analysis decomposes the observed data into three component parts:

$$\text{observed data} = \text{trend} + \text{seasonal effect} + \text{residual}$$

The observed birth rate data and these three component parts are separately plotted in the top panel of Fig. 13.3. This figure and the components can be obtained using the decompose function:

```
NYCd <- decompose(NYCts)
plot(NYCd, xlab = "Year", col = "red")
```

The decompose function takes a ts object and produces a decomposed.ts object with components: $x (original data), $seasonal (the periodic effect), $trend (the trend component of the model), and $random (the residual).

In the upper panel of Fig. 13.3, we can see the trend for a declining birth rate from 1946–8, followed by a sharp increase through 1956 and a leveling off afterward. The seasonal effect shows a repeated pattern for each year: lowest in February (also the shortest month) and highest in July and August. There are no extreme residuals or outliers for us to report in the random plot.

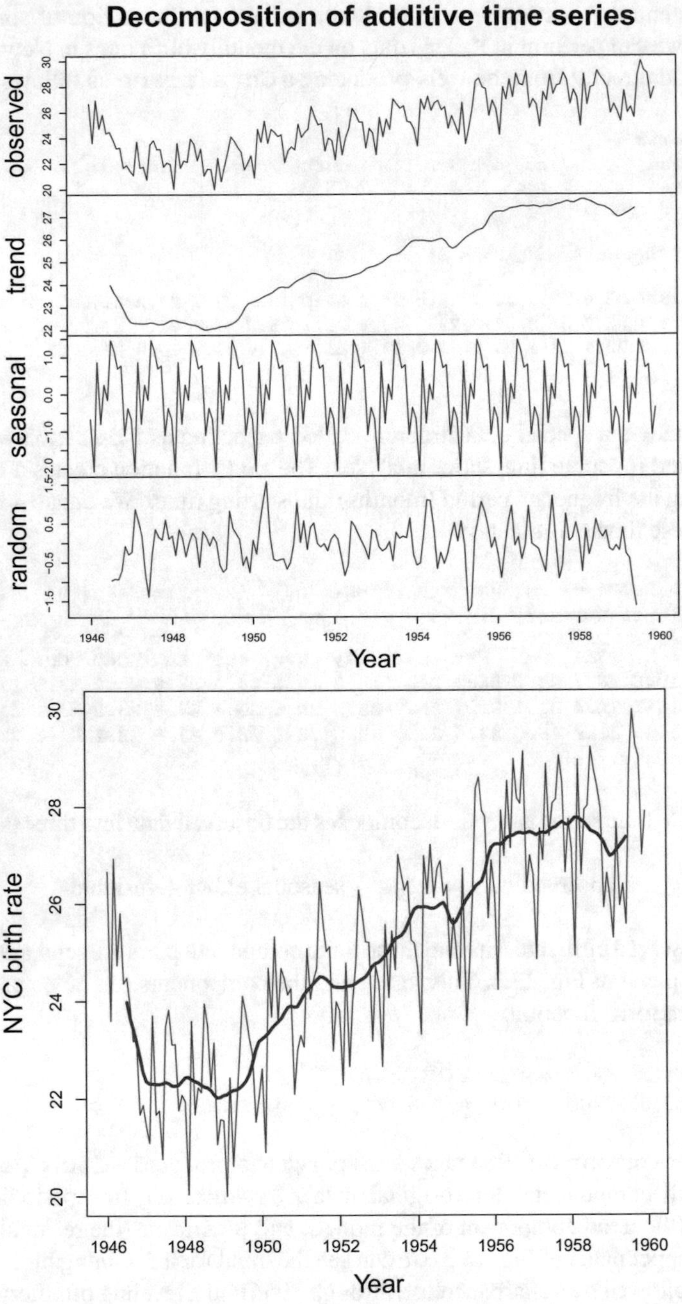

Figure 13.3 Observed New York City birth rates decomposed into trend, cyclical (or seasonal) component, and residual in the top panel, and displayed as superimposed observed and trend (bottom)

Another useful display is to superimpose the observed values and the overall trend, as in the lower panel of Fig. 13.3. This figure was produced using

```
plot(NYCd$x, xlab = "Year", ylab = "NYC birth rate", col = "blue")
lines(NYCd$trend, col = "red", lwd = 3, type = "l")
```

A more sophisticated decomposition of a time series can be performed using the `stl()` function in **R**. This program has more options available including the loess smoothing of the seasonal trend. This smoothing usually produces a better image of the seasonal trend. See Exercise 13.1 for an illustration of its use.

We can control the amount of smoothing in a time series using the `filter()` function which performs a *moving average*. A moving average, as the name implies, is the series of all sequential averages of a number of adjacent observations. The number of points in the moving average is called the *window* or sometimes the *window width*.

As a mathematical example, a moving average m on a time series $x = (x_1, \ldots, x_n)$ with window $w = 5$ is calculated as

$$m_t = (x_{t+2} + x_{t+1} + x_t + x_{t-1} + x_{t-2})/5 \tag{13.1}$$

so every five adjacent observations are averaged.

The moving average is illustrated for the birth rate data in Fig. 13.4 both for the original data and a range of different window widths. Small values of window w remove the short-term noise and emphasize the annual cycles. Values of w greater than 12 will remove much of the annual cycle and leave a smooth image of the overall trend.

In (13.1), we see the moving average m_t is centered around x_t and gives equal weights to all five observations. Some moving averages give greater weight to those observations closer to the center. In (13.1), we see the first and last two m_t's are undefined for $t = 1, 2, n - 1$, and n. Similarly, notice how the different moving averages in Fig. 13.4 become shorter at each end. In some settings where forecasting future trends is the objective, we may want to define moving averages only on the lagging or trailing observations.

In **R**, we calculate moving averages as

```
filter(x, filter = rep(1 / w,  w) )
```

The `filter=rep(1 / w,  w)` parameter specifies the weights in the average are all equal. It is a common practice to give more weight to those observations nearer the center of the window.

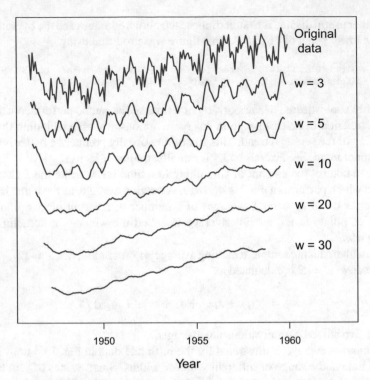

Figure 13.4 Birth rates smoothed with different moving averages of window widths w, as specified

13.2   Autoregressive Models

We begin with an ordered collection of multivariate observations $x(1), x(2), \ldots, x(n)$
taken over a series of evenly spaced time intervals. These observations are correlated
both within the components of $x(t)$ as well as temporally correlated between $x(t)$
and $x(t-k)$. An important assumption we make is the series is *stationary*. This
means the marginal distribution of $x(t)$ does not change over time and is the same
for every value of t. We will explain this point again below and also test its validity.

The models we build will demonstrate the intuitive property observations made
closer in time are more highly correlated than observations made farther apart. Our
interest is to identify trends in the mean of this series of observations but also to
describe regressions modeling later observations from earlier ones. As an example,
can we forecast one year's cancer rates using the data from all previous years?

We can describe the temporal, univariate correlations between other observations
in the same series

$$\widehat{\rho}_k = \mathrm{corr}\{x(t),\ x(t-k)\}$$

for $t = 2, 3, \ldots, n$ and $k = 1, 2, \ldots$.

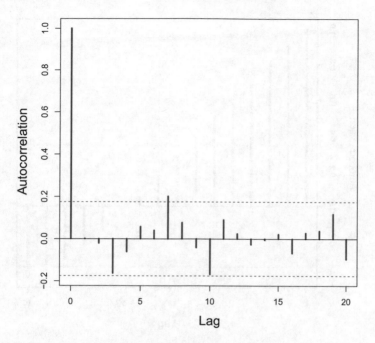

Figure 13.5 Autocorrelation function for random normally distributed data

This is referred to as the *autocorrelation* of *lag k* because it measures the correlation of the data with itself, offset by k observations. The x's in this definition are scalar-valued. If the x's were vector-valued, then the ρ's would be correlation matrices.

The assumption the data is stationary means these correlations are the same for every value of t. Ideally, sufficiently long lags would indicate observations far apart also behave independently. A plot of the autocorrelation $\widehat{\rho}_k$ by the length of the lag k is called the *correlogram, periodogram,* or *variogram.* Useful lag values k are generally much smaller than the sample size n and are rarely larger than 15 or 20.

The acf function in **R** computes autocorrelations of a scalar-values time series and plots the correlogram as a function of the lag for a range of lags. Figures 13.5, 13.6, and 13.7 are examples of these. Figure 13.5 plots the correlogram for a set of randomly distributed standard normal variates. This figure can be obtained with

```
acf(rnorm(125))
```

in **R**.

The autocorrelation with a lag of $k = 0$ is equal to one, corresponding to the correlation of the data with itself. In this example, higher lags have negligible autocorrelations because the data is randomly generated.

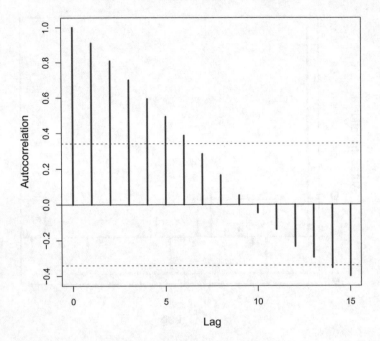

ACF for Overall US Cancer Rates

Figure 13.6   Autocorrelation for US cancer rates for all populations

Figure 13.6 is the estimated autocorrelation function for US total cancer rates, combined over all populations. These correlations are all very high for small lags indicating a high degree of autocorrelation between close years' values. High lags have negative correlations reflecting a regression to the mean for observations far apart.

There is also a cross-correlation function allowing us to measure the lagged correlation of one series with another. That is, we can measure the correlation

$$\text{corr}\{x(t),\, y(t - k)\}.$$

The lag, k, could be either positive or negative depending on which series we can interpret as leading or lagging the other.

The cross-correlation is calculated in **R** using the ccf (x= , y=) function. An example of these appears in Fig. 13.7. In this figure, we see the cross-correlation of cancer rates for white females lagged by the overall US rates. This plot demonstrates there is a high correlation between the two time series.

Figures 13.5, 13.6, and 13.7 include bounds (as dotted lines) for 95% confidence intervals of autocorrelations under the null hypothesis observations are generated independently. The autocorrelation function for the normal random observations are

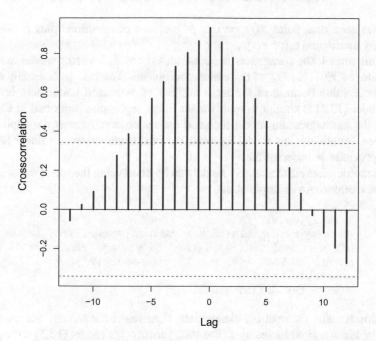

Figure 13.7 Cross-correlation of cancer rates in US White women lagged by total US population

generally within these bounds and those of the cancer rates are well outside their bounds.

The Ljung–Box test (Ljung and Box 1978) is a single test of several autocorrelations that are all zero. In a sample of n observations with estimated autocorrelation $\widehat{\rho}_k$ of order k, then the statistic

$$Q = n(n+2) \sum_{k=1}^{h} \frac{\widehat{\rho}_k^2}{n-k} \tag{13.2}$$

behaves approximately as chi-squared with h df.

In **R**, we compute this test using

```
Box.test(x, lag = 1, type = "Ljung-Box")
```

where x is the time series data and the lag specifies h the number of autocorrelations to be tested. We won't illustrate the use of this statistic at this point: It is better suited to examine the autocorrelations of residuals from the regression models we describe next.

Given a series $\{x(1), \ldots, x(n)\}$ of temporally ordered multivariate observations, the *autoregression model*

$$x(t) = \theta + \Theta_1 x(t-1) + \cdots + \Theta_p x(t-p) + e(t) \qquad (13.3)$$

regresses each data point $x(t)$ on the p previous observations plus multivariate normally distributed error $e(t)$.

In this model, the parameters to be estimated are θ, a vector-valued intercept, and matrices $\Theta_1, \ldots, \Theta_p$ of regression coefficients. The lag, p, is usually chosen as a small value because of the large number of estimated parameters involved. The model (13.3) is similar to multivariate linear regression described in Chap. 9, except the autoregression model included earlier observations as the explanatory variables. Intuitively, this model forecasts the next observation as a linear function of the previous p observations.

The multivariate autoregressive model can be fitted using the VAR (vector autoregressive) routine. An example of this is

```
library(vars)
acan <- read.table(file = "AnnualCancer.txt", header = T)
ofc <- acan[ , c("Overall", "Wfemale", "Bfemale")]
varofc <- VAR( ofc, p = 1, type = "both")
summary(varofc)
res <- residuals(varofc)
```

In this **R** code, we read the cancer data, then select the overall rate as well as those for black and white females. The VAR function fits model (13.3) with $p = 1$. There is a large amount of output from this program and a portion is reproduced in Output 13.1. This includes the estimated regression coefficients in (13.3), their standard errors, and tests of statistical significance. The correlation matrix of the residuals is also included.

At the top half of Output 13.1, see the white female series is highly correlated with its own value from the previous year (Wfemale.l1) and also has a statistically significant regression on black women's cancer rates of the previous year (Bfemale.l1). The fitted regression model for black female cancer rates is statistically significant according to the overall F-test, but no single regression coefficient is significant. The estimated trends are not statistically significant for either of these two populations. The negative values of the estimated trends indicate no overall trend remains after correcting for the regression coefficients.

The multivariate residuals from this regression are plotted in the upper panel of Fig. 13.8. These values have been scaled because the three series have different estimated variances. Scaling each column to zero mean and unit variance is performed using the scale() function. The rug plot on the right margin of this figure does not indicate any deviations from a marginal normal distribution. A test of normality on the residuals can be performed using

```
normality.test(varofc)
```

also in the vars library.

Output 13.1 A portion of the autoregression output for US cancer rates

```
Estimation results for equation Wfemale:
==========================================
Wfemale = Overall.l1 + Wfemale.l1 + Bfemale.l1 + const + trend

            Estimate Std. Error t value Pr(>|t|)
Overall.l1   -0.1081     0.1076  -1.004   0.3243
Wfemale.l1    0.8911     0.1635   5.450 9.12e-06 ***
Bfemale.l1    0.2898     0.1405   2.063   0.0489 *
const       -12.6488    35.6494  -0.355   0.7255
trend        -0.2743     0.2479  -1.107   0.2783
---

Residual standard error: 5.826 on 27 degrees of freedom
Multiple R-Squared: 0.9495,      Adjusted R-squared: 0.942
F-statistic:    127 on 4 and 27 DF,  p-value: < 2.2e-16

Estimation results for equation Bfemale:
==========================================
Bfemale = Overall.l1 + Wfemale.l1 + Bfemale.l1 + const + trend

            Estimate Std. Error t value Pr(>|t|)
Overall.l1   0.27915    0.16816   1.660   0.1085
Wfemale.l1   0.46300    0.25549   1.812   0.0811 .
Bfemale.l1   0.04281    0.21953   0.195   0.8468
const       57.65281   55.70207   1.035   0.3098
trend       -0.04098    0.38728  -0.106   0.9165
---

Residual standard error: 9.103 on 27 degrees of freedom
Multiple R-Squared: 0.8583,      Adjusted R-squared: 0.8373
F-statistic: 40.89 on 4 and 27 DF,  p-value: 4.394e-11


Correlation matrix of residuals:
         Overall Wfemale Bfemale
Overall  1.0000  0.6115  0.4475
Wfemale  0.6115  1.0000  0.4533
Bfemale  0.4475  0.4533  1.0000
```

The `normality.test` computes the multivariate Jarque–Bera test on these data ($p = .80$) and separately for the multivariate skewness ($p = .45$) and kurtosis ($p = .94$). These p-values give us no empirical evidence of a departure from multivariate normal residuals. The details of the Jarque–Bera test are described in Sect. 5.4.

The Ljung–Box test statistic given at (13.2) can be used to detect any autocorrelation in the residuals of a fitted autoregression model, as well. Rejecting the null hypothesis of these residuals is indicative of autocorrelations not accounted for by the autoregression model. This would suggest a larger value of p is needed in (13.3). The lower panel of Fig. 13.8 plots the p-values of these tests for each of the three time

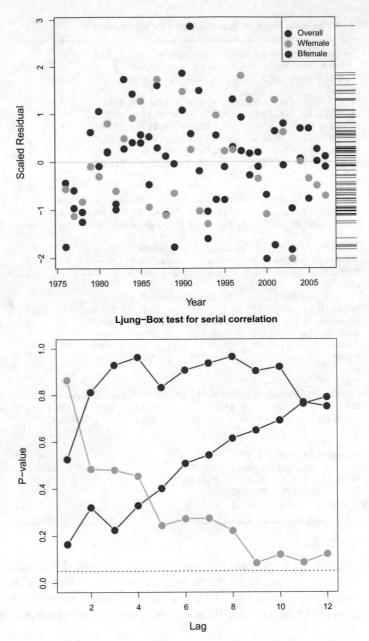

Figure 13.8 Residuals and p-values for the Ljung–Box test from the autoregressive model of US cancer rates in selected populations

series in our model and these give no indication of any inadequacies in the model for $p = 1$.

Another assumption we need to examine is the stationarity of the series. We assume all $x(t)$ have the same distribution, and this assumption can fail in a wide range of ways. There are many possible tests of these departures and several are available in **R**. See Exercise 13.7 for a list of these.

A graphical display of the stationarity assumption appears in Fig. 13.9. Instead of fitting a model with the whole data set, suppose we fit a series of models on a moving window subset $\{x(t + 1), \ldots, x(t + w)\}$ for window width $w > 0$. As the starting value, t, of the window varies, we should not expect to see much difference in the estimated model parameters if the series is truly stationary.

We used a window width of $w = 15$ years in Fig. 13.9 and examined the six estimated model variances, all on a log scale, and the nine estimated regression coefficients Θ, in the bottom panel. The fitted model is the same as in Output 13.1. The overall US cancer rate (in red on the top panel) has a higher estimated variance in the middle years than at either end of the data. A small number of estimated regressions have larger variability at the beginning of the series but otherwise are fairly stable throughout. In conclusion, we see no inadequacies in the autoregressive model for these data with $p = 1$ and the stationarity assumption seems reasonable.

Next, let us introduce a more general model for temporally correlated multivariate data. These models regress on both earlier observations as well as on their model errors. Autoregressive models in (13.3) contain multivariate normally distributed random errors $e(1), e(2), \ldots$ associated with each observation. In autoregressive, integrated moving average (ARIMA) models, these errors are cumulative, and there are additional *moving average* regression coefficients associated with these as well.

Symbolically, the ARIMA model of order (p, q) is

$$x(t) = \boldsymbol{\theta} + \boldsymbol{\Theta}_1 x(t-1) + \boldsymbol{\Theta}_2 x(t-2) + \cdots + \boldsymbol{\Theta}_k x(t-p)$$
$$+ e(t) + \boldsymbol{\Delta}_1 e(t-1) + \boldsymbol{\Delta}_2 e(t-2) + \cdots + \boldsymbol{\Delta}_q e(t-q) \,. \quad (13.4)$$

In the ARIMA model, each observed $x(t)$ is regressed on each of the previous p observed $x(t-1), \ldots, x(t-p)$ as well as on the errors $e(t-1), \ldots, e(t-q)$ associated with the q previous observations.

The parameters to be estimated in the ARIMA model are the vector-valued intercept $\boldsymbol{\theta}$, matrices of autoregressive slopes $\boldsymbol{\Theta}_1, \ldots, \boldsymbol{\Theta}_p$, and matrices of moving average slopes $\boldsymbol{\Delta}_1, \ldots, \boldsymbol{\Delta}_q$. There are a very large number of parameters to be estimated in (13.4). As a consequence, only very long multivariate time series can be fitted. Below, we will illustrate the ARIMA models using only the univariate overall US cancer rate because of the large number of parameters associated with ARIMA models.

ARIMA models can be fitted using

```
arima(x,  order = c(p, 0, q))
```

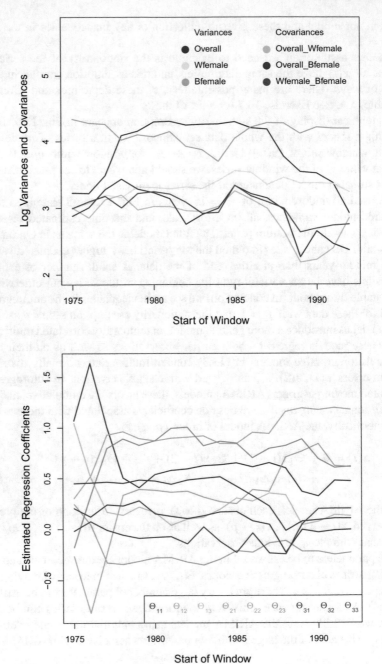

Figure 13.9 Moving window estimates of variances (log scale, at top) and regression coefficients Θ_1 (on bottom) in autoregression model of Output 13.1

for univariate time series (x) and

```
VARMA(y, p = ,  q = )
```

for multivariate data (y). These functions are available in the TSA and MTS libraries, respectively.

The missing option (0) in the order= allows us to change the order of differencing, but it is best set to zero for most applications. When q is set to zero, these programs fit autoregressive models. The arima and VARMA programs have several other options including the ability to regress on other explanatory variables and a choice of whether or not to include an intercept θ.

The details from three fitted ARIMA models are given in Output 13.2. The output includes fitted regression parameters and measures of overall fit, relative to the other models. The three successive models are nested in the sense each subsequent model adds additional parameters to the previous model. We can see the estimated variance of $e(t)$ (denoted by sigma^2) declines with more complicated models indicating a lower degree of uncertainty associated with each subsequent model. Similarly, the log-likelihood increases, also indicating a better fit according to these criteria.

There is also an AIC measure minimizing for the middle of these three models. We will explain this statistic next.

The object of model building is more than maximizing the log-likelihood. This could be accomplished in a complicated model with many parameters, not all of them useful. The AIC, then, charges a penalty to the model log-likelihood for every

Output 13.2 Portions of three ARIMA models of overall cancer rates

```
> arima( acan[ , "Overall"], order = c(1, 0, 0)) # autoregressive (1)
Coefficients:
          ar1   intercept
       0.9709    440.0603
s.e.   0.0297     28.7600

sigma^2 estimated as 66.23:  log likelihood = -117.44,  aic = 238.88
> arima( acan[ , "Overall"], order = c(1, 0, 1)) # ARIMA (1,1)
Coefficients:
          ar1     ma1    intercept
       0.9555  0.3687     441.9634
s.e.   0.0425  0.1480      27.3071

sigma^2 estimated as 56.2:  log likelihood = -114.9,  aic = 235.79
> arima( acan[ , "Overall"], order = c(2, 0, 2)) # ARIMA(2,2)

Coefficients:
          ar1     ar2     ma1     ma2  intercept
       0.7065  0.2170  0.7001  0.3771   444.2845
s.e.   0.4227  0.4051  0.4108  0.3048    25.7473

sigma^2 estimated as 53.34:  log likelihood = -114.17,  aic = 238.34
```

parameter included. The *AIC* is the Akaike[1] Information Criteria and is defined as

$$\text{AIC} = -2 \times \text{Log–likelihood} + 2 \times \text{number of parameters.}$$

In words, every parameter in the model must make a meaningful contribution in order to be included. Maximizing the log-likelihood is one goal, but minimizing the AIC results in simpler models. Other penalized model-building methods are described in Sect. 9.4 for linear regression models.

Specifically, the ARIMA(2,2) model in Output 13.2 has evidence of being *overfitted* or having too many parameters. There is only a modest improvement in reduced `sigma^2`and a slight increase in the log-likelihood ratio between the ARIMA(1,1) and ARIMA(2,2) models. Recall, from Sect. 7.4, twice the difference in the log-likelihood of two nested models should behave as chi-squared when the underlying parameters are zero. In the present case, the ARIMA(2,2) has two more parameters than the ARIMA(1,1) model. At the same time, the AIC has increased indicating the improvement in fit is not enough to warrant an increase in the number of parameters and model complexity.

The ARIMA (1,1) model for the year t of overall US cancer rates $x(t)$ has the smallest AIC of the three models in Output 13.2. The fitted parameters of this model are

$$x(t) = 441.96 + 0.96\,x(t-1) + e(t) + 0.37\,e(t-1)$$

where the e's are normally distributed with mean zero and their estimated variances are 56.2.

There are a number of diagnostics available for the `arima` program. The `tsdiag` program plots residuals and their periodogram and performs tests of different lags in the Ljung–Box test. Exercise 13.7 explores different significance tests of the stationarity assumption. We next examine models to exploit cyclical patterns in the time series.

13.3   Spectral Decomposition

In the previous section, we saw we can build regression models where the observed value in one time period is regressed or explained by observations made at earlier times. In the example of the US cancer rates, we saw reasonable models can be constructed using the previous year's data. Such models are useful when the observed data is relatively smooth but also temporally correlated. The models we examine here are useful for data exhibiting marked cyclical patterns such as those seen in the seasonal variations of the climate data in Fig. 13.2 and, to a smaller degree, in the birth rate data of Fig. 13.3. The approach taken in this section is to decompose the data into its cyclical components of all possible frequencies. We will see simple

---

[1] Hirotugu Akaike (1927–2009). Japanese statistician.

models can be obtained by omitting many terms in the model. In this case, we can delegate many of the high-frequency components to the residuals.

The background theory needed is the *Fourier transform*.[2] Suppose we have a set of numbers $x = \{x_1, \ldots, x_n\}$. Then there is a unique representation of x

$$x_i = \sum_{k=1}^{n/2} a_k \sin(2\pi i k/n) \; + \; b_k \cos(2\pi i k/n) \tag{13.5}$$

in terms of other numbers $a = \{a_k\}$ and $b = \{b_k\}$ for every $i = 1, \ldots, n$.

Briefly, there are sine and cosine cycles with different frequencies and amplitudes in the a and b. The representation of x in terms of its *frequency spectrum a* and b is called the Fourier transform. This is analogous to the way we can use a prism to decompose white light into its component colors.

The representation in (13.5) is unique, in part because there are n numbers on both sides of Eq. (13.5). Further, given a and b, it is possible to invert this relationship using the *inverse Fourier transformation* and obtain the original x again. If n is an odd number, then we set the last b_k to zero in (13.5).

There was a time when calculating (13.5) took a lot of computing power. This changed with the publication of the *fast Fourier transformation* by Cooley and Tukey (1965), although earlier versions were known but not as well utilized. In today's applications, for example, a Fourier transformation can greatly simplify the transmission of video images and audio signals, omitting some of the noise in the high-frequency spectrum, at the expense of losing some fine detail in the picture and sound.

Mathematical models with periodic sines and cosines are most useful when the data x also exhibits strong cyclical patterns. Intuitively, when one a_k and/or b_k are large, then there is a large cyclical effect with period $2\pi k/n$ in x. A useful display, as in Fig. 13.10, is to plot the magnitude of $\{a_k, b_k\}$ against k. The vertical axis in this figure plots values of $\sqrt{a_k^2 + b_k^2}$.

The complete set of magnitudes of all frequencies (expressed in terms of a and b) is referred to as the *spectral decomposition* of the data. These are computed and plotted in Fig. 13.10 using

```
spec.pgram(climate, detrend = TRUE)
```

for the climate data.

The spec.pgram program computes and plots the spectral decomposition for each of the series. The detrend option removes linear trends such as the one apparent in the CO_2 series. The program fits and plots the periodogram in the left panel of Fig. 13.10. The obvious problem is the large amount of noise in the raw periodogram making it difficult to see the underlying pattern in the data.

A *smoothed periodogram* is a much more useful diagnostic. To smooth the periodogram, we add the span option as in

```
spec.pgram(climate, detrend = TRUE, span = c(9, 9))
```

---

[2] Joseph Fourier (1768–1830). French mathematician and physicist.

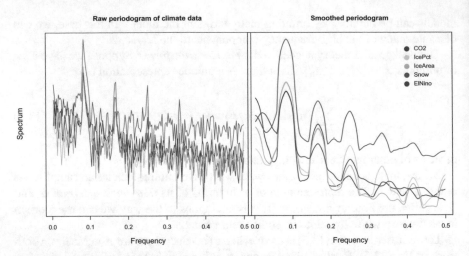

Figure 13.10 Raw and smoothed periodograms of the climate data

The arguments to the span option are a pair of odd integers, where larger values result in greater smoothing and smaller values result in greater fidelity to the original values. This is similar to determining the window width when computing a moving average as seen in Fig. 13.4. The choice of parameter values usually takes some trial and error to produce just the right balance of smoothing and fidelity to the original data.

The vertical axis of the periodogram is called the *spectrum* and is a measure of the strength of each frequency within the series. In Fig. 13.10, the spectrum is given on a log scale. The *frequency* on the horizontal axis tells us how often the cyclical pattern occurs within the data. These patterns are clearer in the smoothed periodogram. The frequencies with the largest values occur at 1/12 = .0833 indicating the twelve-month cyclical pattern in the data. There are also smaller echoes of the twelve-month cycle occurring at 2/12=.1667, 3/12=.25, and so on. We notice how these spectral patterns run parallel for each of the five climate time series.

Smoothing the periodogram cures other problems as well as those seen in Fig. 13.10. The estimate of the spectral density is affected by the abrupt truncation occurring at the beginning and end of the time series. Collecting more data on a longer series does not improve the situation, because a longer series means there are more Fourier coefficients (*a* and *b*) to estimate.

We end this section with a simple, graphical diagnostic for examining the presence of periodicity in the data. This can be accomplished using the *cumulative periodogram*, computed using the cpgram() function in **R**. The individual spectral values are divided by the total, so the cumulative sum increases to one. Two examples are given in Fig. 13.11 for the New York City birth rate data.

The cumulative periodogram includes dotted lines to provide a range of values where the white noise should fall. The original birth rate data jumps outside these

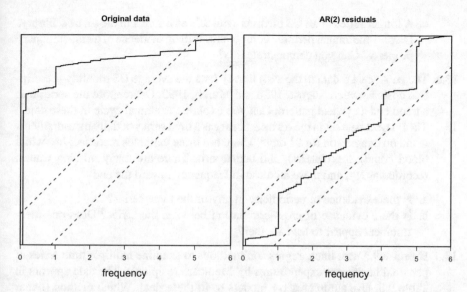

Figure 13.11 Cumulative periodogram of original NYC birth data and residuals from an AR(2) model

bounds for low frequencies corresponding to the strong annual effects. If we fit an AR(2) model to these data and plot the residuals, then there is good evidence there is no periodic effect remaining. These figures were produced using the **R** code:

```
cpgram(NYCts, main = "Original data")
cpgram(ar(NYCts, order.max=2)$resid, main = "AR(2) residuals")
```

In summary of this chapter, time series data can be analyzed using either autoregressive regression models or through their spectral decomposition. The choice of these two different approaches depends on the summary you want to make. Begin by understanding the process giving rise to your data and then draw a few plots to motivate your models.

13.4 Exercises

13.1 Reexamine the New York City birth rate data using `stl`.

 a. Is the loess smoothed seasonal trend more informative than the trend plotted in Fig. 13.3? Or does the loess fit look like one of the moving averages in Fig. 13.4?

 b. Is there evidence the periodic component in this series is not stationary? Does a multiplicative model offer a better fit?

c. A longer series of all US births is available as `birth` in the `astsa` library. Display the annual periodic component. Is there evidence of a non-stationary property? Can you demonstrate this?

13.2 The `prescrip` data in the `TSA` library lists the average US monthly prescription costs between August, 1986 and March, 1992. Decompose the series into a trend and a cyclical pattern. Can you explain the annual cycle in these data?

13.3 The `blood` data set in the `astsa` library is a time series of daily measurements made on one person for 91 days. There are three variables recorded: log(white blood count), log(platelet), and hematocrit. There are many missing values, recorded as `NA`, and these increase in frequency toward the end.

a. Is there evidence of periodicity in any of the three series?
b. Is there evidence of cross-correlation between the series? Does one measurement appear to lead another?

13.4 Exercise 9.3 uses linear regression methods to examine multiple time series of personal healthcare expenditures by Medicare recipients. The data appears in Table 9.3. Use autoregressive models to fit these data. Which method (linear regression or autoregressive) provides a more valid summary of these data? Which method is more consistent with the properties of the sampled data?

13.5 The data set `ambientNOxCH` in the `robustbase` library is another environmental time series, providing 366 daily measurements of air quality in 13 different locations in Switzerland. These locations are very different from each other: one is located along a highway, another in urban areas, and one is on an isolated wooded mountain. There are a number of missing values and linear interpolation between adjacent non-missing values should be a suitable solution to fill these.

a. Apply some graphical techniques to these data. Which of these series exhibit seasonal effects? There is only a little more than a year's worth of data, so we will have to assume seasonal patterns repeat every year. How many of these seasonal patterns appear due to a small number of outlying observations?
b. How do the cross-correlations compare with those in Fig. 13.7?

13.6 The `boardings` data set in the `TSA` library is a bivariate time series measuring the use of public transportation (boardings of bus and light rail services) and gasoline price in the metropolitan Denver, Colorado region.

a. Is there evidence for a seasonal, periodic effect in either of these two series?
b. Does the use of public transportation rise and fall with the price of gasoline?

13.7 Several of the statistical tests of stationarity available in **R** include the Phillips–Perron test (`PP.test`), the Kwiatkowski–Phillips–Schmidt–Shin (KPSS) test (`kpss.test`), and the Augmented Dickey–Fuller test (`adf.test`). Some of these embed the fitted model into a more general model, and others examine the spectral decomposition of the data. Apply these to the `boardings` data of the previous exercise and interpret your findings. Does the boarding data appear stationary? If not, how does it fail this assumption?

Chapter 14
Other Useful Methods

T HIS FINAL CHAPTER provides a collection of useful multivariate methods not fitting into any of the previous chapters. The Bradley–Terry model gives us a way to rank a set of objects examined by pairwise comparisons. Such examples include sports teams playing against each other. Canonical correlations generalize the definition of correlation of a pair of scalar-valued variates to two groups of several variables considered jointly. The study of extremes allows us to examine several of the largest values in a collection of data.

14.1 Ranking From Paired Comparisons

We are familiar with rankings. Headlines proclaim the best city to live in or the best university to attend. There is a lot of quantitative data behind such rankings, but of course, the results depend highly on the relative weights we give to each measurement. Principal components may be helpful, but the interpretation of the weights and loadings may not correspond to any useful sense of ranking the observations.

We can easily rank one-dimensional data. For instance, there is a tallest and a shortest person in the room. We can easily make pairwise comparisons of the heights of any two persons, and the random variability of such a comparison is negligible. We are also familiar with pairwise comparisons between sports teams. At the end of the season, we can rank the teams on the basis of their record of wins and losses. Taken to a light-hearted extreme, the website http://william.hoza.us/rank/ attempts to rank *everything* by means of asking viewers to make pairwise comparisons between two seemingly unrelated things.[1]

---

[1] A recent visit to this website asked the viewer to choose the better of "pig" or "castanet".

© Springer Nature Switzerland AG 2022
D. Zelterman, *Applied Multivariate Statistics with R*, Statistics for Biology and Health,
https://doi.org/10.1007/978-3-031-13005-2_14

Table 14.1 Cross-citation rates among selected probability journals in 1987–8

Cited journal	Citing journal					
	AnnPr	PrTh	StochPr	JAppPr	ThPrApp	AnnSt
AnnPr	468	255	33	46	72	74
PrTh	333	322	47	47	72	76
StochPr	208	155	93	76	40	41
JAppPr	121	31	37	283	26	35
ThPrApp	101	60	23	38	344	63
AnnSt	76	81	13	14	50	1009

Source Stigler (1994). Used with permission

As a specific example, consider the problem of associating a level of prestige associated with academic journals. Academic faculty need to publish their results and want to have these appear in the highest-impact journals. At the same time, we need a way of performing a pairwise comparison. A solution, presented by Stigler (1994), was to count the number of times articles in one journal cite articles in the other journal. The premise is a journal tending to be cited more often is also viewed as the source of the newest and best ideas. There are flaws in this argument, of course, but perhaps we can think of information flowing between the journals. It would be useful to have a measure of the directions of these flows.

The data in Table 14.1 is part of Stigler's article.[2] The names of the citing journals are listed as the columns and the names of the journals being cited are the rows. As an example, in 1987–8, the *Annals of Probability* (AnnPr) was cited 74 times in the *Annals of Statistics* (AnnSt).

In our model of ranking, we will consider the event journal i is cited by journal j at a greater rate by journal j than journal j is cited by journal i. As a shorthand, we will use the notation "$i > j$" to signify journal i has a greater impact than journal j, consistent with our goal of ranking. See Exercise 14.8 for details of this notation.

The pairwise comparisons do not allow for *ties*, so we make no provision for the event "$i = j$" where the journals have equal rankings. Similarly, the probability i beats j is complementary to the probability j beats i and we have

$$\Pr[\,i > j\,] = 1 - \Pr[\,i < j\,].$$

A journal citing itself provides no information in its ranking among others. Let n_i denote the number of citations in journal i to a journal other than itself. A journal with many citations, for example, is more likely to have many citations to other journals, and we need to adjust for this. Similarly, the rate of $i > j$ (versus $i < j$) should be in the ratio n_j/n_i if the citation rates are equal.

Written in another way, we expect

---

[2] A smaller subset of Stigler's data is also available in **R** as the citation data in the BradleyTerry2 library. The interested reader can build comparisons between other journals and years using *Journal Citation Reports*.

$$\text{logit} \Pr[\, i > j \,] = \log(n_j/n_i) \tag{14.1}$$

if the citation rates were the same between the journals i and j.

Recall from (10.1) the logit is shorthand for "log-odds" so (14.1) models

$$\text{logit} \Pr[\, i > j \,] = \log\left\{ \frac{\Pr[\, i > j \,]}{1 - \Pr[\, i > j \,]} \right\} = \log\left\{ \frac{\Pr[\, i > j \,]}{\Pr[\, i < j \,]} \right\}.$$

One way to think about (14.1) is to consider a randomly chosen citation between journals i and j. We want to model the probability this citation represents a citation of journal i by journal j. The number of citations n_i made by journal i counts against it in this competition for ranking and prestige.

Bradley and Terry (1952) proposed a method for modeling comparisons of this type also used for ranking purposes. Suppose the i−th journal has a prestige or influence score λ_i we will estimate. The Bradley–Terry model comparing journals i and j is

$$\text{logit} \Pr[\, i > j \,] = \lambda_i - \lambda_j + \log(n_j/n_i) \tag{14.2}$$

after taking into account the marginal numbers of citations as in model (14.1).

Larger values of λ_i correspond to greater strength in the pairwise comparisons of journal i with all other competitors. Given the estimated values $\widehat{\lambda}_i$, then we can rank but also assign a relative strength to each journal.

Before we fit the Bradley–Terry model (14.2) in **R**, let us point out two features of this model. First, notice how we can add a constant to all of the λ's and still obtain the same model. Such a model is said to be *non-identifiable*. A non-identifiable model is one in which different parameter values give rise to the same model.

A simple solution to make model (14.2) identifiable is to arbitrarily set λ_1 equal to zero. Then all λ's are interpreted as comparisons with this item. The item associated with λ_1 is then referred to as the *reference category*. This choice of reference category can be changed in the **R** program to fit the Bradley–Terry model, as described below.

A second feature of model (14.2) is the inclusion of the $\log(n_j/n_i)$ term. We see this term is included in the model, but there is no associated parameter to estimate with it. Such a term in a model is called an *offset*. In the present example, the offset adjusts for the different underlying numbers of citations with no additional estimation necessary.

Output 14.1 shows how we can fit the Bradley–Terry model given at (14.2). This code includes some of the output from **R**. The `countsToBinomial` routine is a handy feature to convert a contingency table format as in Table 14.1 to a list of all pairwise comparisons. A portion of the output from this routine is given to illustrate this feature. The values `win1` and `win2` list how many times each pair of journals cites each other.

The `BTm` routine fits the model, and the output in Output 14.1 lists the different estimated λ's along with their standard errors and significance levels. The first listed journal, *Annals of Probability* (`AnnPr`), is the reference category and has an assigned $\lambda = 0$ for identifiability.

Output 14.1   Program and selected output fitting Bradley-Terry model to journal data

```
> prcite <- read.table(file = "probcite.txt", header = TRUE,
+     row.names = 1)
> prcite <- prcite[-7, -7]      # remove Totals in margins
>                               # number of non-self citations
> ns <- colSums(prcite) - diag(as.matrix(prcite))
> library(BradleyTerry2)        # necessary package
> # convert contingency table to list and remove self reference
> clist <- countsToBinomial(prcite)
> names(clist)[ 1 : 2] <- c("journal1", "journal2")
> clist

     journal1 journal2 win1 win2
1       AnnPr     PrTh  255  333
2       AnnPr  StochPr   33  208
3       AnnPr   JAppPr   46  121
     .   .   .                .   .
14     JAppPr    AnnSt   35   14
15    ThPrApp    AnnSt   63   50

> ni <- ns[match(clist$journal1, names(ns))]
> nj <- ns[match(clist$journal2, names(ns))]
> os <- log(nj / ni)            # offset
> clist <- cbind(clist, os)
>
> fitBTo<- BTm(cbind(win1, win2), journal1, journal2,
+        offset = os, data = clist)
> summary(fitBTo)
     .   .   .      .   .   .      .   .   .
Coefficients:
           Estimate Std. Error z value Pr(>|z|)
..PrTh     -0.01349    0.06878  -0.196    0.845
..StochPr  -0.19659    0.10159  -1.935    0.053 .
..JAppPr   -0.71494    0.10458  -6.836 8.13e-12 ***
..ThPrApp  -0.71571    0.09739  -7.349 1.99e-13 ***
..AnnSt    -0.87605    0.09925  -8.826  < 2e-16 ***
---
Signif. codes:  0 '***' 0.001 '**' 0.01 '*' 0.05 '.' 0.1 ' ' 1
```

All of the estimated λ's are negative indicating the *Annals of Probability* has the highest citation rate. Each successive journal has lower rates of citation as we read down the list of estimated coefficients in Output 14.1. The third and fourth journals have the word "Applied" in their titles and the last, *Annals of Statistics* (AnnSt), is very mathematical but not primarily a journal of research in probability. This conclusion agrees with the finding of Stigler (1994) who reports the citations of the newest ideas appear to flow from the theoretical journals to the more applied journals and not as much in the other direction.

Exercise 14.8 asks you to compare the citation rates of other statistics journals. Exercise 14.8 shows how we can assign relative strength to different sports teams.

14.2   Canonical Correlations

Correlations are defined between pairs of column vectors of data x and y. How can we generalize this concept to the correlation between sets of several columns $X = \{x_1, x_2, \ldots, x_n\}$ and $Y = \{y_1, y_2, \ldots, y_m\}$? As an example, consider the BRFSS health survey data introduced in Sect. 9.3. We want to identify a relationship between several measures of behaviors with several measures of health outcomes. Is there anything we can say about the group of behaviors having any relationship with the group of health outcomes?

The idea of *canonical correlations* is attributed to Hotelling (1935). He proposed methodology to find a pair of weights a and b in a way the correlation of the linear combinations $a'X$ and $b'Y$ is maximized.

The values of $a'x_i$ and $b'y_i$ are called *canonical scores* for the i-th individual. These scores serve to reduce this individual's multivariate data (x_i, y_i) to a pair of scalars capturing much of the information needed to compute the correlation. The weights a and b are the same for every individual and need to be estimated.

This approach is analogous to principal components in which a weighted average of every individual's complete data captures the maximum variability. By further analogy to principal components, the first, second, and subsequent canonical scores

$$(a_1'x_i, \ b_1'y_i), \ (a_2'x_i, \ b_2'y_i), \ \ldots$$

are highly correlated and also mutually orthogonal with the other canonical scores.

How is this approach different from multivariate linear regression? Multivariate linear regression, described in Sect. 9.2, expresses the mean of each column of Y as a separate linear combination of the columns in X resulting in a set of separate regression coefficients. We then examine the set of multivariate residuals in a principal component analysis, looking for additional explanatory value among the Y after having corrected for the X.

In canonical correlation, we seek linear combinations of columns in X and Y resulting in separate, respective univariate measures highly correlated with each other. The idea is to distill all of the linear information in X and Y resulting in highly correlated, scalar-valued canonical scores.

As an example of how we use this method, consider the car data examined in Sect. 9.2. Every car has 11 different attributes, each of which we described as either being a design feature built into the car by the engineers at the factory or else an empirical feature, readily experienced by the driver.

How can we combine all of the design features and show how these are related to a combination of the driver features? Further, can we assess the relative importance of each of the design features equally important in creating the driver experience? Equivalently, which driver experiences dominate, or summarize the others? Finally, which cars appear on different ends of this scale?

Table 9.1 lists the variables in the mtcars data set. Variables considered as user features are cylinders, displacement, rear axle ratio (drat), forward gears, "v", or

Output 14.2 Program to compute canonical correlations and plot the loadings in car data

```
require(datasets, CCA)
design <- mtcars[ , c(2, 3, 5, 8, 10, 11)]# cyl, disp, carb, drat, gear,vs
driver <- mtcars[ , c(1, 4, 6, 7, 9)]      # mpg, hp, wt, qsec, am

cancor(design, driver)
cc(design, driver)    # CCA package enhancement
ccs <- cc(design, driver)

desccl  <- ccs$scores$xscores[ , 1]
drivcc1 <- ccs$scores$yscores[ , 1]

sdr <- sort(drivcc1)
sdr <- sdr[c(1, length(sdr))]    # first and last
ext <- match(sdr, drivcc1)

plot( desccl, drivcc1,
   xlab = "Design canonical scores",
   ylab = "Driver canonical scores")
text(desccl[ext], drivcc1[ext], labels = rownames(mtcars)[ext],
   pos = c(4, 2), cex = .8)
```

straight arrangement of the cylinders. Driver features are miles per gallon, horse-power, weight, 1/4 mile time, and automatic or manual transmission.

The program to compute the canonical correlations and plot loading of the first coefficients is given in Output 14.2. The plot of the first canonical correlation loadings appears in Fig. 14.1. Two of the extremes are identified. Large luxury cars appear in the lower-left corner, and smaller economy cars are in the upper right. Overall, there is a very high correlation between these scores. These correspond exactly to the first canonical correlation, which we can verify as follows:

```
> cancor(design, driver)$cor

[1] 0.9850787 0.8471577 0.5796657 0.4137175 0.2548956

> cor(desccl, drivcc1)

[1] 0.9850787
```

The additional $cor values correspond to the second and subsequent canonical correlations.

We see the canonical correlation scores in Fig. 14.1 correspond, roughly, to the size and weight of the car. The compact Honda Civic in one corner and the Chrysler Imperial in the other. There is some evidence there are groups of individual cars on this scale. There are four cars located near the Imperial. The other three are Cadillac Fleetwood, Lincoln Continental, and Maserati Bora.

In summary, the canonical correlations can be used similarly to the way we used principal component analysis to identify and distinguish between groups of individuals. See Exercise 14.8 for more on this interpretation. In the following example,

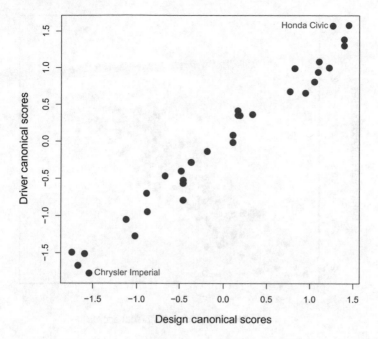

Fig. 14.1 Loadings of canonical correlation analysis of car data

the canonical correlation does not separate individuals well but identifies groups of variables that work together or against each other.

The BRFSS data is introduced and explained in Sect. 9.3. We examined the health characteristics of these US cities in terms of behavioral measures and the corresponding health outcomes. In the present analysis, we will use canonical correlations to find linear combinations of behavior rates having a high correlation with a linear combination of health outcomes.

The plot of canonical correlations for behaviors and health outcomes is given in Fig. 14.2. The most extreme cities identified in this plot are Provo, Utah, and Arcadia, Florida. These cities are not the same extremes identified using multivariate linear regression methods in Sect. 9.3. It is not obvious how these cities are remarkably different. A better summary of this analysis is to examine the weights given to each of the survey questions, as we show next.

The CCA library contains a number of useful enhancements to the basic canonical correlation program offered in **R**. The plt.cc program provides a graphical display of the variable weights going into each of the first two canonical correlations. An example of the use of this program is

```
library(CCA)
out <- c(2, 3, 5, 6, 7, 8, 11, 14)     # health outcome variables
beh <- c(1, 4, 9, 10, 12, 13, 15, 16, 17, 18) # behavioral measures
ccs <- cc(BRFSS[,out], BRFSS[,beh])
plt.cc(ccs, d1 = 1, d2 = 2, type = "v", var.label = TRUE)
```

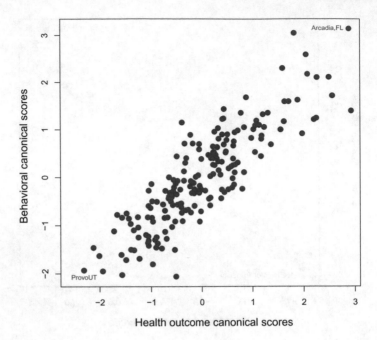

Fig. 14.2 Loadings of canonical correlation analysis of BRFSS survey data

and this code produces Fig. 14.3.

The weights for the first two canonical correlations are plotted in this figure: red for health outcomes and blue for behavioral variables. Variables listed within the inner target have low weight and are generally not useful in performing the canonical correlation. Specifically, the binge drinking, prostate test, flu shot, or PAP test are not useful in describing the canonical score for behaviors. Similarly, pregnancy diabetes or pre-diabetic conditions are not useful in summarizing health outcomes in a canonical correlation analysis. Health outcomes and behavioral variables appearing in the outer doughnut shape are more important to the canonical correlation summary of these data.

Important behavior measures include visiting a dentist, body mass index, exercise, health care coverage, and smoking. Important health outcomes are general health perception, asthma, and negative weights on each of disability, heart attack, and tooth loss. Notice also, asthma is an important health outcome in the second canonical correlation but not the first. In words, asthma is a separate or *orthogonal* outcome and is different from the others.

In summary, the canonical correlation analysis of multivariate data is useful when all variables can be classified into two groups: driver and design features for the car data, or the behavioral measures and health outcomes for the BRFSS data, for example. The canonical correlation approach creates a linear combination of variables in the separate groups having high correlation with each other. In the car data, we see

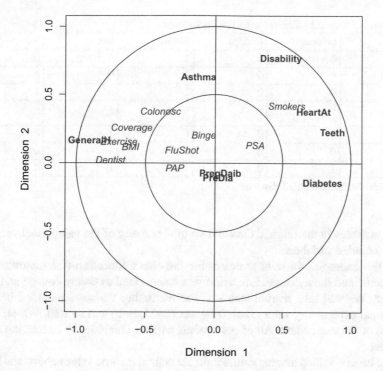

Fig. 14.3 Variable weights for the first two canonical correlations in the BRFSS data

how canonical correlations can help identify groups of individuals, as in a factor analysis or clustering. In the BRFSS, we see canonical correlation can be used to identify variables more (and also less) important in reducing multivariate data into scalar-valued linear combinations or variables.

14.3 Mediation

Mediation is part of the larger class of models where we want to identify *causal* relationships. Correlation, for example, identifies how two measurements jointly change in value but fails to identify causation. Correlation being symmetric in its arguments is unable to identify the direction of the relationship. Similarly, regression models suggest how one variable might explain the values of another, but again, this method avoids any discussion of a causal relationship. Mediation attempts to get at the causal relationship through the use of a mediating variable.

Let us illustrate the use of mediation with an example. A large sample from the 1994 US census of adults included income data. In this example, we want to determine the effect of education on income. The data in Table 14.2 omits many

Table 14.2 Excerpted values from the 1994 US census

	Income	College	Married	Sex	Race
1	0	0	1	0	0
2	0	0	0	0	0
3	0	0	1	0	1
$\vdots$	$\vdots$	$\vdots$	$\vdots$	$\vdots$	$\vdots$
32558	0	0	0	1	0
32559	0	0	0	0	0
32560	1	0	1	1	0

https://archive.ics.uci.edu/ml/datasets/

other variables in the original data and simplifies many of the categorical values of those included variables.

In this example, we want to determine the effect education (the treatment) has on income and the outcome. Education was categorized as 0=any college and 1=no college. We will take marital status as the mediating variable. Included here are additional explanatory values indicating sex (0=M, 0=F) and race (0=White, 1=All others) of the respondent. All of our models will also include the interaction of sex and race.

The binary-valued income values indicate annual income values above and below $50K. In 1994, the median US income was about $34K per year so the indicators represent amounts almost 50% above the median. The whole data set is very large and we chose to examine a 10% sample.

To illustrate the effect of mediation, let us first perform three regressions and compare the relevant estimated regression coefficients.

Initially, the marginal effect of any college experience on income we have

$$\text{logit(Income)} = \alpha_1 + \beta_1 \, \text{College} \quad + \quad \text{effects of sex} * \text{race}$$

where $\widehat{\beta_1} = -.368 \, (p = .004)$ so, marginally, education has a large effect on income.

When we perform the regression of college education on marriage

$$\text{logit(Marriage)} = \alpha_2 + \beta_2 \, \text{College} \quad + \quad \text{effects of sex} * \text{race}$$

we obtain $\widehat{\beta_2} = -.287 \, (p = .002)$. Clearly, education has a strong effect on marital status as well.

In the third regression

$$\text{logit(Income)} = \alpha_3 + \beta_3 \, \text{College} + \beta_3' \, \text{Marriage} \quad + \quad \text{effects of sex} * \text{race}$$

where $\widehat{\beta_3} = -.292 \, (p = .009)$ and $\widehat{\beta_3'} = 2.10 \, (p < .001)$.

When we compare $\widehat{\beta}_1 = -.368$ in the marginal regression of education on income, we see it is smaller in (absolute) magnitude than $\widehat{\beta}_3 = -.292$ in the third regression model which includes marriage. That is, the effect of education on income is attenuated or mediated by marriage.

Mediation attempts to get at a causal relationship through the use of a mediating variable. Treatment affects the outcome directly. In the example we just discussed, the outcome is income and the treatment is college education. The mediating variable is marital status. In the second of these three regressions, marriage is also related to education. So education is related to income. But education also has a strong relationship to marriage, and marriage, in turn, is also a strong determinant of income.

We want to partition these two effects of education on income. Specifically, how much of the effect of education is due directly to income as opposed to indirectly, through the effect of education on marriage and then marriage on income?

In mediation analysis, the treatment affects the outcome, both directly and also through the mediating variable. In some cases, it is possible to measure the separate effects of treatment on outcome directly and also through the mediating variable.

Let us introduce some of the language and notation used in mediation. Suppose there is a treatment t_i which is randomized to the i-th subject. For the moment, let us assume t_i only takes on the value 0 or 1.

There is a mediating variable $m(t)$ which depends on the treatment. We can pose a mathematical model for this relationship, referred to as the *mediator model*. There may be other explanatory variables x available to us so we might also write the mediator model as $m(t, x)$.

The outcome of interest is y and its value depends on both the treatment and mediating variable. We can pose a model for this relationship as well. The *outcome model* is written as $y(t, m)$ or perhaps as $y(t, m, x)$. The mediating variable m depends on the treatment t so the outcome model is also written as $y(t, m(t), x)$.

What is the effect of treatment t on the outcome y? There are two ways to describe this. The *total effect* of treatment is the difference in the outcome when $t = 0$ and $t = 1$. That is

$$\text{Total effect} \ = \ y(1, m(1)) \ - \ y(0, m(0))$$

noting the same treatment value associated with both the outcome y as the mediator m.

The central idea behind mediation analysis is our ability to partition the total effect into two components. These are the *direct effects*:

$$\text{DE}(t) \ = \ y(1, m(t)) \ - \ y(0, m(t))$$

and the *causal mediation effects*:

$$\text{CME}(t) \ = \ y(t, m(1)) \ - \ y(t, m(0))$$

so together, these add up

$$\text{Total effect} = \text{CME}(t) + \text{DE}(1 - t)$$

for any treatment $t = 0, 1$.

Informally, the direct effect measures the change in outcome when the treatment changes but the mediating variable remains the same. Similarly, the mediating effect measures the change in outcome when the treatment is unchanged but only the mediating variable varies.

In this manner, we are able to express the direct effect treatment has on the outcome (DE) separately from the effect of the outcome through the mediating variable (CME). Visually, we can describe these relationships as

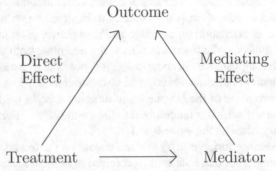

where the treatment effect is measured as the sum of its separate effects on outcome directly and also through its effect through the mediating variable.

In Output 14.3, we present the **R** program and selected output for the mediation analysis. Briefly, the analysis consists of separate logistic regressions for income and marital status, both binary-valued. The `mediate` statement, in the **R** package `mediation`, combines the output of these two logistic regressions and performs the mediation analysis.

More specifically, Output 14.3 begins with a logistic regression in `glm` for marital status as a linear function of any college, sex, race, and the sex–race interaction term. The women appear to be very unlikely to be married. Presumably, the Census considered the male partner in a marriage to be the head of the household so the women answering the survey were single. The race is also a strong determinant of marital status, as is its interaction with sex.

The direct effect model is another logistic regression performed in `glm`. This model shows marriage is strongly associated with income. College education has a smaller effect. Sex, race, and their interaction are not statistically significant in this model.

The `mediate` program in the `mediation` package takes the output of these two separate logistic regressions and estimates the separate direct and mediation effects, both analytically and through a simulation. These separate effects and their confidence intervals are plotted in Fig. 14.4.

Overall, there is a large statistical effect of education on income. This is measured as the total effect. The separate direct effects and mediation effects of marriage are also both statistically significant. The direct effect is about twice as large as the

Output 14.3 Selected output for the mediation analysis of 1994 census data

```
mediation.model <- glm(married
~ college + sex + race,
                        family = binomial, data = adult)
summary(mediation.model)

Coefficients:
            Estimate Std. Error z value Pr(>|z|)
(Intercept)  0.64532    0.05448  11.844  < 2e-16 ***
college     -0.28714    0.09194  -3.123  0.00179 **
sex         -2.16841    0.10499 -20.654  < 2e-16 ***
race        -0.74830    0.13530  -5.531 3.19e-08 ***
sex:race     0.62544    0.25988   2.407  0.01610 *

outcome.model <- glm(income ~ college + married + sex * race,
                    family = binomial, data = adult)
summary(outcome.model)

Coefficients:
            Estimate Std. Error z value Pr(>|z|)
(Intercept) -2.27640    0.11602 -19.621  < 2e-16 ***
college     -0.29150    0.11141  -2.616  0.00888 **
married      2.10233    0.11709  17.954  < 2e-16 ***
sex         -0.29625    0.13674  -2.167  0.03027 *
race        -0.07833    0.17086  -0.458  0.64662
sex:race    -0.13439    0.33344  -0.403  0.68693

med.out <- mediate(mediation.model, outcome.model, treat = "college",
                mediator = "married", robustSE = TRUE, sims = 100)
summary(med.out)

                          Estimate 95% CI Lower 95% CI Upper p-value
ACME (control)             -0.0211      -0.0347      -0.01   0.008 **
ACME (treated)             -0.0181      -0.0316      -0.01   0.008 **
ADE (control)              -0.0443      -0.0760      -0.01   0.008 **
ADE (treated)              -0.0413      -0.0694      -0.01   0.008 **
Total Effect               -0.0623      -0.0943      -0.03  <2e-16 ***
Prop. Mediated (control)    0.3451       0.1072       0.68   0.008 **
Prop. Mediated (treated)    0.2846       0.0871       0.66   0.008 **
ACME (average)             -0.0196      -0.0323      -0.01   0.008 **
ADE (average)              -0.0428      -0.0726      -0.01   0.008 **
Prop. Mediated (average)    0.3149       0.0972       0.67   0.008 **

plot(med.out)
```

mediation effect. The mediation effect could also be explained when married couples combine their separate incomes.

The mediation package allows for generalities such as multiple mediating variables and non-binary-valued treatments. There are also assumptions concerning the methodology used and these assumptions can be tested as well in this package. Finally, there is a sensitivity analysis to see how much the mediation estimates change when these assumptions are violated.

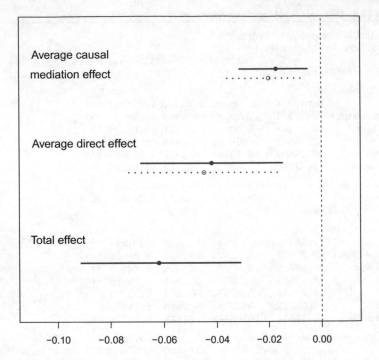

Fig. 14.4 Average direct and mediation effects of education on income

14.4   Counterfactuals

Along with mediation, covered in the previous section, another topic in causality is the counterfactual approach. Counterfactuals ask what might have happened under different circumstances. The estimation is not simply extrapolation, but rather a mathematical argument using the existing data.

Let us start with a simple example involving a clinical trial. Every patient received either a placebo ($j = 0$) or else the active drug ($j = 1$). These two groups of patients might be different in other ways as well. The data is observed in a retrospective manner with all treatments and outcomes known to us. The counterfactual analysis asks how different the outcomes would have been had the treatments been reversed.

We can talk about the characteristics of the treated patients X_1 and placebo patients X_0. The patients might be different in terms of demographic or clinical characteristics. Proper randomization may serve to reduce some of these differences but many are unavoidable. These characteristics will have different distribution functions, denoted F_{X_1} and F_{X_0}, respectively.

Every patient has a measured outcome. The outcome might measure survival time, the percent reduction in symptoms, or other useful clinical endpoints. We can speak about the outcomes Y_1 of the treated patients and the distribution $F_{Y_1(X_1)}(y)$ of these outcomes. Specifically, this is the distribution of outcomes of treated patients with the characteristics of treated patients. Similarly, there are placebo outcomes Y_0 and their distribution $F_{Y_0(X_0)}(y)$ as well.

There are also conditional distributions for outcomes of treated patients $F_{Y_1 X_1}(y \mid x)$ and placebo patients $F_{Y_0 X_0}(y \mid x)$. These are conditional distributions of outcomes of treated patients given characteristics of those treated patients.

The counterfactual argument allows us to derive the marginal distribution of treated outcomes Y_1 when the patients have placebo characteristics X_0. That is,

$$F_{Y_1(X_0)} = \int F_{Y_1(X_1)}(y \mid x) \, dF_{X_0}(x)$$

with a similar expression for $F_{Y_0(X_1)}$.

This result is purely mathematical and is not observable in practice. In order for it to work properly, the distributions of X_0 and X_1 cannot be very different. As long as there is a large overlap in values of characteristics X_0 and X_1, then, intuitively, we can move some of the emphasis around to obtain the counterfactual distribution.

There is a useful partitioning we can see by writing

$$F_{Y_1(X_1)} - F_{Y_0(X_0)} = \left\{ F_{Y_1(X_1)} - F_{Y_0(X_1)} \right\} + \left\{ F_{Y_0(X_1)} - F_{Y_0(X_0)} \right\}.$$

The interpretation here is the overall difference in outcomes we observe is the sum of differences in outcomes under the same patient characteristics plus the differences in characteristics for the same outcome.

In most of the discussion so far about counterfactuals, the distributions F could also be replaced by their inverse functions F^{-1} and statements could be made about the *quantiles* of the various distributions. As a result, many statements and models for counterfactuals are concerned with the quantiles of distributions, rather than the distribution functions themselves. Specifically, the `counterfactual` program, illustrated below, computes the counterfactual distribution in terms of the `quantile effects` often abbreviated as QE.

Let us illustrate a counterfactual analysis and show how we perform this in **R**. Consider the data in Table 14.3 published by Engel[3] in 1857. *Engel's law* states the percent of one's income spent on food will decrease with income. As one's income rises, a smaller percent will be spent on necessities such as food and more money is available to spend on luxury goods. This data set is available as `engel` in the quantreg library.

Engel's data is plotted in Fig. 14.5. The income is transformed to a log scale. The *loess* fit confirms Engel's theory: percent of food expenditure decreases with income. The `loess` fit is non-linear, almost constant for the lowest half of income levels but decreasing more steeply as income increases.

Suppose we propose a hypothetical tax policy and use counterfactual methods to estimate the resultant percent income spent on food. We can make the proposed taxation progressive, where higher incomes are more heavily taxed and the lowest

---

[3] Ernst Engel (1821–1896). German statistician and economist.

Table 14.3 The `engel` data measuring income and food expenditures for 235 Belgian families

	Income	Food expenditure
1	420.1577	255.8394
2	541.4117	310.9587
3	901.1575	485.6800
	⋮	⋮
233	581.3599	468.0008
234	743.0772	522.6019
235	1057.6767	750.3202

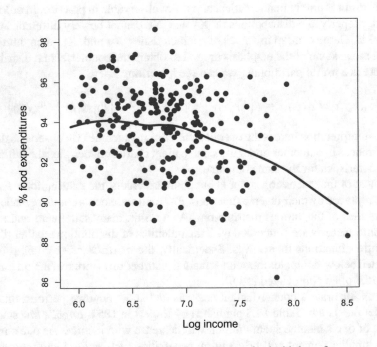

Fig. 14.5 Engel's data describing percent of income spent on food with *loess* fit

incomes are supplemented. Specifically, let us propose a 5% tax for every standard deviation the citizen's income is above the mean income, all on a log scale. Similarly, we can also propose a 5% supplement for every standard deviation below the mean income, again on a log scale.

The **R** code is given in Output 14.4. This code begins by obtaining the data and creating the *loess* fit given in Fig. 14.5.

The counterfactual `taxed_income` values are created and their cumulative distribution is plotted in Fig 14.6. The original, observed, values and these counterfactual

Output 14.4 R code for counterfactual analysis of Engel's data

```
library(Counterfactual, quantreg)
data(engel)

engel <- engel[order(engel$income), ]        #  sort by income values
pctfd <- 100 * log(engel$foodexp) / log(engel$income) #  percent food
                                                       #       expenditure
loginc <- log(engel$income)                   #  log income scale
food.lo <- loess(pctfd ~ loginc)              #  fit loess model
food.lo <- predict(food.lo)                   #  loess values to plot
                                              #  draw Figure 15.5
plot(loginc, pctfd, xlab = "Log income", ylab = "% food expenditures",
     cex.lab = 1.25, col = "blue", pch = 19, cex = 1.25)
lines(loginc, food.lo, lwd = 4, col = "red")


#              Counterfactual values of taxed income
taxed_income <- loginc - .05 * (loginc - mean(loginc)) / sd(loginc)


#              Counterfactual analysis of taxed log(income)
quants <- c(1:99)/100                         #  quantiles to examine
prange <- 5 : 95                              #  plotting range of these
                                              #     values
cfres <- counterfactual(pctfd ~ loginc,
              counterfactual_var = taxed_income, printdeco = FALSE,
              quantiles = quants, transformation = TRUE)
cf <- (cfres$resCE)[,1]                        #  estimated quantiles
cflow <- (cfres$resCE)[,3]                     #  lower confidence intervals
cfhigh <- (cfres$resCE)[,4]                    #  upper confidence intervals
                                               #  draw Figure 15.7
plot(c(0, 1), range(c(min(cflow[prange])), max(cfhigh[prange])),
       xlim = c(0, 1), type = "n", xlab = "Income quantile",
       ylab = "Difference in food expenditure", cex.lab=1.25)
polygon(c(quants[prange], rev(quants[prange])),
        c(cfhigh[prange], rev(cflow[prange])),
        density = -100, border = FALSE, col = "grey90")
lines(quants[prange], cf[prange], col = "red", lwd = 2)
abline(h = 0, lty = 2)
```

values have the same mean but the counterfactual values have a smaller standard deviation. Specifically, we can see both the tails of the observed income distribution are shortened in Fig. 14.6. That is, the proposed taxation program reduces the extremes in income but keeps the mean the same. Otherwise, these two distributions are not too different, a requirement for the counterfactual argument to work properly.

The remainder of Output 14.4 is concerned with estimating the counterfactual distribution and plotting it in Fig. 14.7. Specifically, the `counterfactual` statement requires we specify the model (`pctfd~loginc`) for the observed data, just as we would in `glm`. The other requirement is to specify the counterfactual variable to be substituted for the observed values. The specific quantiles of the counterfactual distribution we require are specified as `quantiles` = and the `printdeco` = controls the amount of output produced. The `transformation` = option specifies the counterfactual income values are a function of the original values. Finally,

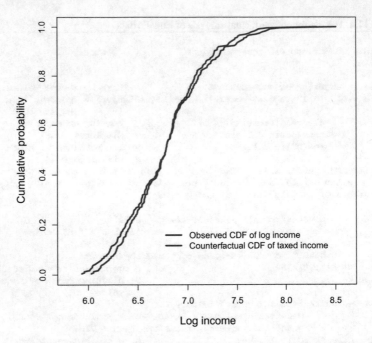

Fig. 14.6 Cumulative distributions of observed and counterfactual taxed incomes, all on a log scale

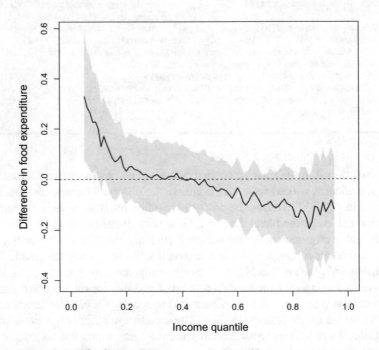

Fig. 14.7 Counterfactual food expenditures on proposed taxed income

Output 14.4 provides the code to produce Fig. 14.7 including the shading of confidence intervals.

In contrast to the food expenditures estimated in Fig. 14.5, we see the counterfactual estimates in Fig. 14.7 fall off even at the lowest income levels. From this exercise, we conclude income supplements at the lowest income levels reduce the rates of food expenditures. At higher incomes, the rate of food expenditures levels off with a somewhat larger confidence interval.

Of course, many assumptions have been made in order to use this statistical method and to come to these conclusions. In individual cases, there is no telling how an income supplement might be spent. The counterfactual method assumes households with a hypothetical, supplemented income would behave as an observed household with higher incomes. Similarly, we are anticipating taxed individuals would behave as observed individuals with corresponding lower incomes. In this example, it is reasonable to ask what may have happened if some of the subjects were able (or forced to) to act as others in the same data set.

Counterfactual analysis has its critics. It is possible to consider what might have happened under totally unreasonable, unobservable circumstances. In the example of this section, it is possible to consider the outcomes if income values were extrapolated beyond those observed in the original data. Instead, we considered pulling extreme values closer to the center of the observed distribution and assumed such individuals would behave as those in the observed sample. Extrapolation is a common danger in many statistical methods.

14.5 Methods for Extreme Order Statistics

Statisticians are prone to looking at measures of central tendency such as the mean or the median. But it is often the extremes in the data grabbing the attention of the public. We talk about the worst flood, instead of the typical rainfall. Headlines shout about the largest clusters of cancer cases, not the average morbidity rate. The extremes cause us to sit up and notice the best and worst of things.

Nobody much cares about the average marathoner's record, for example. In a race, somebody has to be fastest, and we usually only care about the winner. Are the first few finishers so much stronger than the rest of the pack or are they all about the same in their abilities? In athletic endeavors, to continue this example, we may point to one extraordinary individual achievement but then ask whether this one person is much stronger than the second—and third—place finishers. Some runners will finish faster, but do their abilities outshine the others? Is it possible to identify a small number of outstanding athletes whose performance is completely beyond the rest of the pack?

The study of extremes is also tantamount to asking where the tail of the distribution begins. Sometimes we just want to know about the approximate distribution of the single, largest value, but there are situations where the joint, multivariate distribution of several of the largest values is also of interest.

Table 14.4 Largest financial advisors in first half of 2012

Advisor	Number of deals	Value in $B	Market share in %
Goldman Sachs	190	279	25
Morgan Stanley	170	249	22
JPMorgan Chase	138	221	20
Deutsche Bank	116	214	19
Barclays	146	195	18
Credit Suisse	117	184	17
Citigroup	100	152	14
Bank of America	95	140	13
Lazard	111	116	10
Nomura	89	105	9
Rothschild	116	89	8
BNP Paribas	35	75	7
UBS	82	68	6
RBC	91	53	5
M Klein	1	49	4

Source NYTimes (July 3, 2012) and
Thompson Reuters

For another example, consider the 15 largest financial advisors, ranked by the
value of the deals they brokered in the first half of 2012. The data in Table 14.4
includes the number of merger and acquisition deals brokered and percentage of
market share.

It is easy to identify the largest deal-makers, but are their numbers completely
out of line relative to the other numbers in this table? After all, some advisory firms
have to be the largest. One could argue a firm with familiarity in negotiating large
transactions would be best suited for conducting more of the same.

In this section, we want to describe a model for the tail behavior of several of the
most extreme order statistics. Define $x_{(1)} \geq x_{(2)} \geq \cdots$ as the ordered data values,
in decreasing order. The usual notation for order statistics is to put the subscripts in
parentheses. We do this to distinguish the ordered values from a random list of the
data.

Let us introduce some theory for the behavior of extremes. The *standardized
extreme values* z_i are defined as

$$z_i = \left(x_{(i)} - b \right) / a$$

for $i = 1, 2, \ldots, k$.

These values are ordered $z_1 \geq z_2 \geq \cdots \geq z_k$ and standardized by the location
parameter b and scale parameter $a > 0$. We will show how to estimate a and b,
below.

The literature on extreme order statistics talks about the extreme tail behavior of a distribution in terms of its *domain of attraction*. The domain of attraction is shorthand for how fast the upper tail of the distribution tapers off. Specifically, we will assume the population we are sampling from is in the domain of attraction of the Type I or Gumbel[4] distribution. This means that, when properly normalized, z_1 behaves as an observation from the Gumbel distribution with cumulative distribution function

$$F(z) = \exp(-e^{-z}).$$

This assumption holds for a variety of commonly encountered distributions including the normal, gamma, log-gamma, Weibull, logistic, as well as the Gumbel distribution itself, but not the uniform or Cauchy distributions.

Under the assumption of a Type I domain of attraction, the joint distribution of $z_1, z_2, \ldots, z_k$ has an approximate density function

$$f(z_1, z_2, \ldots, z_k) = \exp\left(e^{-z_k} - \sum z_i\right) \tag{14.3}$$

for $z_1 \geq z_2 \geq \cdots \geq z_k$.

In order for (14.3) to hold, we will also assume that the sample size n is very large, but the number of observations in the tail k is modest. It is not necessary to know the value of the full sample, n. In the data of Table 14.4, for example, the full census of all financial advisors is likely to be very large, but we only observe the largest of these. Below, we will also demonstrate a method for estimating the values of k in the data where (14.3) appears to be valid.

When (14.3) holds, the marginal distribution of z_i has density function

$$f_i(z) = \exp\left(-e^{-z} - iz\right) / (i - 1)!.$$

Figure 14.8 plots the first five extreme value marginal densities. The largest value z_1 has a skewed distribution. Order statistics, with larger values of i, are nearer the center of the population. Those closer to the center will have less skewed and more nearly normal distributions.

The mean of the marginal distribution z_1 of the largest extremal distribution is γ where

$$\gamma = 0.577216\ldots$$

is the *Euler constant*.[5]

The mean of z_i for $i = 2, 3, \ldots$ is $\gamma - S_i$ where

$$S_k = 1 + 1/2 + \cdots + 1/(k - 1).$$

The variance of z_1 is $\pi^2/6$ and the variance of z_i is

---

[4] Emil Julius Gumbel (1891–1966). German mathematician and political writer.
[5] Leonhard Euler (1707–1783). Swiss physicist and mathematician.

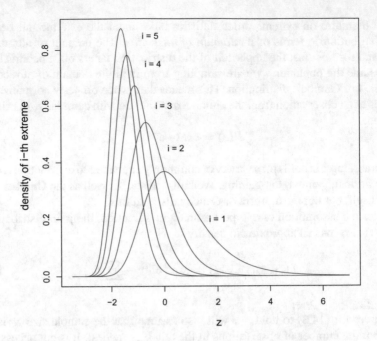

Fig. 14.8 The density functions of the first five extremal value distributions

$$\pi^2/6 - 1 - 1/2^2 - \cdots - 1/(i-1)^2)$$

for $i = 2, 3, \ldots$.

In words, the mean and variance of extreme order statistics become smaller as we consider order statistics farther below the largest. The distributions farther from the largest are also more symmetric and look more like normal. We will use these expressions for the means and variances of z_i in the construction of Fig. 14.10, below.

The parameter values for scale a and location b are estimated as follows. Define

$$\overline{x}_k = k^{-1}(x_{(1)} + \cdots + x_{(k)})$$

as the average of the k largest observations.

Then we estimate a as

$$\widehat{a}_k = \overline{x}_k - x_{(k)}$$

and

$$\widehat{b}_k = \widehat{a} + k(S_{k-1} - \gamma) + x_{(k)}.$$

The estimates of a and b depend on the choice of k so it is useful to write these estimates as $\widehat{a}_k$ and $\widehat{b}_k$.

The discussion so far shows how we can fit models of extremes and describe their approximate density function. We still need a way to determine whether these models are appropriate for our data. A useful approach to studying goodness of fit is to examine the spacings, or differences between adjacent ordered values. Spacings were introduced in Sect. 2.5.

Define the *normalized spacings* as

$$d_i = i \left(x_{(i)} - x_{(i+1)} \right)$$

for $i = 1, 2, \ldots, k$.

The theory of extremes (see Weissman 1978, or Zelterman 1993, for examples) is these normalized spacings will all be approximately independent, and all have the same exponential distribution. The farther out in the tail we go, the farther apart the observations should be from each other. This helps explain the "i" multiplier in the definition for d_i.

Several assumptions go into this claim, of course. We need statements about the actual shape of the tail (domain of attraction) of the parent distribution giving rise to $x_1, x_2, \ldots, x_n$. The conditions on the actual shape of the tail are harder to describe in mathematical terms, but usually appear in practice. Next, we will show how to estimate the value of k where this approximation works.

Where does the tail of the distribution begin, and what is an appropriate value of k for the data? To answer this question, we will consider a test for independent, exponentially distributed observations based on the Gini[6] statistic. Gail and Gastwirth (1978) describe the Gini statistic in this context.

The Gini statistic is

$$G_k = \sum_{i=1}^{k-1} i(k-i) \left(d_{(i)} - d_{(i+1)} \right) \Bigg/ (k-1) \sum_{i}^{k} d_i \ . \qquad (14.4)$$

This statistic behaves approximately as normal with mean $1/2$ and variance $12(k-1)$ when the spacings d_i are approximately distributed as exponential. Notice there is no need to estimate the mean parameter of these exponential variates. The test of the exponential character of the spacings of the original data is based on the spacings of those spacings. Let us show how to use this statistic to estimate where the tail of the distribution of the x's begins for the corporate asset data.

For each of the $k = 2, 3, \ldots, 15$ financial advisors in this data set, we calculated the Gini statistic G_k and plotted the p-value for each in Fig. 14.9. In this figure, we see the largest 10 values in this data set jointly follow the model of extreme values but the largest 12 (or more) of these start to fail the assumptions. Even so, there is good evidence in Fig. 14.10 for using all of the extreme data in Table 14.4.

The observed and fitted density functions are displayed in Fig. 14.10. The observed values are given as large red dots in this figure, plotted against their ordered values on the vertical axis. The thin black lines are central 95% of the marginal (individual)

---

[6] Corrado Gini (1884–1965). Italian statistician, demographer, and social theorist.

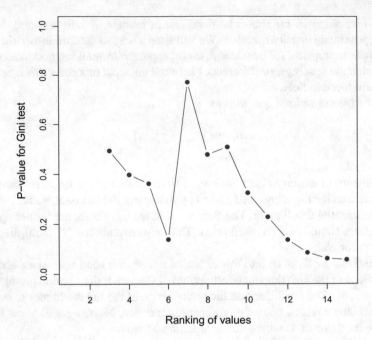

Fig. 14.9 P-values of Gini statistic (14.4) for the deal values in Table 14.4

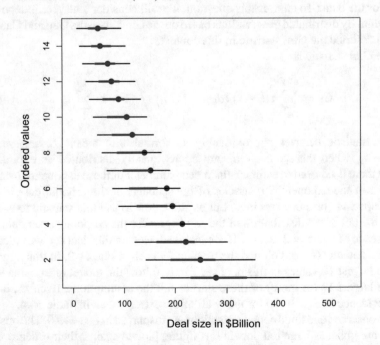

Fig. 14.10 Largest financial deals brokered in the first half of 2012 (in red) and fitted extreme value distributions. The central 50% of each distribution is in blue and 95% in black

distributions f_i, and the thick blue lines are the central 50%. The ordered values $x_{(i)}$ appear to be where the extreme value distributions would expect them to occur. In summary, the extreme values in this data set do not appear to be out of line. There are many other companies not listed in these data, and the present sample is within the expectation of the extreme value theory.

In Fig. 14.10, we used all of the data to estimate values of a and b. See Exercise 14.8 for a discussion of the choice of k in estimating these parameters. Other exercises examine extremes in salaries, oil spills, and votes for candidates in a primary election.

14.6 Methods for Overdispersion

A model may fail to explain the data adequately or fail to fit the data in a certain region. We usually point to problems in the specification of the mean for these shortcomings. Any lack of fit may also be due to an unexplained increase in the variability. We plot residuals, for example, but these alone are unable to distinguish these separate situations in practice. This section develops a different set of diagnostic measures especially suited for detecting an increase in variability. As with shortcomings in the mean parameter to explain the data, these are methods to model differences in the variances.

Let us begin with a small example to illustrate and motivate the methods we develop in this section. Many of the details are given in Exercise 14.8 in order to simplify the narrative here.

Suppose we have a sample from a Poisson distribution with mean parameter $\lambda > 0$. We will attribute an increase in the Poisson variability due to the values of λ varying from one observation to another. That is, we want to compare a situation where λ is the same for every observation versus a different model where the values of λ vary slightly between every observation. If the behavior of λ under this model can be described by a gamma random variable, then the marginal distribution of the observations will follow the negative binomial distribution. The details are given in Exercise 14.8.

Figure 14.11 plots the deviances for the Poisson distribution (in red) and different negative binomial models (in blue). In all of these models, the means of the distributions are the same and only the variances change. Increasing the variability induced by the gamma mixture results in the deviances flattening out in the neighborhood of the maximum likelihood estimator of the mean parameter. This flattening of the likelihood function is the result of overdispersion or extra-variability. The change in curvature can be expressed in terms of the second derivative of the likelihood, as we will demonstrate next.

Let us first give some background of the methods, in general terms, and then work out a specific example for a linear model. Let $x_1, x_2, \ldots, x_n$ denote independent observations sampled from the same density function $f(x \mid \theta)$ indexed by parameter θ.

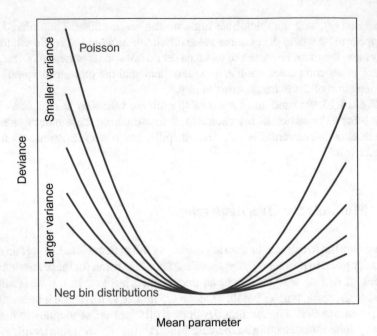

Fig. 14.11 Deviances for the Poisson distribution *in red* and for the negative binomial *in blue*. The means are the same for all of these distributions. The variances of these distributions increase from top to bottom

The question of overdispersion hinges on whether or not the values of θ are the same for every value of x. If θ is the same or *homogeneous* for every observation, then the model is not overdispersed. In this section, we suggest overdispersion or excess variation results from θ varying between observations.

Lambert and Roeder (1995) proposed a *convexity plot* as a means of detecting overdispersion.[7] They propose plotting $C(\theta)$ against θ where

$$C(\theta) = n^{-1} \sum_{i=1}^{n} f(x_i \mid \theta) / f(x_i \mid \widehat{\theta})$$

where $\widehat{\theta}$ is the maximum likelihood estimate of θ. If this plot exhibits convexity, then there is evidence of overdispersion.

The test of heterogeneity proposed by Zelterman and Chen (1988) is based on a flattening of the log-likelihood function and rejects the null hypothesis of parameter homogeneity for large values of the statistic $\sum H(x_i)$ where

$$H(x_i) = f''(x_i \mid \widehat{\theta}) / f(x_i \mid \widehat{\theta}) \tag{14.5}$$

---

[7] This diagnostic is unrelated to the convexity plot used in finance to describe the price of a bond.

where f'' is the second derivative of f with respect to θ.

The overdispersion residuals $H(x_i)$ examine the apparent change in curvature of the likelihood function. Such change in curvature is illustrated in Fig. 14.11. See Exercise 14.8 for details and applications of this statistic.

To illustrate these methods, let us return to the large BRFSS survey data described in Sect. 9.3. Let us perform a linear regression, fitting exercise rates as a linear function of other measures of self-care. The specific model of interest is

$$\texttt{Exercise} = \beta_0 + \beta_1 \,\texttt{Dentist} + \beta_2 \,\texttt{Teeth} + \beta_3 \,\texttt{BMI} + \beta_4 \,\texttt{Smokers} \quad (14.6)$$

plus normally distributed errors.

This model has five parameters $\beta = \{\beta_j\}$: an intercept plus four slopes. These can be estimated in $\texttt{glm}$. The overdispersion diagnostics provide evidence of whether these parameters are constant throughout the data and possibly where these appear to vary.

To develop the diagnostics for linear models, let us provide some useful notation. There are n residuals r_i ($i = 1, \ldots, n$) with estimated standard error s. The maximum likelihood estimates $\widehat{\beta}_j$ have estimated standard errors σ_j for $j = 0, 1, \ldots, p$. The j−th covariate value (independent variable) measured on the i−th city is x_{ij}. Let $\phi(z)$ denote the density function of the standard normal distribution.

The likelihood function for the i−th subject is $\phi(r_i/s)/s$ so the convexity plot for the β_j parameter plots values of z for values of

$$C_j(z) = n^{-1} \sum_{i=1}^{n} \phi(r_i/s \mid \beta_j = \widehat{\beta}_j + z\sigma_j)/\phi(r_i/s \mid \widehat{\beta}) \,.$$

A change in the estimated parameter value can be expressed in terms of the residual giving us

$$C_j(z) = n^{-1} \sum_{i=1}^{n} \phi\{(r_i - z\sigma_j x_{ij})/s\}/\phi(r_i/s) \,.$$

These values are plotted in Fig. 14.12 for each of the covariates in the linear model (14.6). The **R** code to produce this figure is given in Output 14.5, illustrating how to extract the necessary fitted parameters and statistics from the $\texttt{glm}$ output.

This figure indicates a clear overdispersion in the covariate for the missing teeth covariate. To confirm this finding, the plot of exercise rates by tooth loss given in Fig 14.13 clearly exhibits a larger amount of variability of exercise for larger rates of tooth loss.

The intercept in Fig. 14.12 shows some evidence of overdispersion, perhaps in certain circumstances or regions of the data. The other covariates in the linear model ($\texttt{Dentist}$, $\texttt{Smokers}$, $\texttt{BMI}$) do not exhibit overdispersion.

Finally, we can identify individual observations contributing to overdispersion. The overdispersion residuals, H_i given in (14.5) are weighted functions of $r_i^2 - s^2$ or the difference between squared residuals and their expected values. These

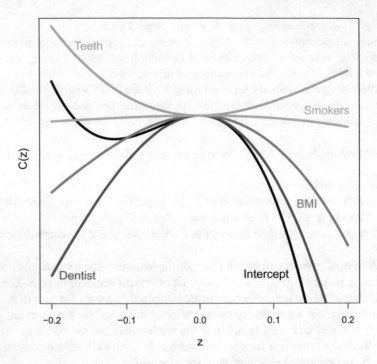

Fig. 14.12 Convexity plots for each of the covariates in the linear model (14.6)

weights are proportional to the square of the covariate values. We then can define the overdispersion residuals

$$H_{ij} = x_{ij}^2 \ (r_i^2 - s^2) \ \bigg/ \ 3^{1/3} \ s^2 \ n^{-1} \sum_k x_{ki}^2 \ .$$

Large overdispersion residuals will result from a combination of large covariate absolute values and large residual absolute values. Negative overdispersion residuals indicate observed data close to the fitted regression line. These negative overdispersion residuals are usually not of concern unless there are too many of them, perhaps indicating artificial data fitting the model too well.

These overdispersion residuals for model (14.6) appear in Fig. 14.14. A few remarkable cities are identified in this figure. Midland, TX has extreme values for all five of its overdispersion residuals making it the real standout among these cities.

Output 14.5 R code to produce convexity plot in Fig. 14.12

```
overlinear <- function(z, resid, ses, xmat, sighat) {
    #  convexity plots C(z) for overdispersion in linear models
    N <- dim(xmat)[1]
    p <- dim(xmat)[2]                          #  includes intercept
    rmat <- matrix(resid, N, p)                #  p column copies of residuals
    den <- dnorm(resid, sd = sighat)           #  denominators
    den <- matrix(den, nrow = N, ncol = p,     #  as matrix, with p columns
                  dimnames = list(row.names(xmat), colnames(xmat)))
    xs <- xmat * t(matrix(ses, nrow = p, ncol = N))  # X matrix * se's
    build <- NULL
    for (i in 1 : length(z) ) {                #  for each value of z
        difm <- as.matrix(rmat - z[i] * xs)    #  difference, as matrix
        difm <- dnorm(difm, sd = sighat)       #  terms in numerators
        difm <- difm / den
        cm <- colMeans(difm)                   #  C(z) for each covariate
        colnames(cm) <- NULL
        build <- rbind(build, c(z[i], cm))          }
    colnames(build) <- c("z", colnames(xmat))
    build }
BRFSS <- read.table(file = "BRFSS.txt",        #  example data
                header = T, row.names = 1)[, c(9, 13: 15, 17)]
BRFSS[1:2, ]                                    #  look at some values
            Exercise Dentist Teeth  BMI Smokers
Akron,OH        77.4    75.6 46.9 38.2    25.5
Albuquerque,NM  82.0    70.4 39.0 43.3    19.4

glm.out <- glm(Exercise ~ Dentist + Teeth + BMI + Smokers, data = BRFSS)
sum.out <- summary(glm.out)
xB <- cbind(1, BRFSS[, -1])                    #  omit response, add "1" column
xB[1:2, ]                                       #  independent variables
            1 Dentist Teeth  BMI Smokers
Akron,OH        1   75.6  46.9 38.2    25.5
Albuquerque,NM 1   70.4  39.0 43.3    19.4

Cz <- overlinear(z = (-50 : 50) / 250, resid = glm.out$residuals,
    sighat = sigma(glm.out), ses = sum.out$coefficients[,2], xmat= xB)
Czr <- range(Cz[,-1])
plot(Cz[,1], Cz[, 2], type = "l", ylab = "C(z)", xlab = "z", yaxt = "n",
    cex.lab = 1.25, lwd = 4, col = 1, ylim = c(.999, 1.0005))
for(i in 3: dim(Cz)[2])
    lines(Cz[,1], Cz[,i], type = "l", lwd = 4, col = i - 1)
```

14.7 Big Data and Wide Data

As we come to the end of this book, we should ask: Where is all of this going next? The short answer is we are headed toward larger and more massive data sets than were considered in this volume. The advantage of the modest-sized data sets considered here is they are useful for illustrating the statistical methods. However, the real application of the methods is to summarize the large data sets being collected today.

Computing power needs to keep up. We should look back at Table 1.7 comparing SAS and R. Perhaps we should have been discussing SAS all along, in order to make

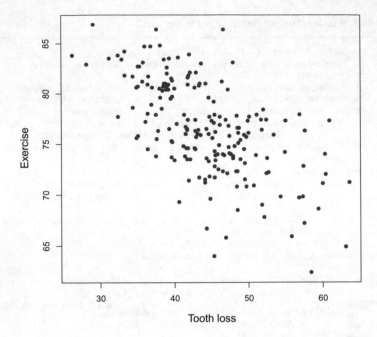

Fig. 14.13 Plot of exercise and tooth loss in BRFSS data exhibits non-constant variability

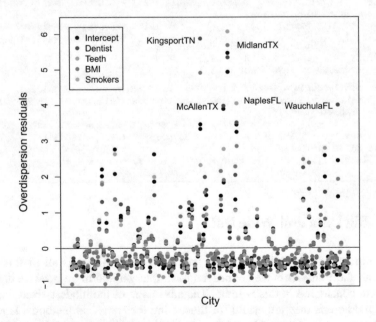

Fig. 14.14 Overdispersion residuals H_{ij} with selected cities identified

use of its data handling capacity. If the data doesn't fit into the software package then of what use is it? There are versions of **R** being developed to address this shortcoming, but they are arriving late to the party.

Many of the methods described in this book are easily scalable to ever larger sizes of data. We pointed out that histograms and boxplots are scalable but scatterplots are not. Similarly, principal components rely only on data being reduced to a matrix of covariances. If this matrix is not too large, then it doesn't matter how many observations there were in the original data. As another example, we can perform linear regressions because these also only require the covariance matrices. Again, this works as long as we don't have too many covariates to examine. Looking for outliers in linear models may be difficult in huge data sets however.

Here are some examples of where the analysis of big data has been successful. *Google Flu Trends* follows Internet searches to detect an epidemic. If many people are suddenly searching on the keyword *fever*, for example, then there must be something going around. But Google's search algorithm changes, so one year is not comparable to the searches conducted at the same time in previous years. Even so, commercial gains can be made by exploiting the search algorithm. Pharmaceutical manufacturers may abruptly increase their advertising budget to associate their product with the treatment of the flu. Drug companies already have years of experience with sales of their products so their Bayesian prior knowledge may be as good or better than the search data can tell us.

Big is not necessarily better. We may need to combine large data sets collected at different times, under different conditions. Suppose we had all of the weather data or baseball statistics in one place: Would we be able to make better predictions? Weather forecasting is useful to all of us, but for what purpose would baseball predictions serve, outside of the specialized groups of gamblers or coaches?

Wide data is another interesting development. Instead of a relatively small amount of data collected on each of many patients, medical studies in genetic markers and *micro-arrays* allow us to collect huge amounts of data on a relatively small number of subjects. For each marker, we need to identify the associated genetic pathway. These markers sometimes work in parallel with others, or as a single road block, shutting down the whole process. This suggests the measurements are associated with each other and *a priori* need to be considered collectively.

The reader who has worked out many of the exercises here has benefited by not being concerned with the huge data cleaning tasks preceding the statistical analysis. The data cleaning and concern for missing values are much more time-consuming than setting up and running the computer program summarizing these. What's more, the proper planning for collecting the appropriate data can be quite involved as well.

There is much work yet to be done.

14.8   Exercises

14.1 In the housing data of Table 1.1, are the extreme housing prices and apartment rents completely out of line with the remainder of the data? Examine a plot, similar to Fig. 14.10, to make a case of whether or not the extremes in Fig. 3.10 could be called outliers.

14.2 The data set `planets` in the HSAUR2 library lists properties of known *exoplanets*. These are known planets which orbit stars other than our sun. The first column is the estimated mass, in multiples of Jupiter. Let us concentrate on the mass values, specifically the largest of these. Is there evidence of *size bias*, meaning only some of the largest exoplanets have been discovered? Or does our current knowledge look more like a representative random sample of what is lurking in outer space? What do we need to assume about the underlying distribution of exoplanet masses? Do the largest of these follow the distributions of extremes?

14.3 Table 14.5 lists the sizes of the largest oil spills, along with their dates and locations. The estimated amounts of oil spilled are given in thousands of tons, barrels, and US gallons. Many of these data values are rough estimates. The units may not be precisely convertible from one to another, but are close to being constant multiples of each other. If a range is provided, the midpoint of the interval is given here.

  a. Use the extreme value methods of Sect. 14.5 to show the largest of these was a far greater environmental disaster than expected, relative to the others on this list.

  b. If we exclude the single largest of all oil spills, use the Gini statistic (14.4) to show several of the remaining largest spills are not out of line with what we would expect to see. Estimate the number of largest observations following the extremal value distribution.

14.4 In Sect. 14.5, how much do the estimates of a_k and b_k depend on the value of k? Specifically, take the corporate asset data in Table 14.4 and calculate estimates of these two parameters for a range of values of k providing reasonable p-values for the Gini statistic in Fig. 14.10. Describe how these estimates change when the value of k varies. How critical is the value of k when estimating these parameters?

14.5 The data set `schizophrenia` in the HSAUR2 library lists the age at onset of schizophrenia, separately for male and female patients. Show that, overall, the age is skewed but there are no extreme outliers among the oldest and youngest patients. In both tails, the 15 most extreme observed values are largely where we would expect them to appear. *Hint:* To examine the *lower* tail, we can reverse the tails by transforming the data with a minus sign, as in $70 - age$.

14.6 a. Table 14.6 lists the highest compensation for the chief executive officer (*CEO*) among all non-profit groups. Is there evidence the highest paid among

Table 14.5 Largest oil spills

Name	Location	Year	Estimated size of spill in thousands:		
			Tons	Barrels	Gallons
Kuwaiti oil fires	Kuwait	1991	170,500	1,250,000	52,500,000
Kuwaiti oil lakes	Kuwait	1991	5,114	37,500	1,575,000
Lakeview Gusher	California	1910–11	1,200	9,000	378,000
Gulf War oil spill	Persian Gulf	1991	955	7,000	294,000
Deepwater Horizon	Gulf of Mexico	2010	573	4,500	176,000
Ixtoc I	Gulf of Mexico	1979–80	467	3,425	143,829
Atlantic Empress/ Aegean Captain	Trinidad & Tobago	1979	287	2,105	88,396
Fergana Valley	Uzbekistan	1992	285	2,090	87,780
Nowruz Field	Persian Gulf	1983	260	1,907	80,080
ABT Summer	Angola	1991	260	1,907	80,080
Castillo de Bellver	South Africa	1983	252	1,848	77,616
Amoco Cadiz	France	1978	223	1,635	68,684
MT Haven	Italy	1991	144	1,056	44,352
Odyssey	Canada	1988	132	968	40,656
Sea Star	Iran	1972	115	843	35,420
Irenes Serenade	Greece	1980	100	733	30,800
Urquiola	Spain	1976	100	733	30,800
Torrey Canyon	UK	1967	100	730	30,660
Greenpoint spill	New York City	1940s	76	555	23,500

Source Wikipedia

Table 14.6 Highest paid CEO's of non-profit organizations

Organization	Compensation	Total revenue in $ m	
		Total	Gov't
American Cancer Society	$1,045,887	429	9
American Heart Association	995,424	645	0
Boys & Girls Clubs of American	988,591	107	41
March of Dimes	627,104	237	10
American Red Cross	455,690	3,300	125
Big Brothers, Big Sisters	349,563	33	11
Mothers Against Drunk Driving	256,380	41	9

Source NYTimes July 27, 2010, page A12

Table 14.7 Wealthiest individuals in the world. Net worth is measured in billions of US dollars

Rank	Name	Net worth	Age	Nationality	Source
1	J Bezos	$177	57	US	Amazon
2	E Musk	151	49	US	Tesla
3	B Arnault	150	72	France	LVMH
4	B Gates	124	65	US	Microsoft
5	M Zuckerberg	97	36	US	Facebook
6	W Buffett	96	90	US	Berkshire
7	L Ellison	93	76	US	Oracle
8	L Page	92	48	US	Alphabet
9	S Brin	89	47	US	Alphabet
10	M Ambani	85	63	India	Reliance

Source Wikipedia, as of August, 2021

these executives is over-compensated? What use can you make of the additional data in this table on total revenue for the organization?

b. What can we do about the net worth of the richest individuals in the world? These are listed in Table 14.7. Are there any who stand out from the rest or do these measures of net worth appear about where we expected them to be?

14.7 Repeat the analysis of the data in Table 14.4 for the *number* of deals and percent of market share. Do these extreme values seem out of line or consistent with what we would expect of the several most extreme observations?

Table 14.8 US counties with the greatest rates of COVID-19 cases as of May 24, 2020. *Source* NYTimes, May 25, 2020

County	Total Cases	Cases per 100,000
Trousdale, Tenn	1393	14,551
Dakota, Neb	1596	7,855
Lincoln, Ark	974	7,112
Nobles, Minn	1457	6,672
Colfax, Neb	599	5,567
Lake, Tenn	409	5,434
Ford, Kan	1558	4,518

Table 14.9 Votes earned by the top candidates in a primary election

Candidate	Votes
Bill de Blasio	130,008
Wm C. Thompson Jr.	85,506
Christine C. Quinn	51,059
John C. Liu	27,349
Anthony D. Weiner	17,356
Erick J. Salgado	8,470
Randy Credico	6,289
Sal F. Albanese	3,444
Neil Grimaldi	2,757

Source NY Times

14.8 The New York City mayoral primary was held on September 10, 2013. With 55% of the precincts reporting, the results for the top candidates in the Democratic Party are given in Table 14.9.

a. Fit an extremal distribution to these values. Is there evidence of a group of leaders who received votes far above those of the rest of the "also rans?"

b. The law requires a second, run-off election if no candidate receives 40% of the vote. At this point in the vote tabulating, what probability can you assign to the need for a run-off?

14.9 During the global pandemic, the number of COVID-19 cases was carefully watched and reported. Table 14.8 lists the US counties with the highest rates per 100,000 population. Does the county with the highest rate stand out from the rest? Use extreme value methods to see if the counties with the highest rates were exceptional.

14.10 Consider the notation of ranking academic journals where "$i > j$" means journal i is cited at a greater rate by journal j than journal j is cited by

Table 14.10 Cross-citation of statistics journals 1987–9

Citing	Cited journal								
Journal	AnnSt	Biocs	Bioka	ComSt	JASA	JRSSB	JRSSC	Tech	Totals
AnnSt	1623	42	275	47	340	179	28	57	2591
Biocs	155	770	419	37	348	163	85	66	2043
Bioka	466	141	714	33	320	284	68	81	2107
ComSt	1025	273	730	425	813	276	94	418	4054
JASA	739	264	498	68	1072	325	104	117	3187
JRSSB	182	60	221	17	142	188	43	27	880
JRSSC	88	134	163	19	145	104	211	62	926
Tech	112	45	147	27	181	116	41	386	1055
Totals	4390	1729	3167	673	3361	1635	674	1214	16,843

Source Stigler (1994). Used with permission

journal i. We can also write $i = j$ if journals i and j cite each other at the same rate. Prove the following relationships, or provide counter-examples:

a. If $i > j$ and $j > k$ then $i > k$.
b. If $i = j$ and $j = k$ then $i = k$.

14.11 Table 14.10 summarizes cross-citation of statistical journals for the years 1987–9. Repeat the analysis from Sect. 14.1 for these journals and see if you reach the same conclusion, namely, ideas appear to flow from the theoretical journals to the applied ones. The four most theoretical journals are *Annals of Statistics* (AnnSt), *Biometrika* (Bioka), *Journal of the American Statistical Association* (JASA), and *Journal of the Royal Statistical Society*, Series B, (JRSSB). The other four are generally considered to be more applied.

14.12 The `baseball` data set in the `BradleyTerry2` library contains the win/loss records of seven baseball teams who played each other several times throughout the 1987 season. Fit a Bradley–Terry model for the paired comparisons in this data and provide a ranking of the teams.

a. Is the offset necessary to account for the different number of games played by each team?
b. Do the fitted λ's in the Bradley–Terry model coincide with the win–loss records of these teams?
c. The data includes an indication of which games were played at home or away. How much of a home-field advantage is there?

14.13 Repeat the canonical correlation analysis of the car data.

a. Interpret the loadings for the driver features.
b. Perform a principal components analysis for the driver features. Are the loadings comparable to those of the canonical correlations in part a?
c. Repeat this comparison for the design features.

14.14 Provide the details to produce Fig. 14.11.

    a. The Poisson distribution has the mass function

$$p(x, \lambda) = \exp(-\lambda)\, \lambda^x / x!$$

    for mean parameter $\lambda > 0$ and $x = 0, 1, \ldots$.
Show this function is maximized at $\lambda = x$ (for $x > 0$). Find a simpler expression for the deviance:

$$\log\{\, p(x, \lambda = x)/p(x, \lambda)\, \}.$$

    b. The gamma density with shape $k > 0$ and scale $\theta > 0$ has density function

$$f(t \mid k, \theta) = \frac{1}{\Gamma(k)\, \theta^k}\, t^{k-1}\, \exp(-t/\theta)$$

    for $t > 0$. Show this distribution has mean $\mu = k\theta$.

    c. Show how, in an overdispersed Poisson distribution, if the mean behaves as a gamma random variable then this can be expressed as a negative binomial distribution. Specifically, demonstrate

$$\mathrm{NB}(x \mid k, \mu) = \int p(x, \lambda) f(\lambda \mid k, \theta)\mathrm{d}\lambda = \binom{x+k-1}{k-1} \left(\frac{k}{\mu+k}\right)^k \left(\frac{\mu}{\mu+k}\right)^k.$$

    d. Show this function is maximized at $\mu = x$ and simplify an expression for the deviance

$$\log\{\, \mathrm{NB}(x \mid k, \mu = x)/\mathrm{NB}(x \mid k, \mu)\}$$

14.15 a. Fit a bivariate normal distribution to the Swiss development data plotted in Fig. 6.1.

    b. Construct a convexity plot for these data. Compare this plot to Fig. 3.11. Both sets of data have about the same number of observations and are fitted to the same model. How are these figures similar or different?

    c. Which observations do the overdispersion residuals identify as unusual? Explain why these observations stand out.

14.16 Leading up to the 2020 US presidential election, several members of the Democratic party announced their candidacy and began fundraising to support their campaign. Table 14.11 summarizes fundraising results as of June 30, 2019. Some candidates received most of their contributions from selected demographics of the population or primarily from certain parts of the country. As a result, the individual contributors in Table 14.11 can represent very different sources of contributions.

Table 14.11 Fundraising results of leading Democratic candidates for the 2020 presidential election as of June 30, 2019

Candidate	Individual contributors (in 1000's)	Amount raised (in $ million)
Bernie Sanders	746	36
Elizabeth Warren	421	25
Pete Buttigieg	390	32
Kamala Harris	277	24
Joseph Biden	256	22
Beto O'Rourke	188	13
Andrew Yang	133	5
Julian Castro	110	4
Cory Booker	100	10
Tulsi Gabbard	88	4
Amy Kloobuchar	79	9
Jay Inslee	78	5
Kirsten Gillibrand	77	5
Marianne Williamson	75	3
Michael Bennet	28	3
Steve Bullock	17	2
Seth Moulton	14	1
John Hickenlooper	14	3
Tim Ryan	10	1
John Delaney	8	2
Bill de Blasio	7	1

Source NYTimes, Aug. 2, 2019

Use extreme value methods to show there were a small number of candidates who stood out from the rest in terms of funds raised. Also, show one candidate had an unusually large number of individual contributors.

14.17 a. Show the statistic (14.5) has zero mean under the null hypothesis of no parameter heterogeneity.

b. Suppose θ has a distribution with density function $g(\theta)$ with mean θ_0 and small variance denoted σ^2.

Find the log-likelihood ratio to test null hypothesis $x_1, \ldots, x_n$ are independently sampled from $f(x \mid \theta_0)$ against the alternative the x's are sampled from $\int f(x \mid \theta) g(\theta) d\theta$. *Hint:* Write a Taylor series under the integral sign in $f(\theta)$ about θ_0 and then integrate each term to obtain

$$\int f(x \mid \theta)\, g(\theta)\, d\theta \,/\, f(x \mid \theta_0) = 1 + \sigma^2 f''(x \mid \theta_0) \,/\, 2 f(x \mid \theta_0)$$

Table 14.12 Breast cancer recurrence

	Recurrence	Radiation	Degree	Nodes	Caps
1	0	0	0	1	0
2	0	0	0	1	0
3	0	0	0	1	0
⋮					⋮
283	1	0	0	1	0
284	1	0	1	2	0
285	1	0	1	2	0

Source https://archive.ics.uci.edu/ml/datasets/

plus smaller terms. Then write $\sum \log(1 + \epsilon_i) = \sum \epsilon_i$ for small values of ϵ_i to obtain (14.5).

14.18 Consider a linear regression model

$$y_i = \alpha + \beta x_i + \epsilon_i$$

where the ϵ_i are independently distributed as normals with mean zero and variance σ^2. Use (14.5) to derive tests of overdispersion for each of the parameters α, β, and σ. Interpret each of these three test statistics in simple terms.

14.19 The excerpted and edited data in Table 14.12 summarizes the treatment and outcome histories of 285 women diagnosed with breast cancer in Yugoslavia. There were many other variables in addition to those given here but we chose to keep this example simple for illustration.

The outcome of interest is binary-valued, whether the disease recurs (1) or not (0). The treatment of interest was whether radiation was used (1) or not (0) in the patient's care. The mediating variable is the degree of disease severity, also coded as binary, with the value 0 indicating less severe cases and 1 for these more severe.

Use these data to determine the usefulness of radiation in preventing disease recurrence including the mediating effect of disease severity. The treatment was not randomly assigned because the disease severity probably dictated the treatment chosen by the physician.

Additional explanatory values include the number of nodes involved (coded as 0 for 0–2; 1 for 3–5; and 2 for more than 5 modes) and whether the nodes were capped. Nodes are said to be "capped" when the tumor metastasizes and is contained in the capsule of the lymph node.

Appendix A
R Libraries Used

Name	First page cited
ape	307
aplpack	57
astsa	390
boot	56
BradleyTerry2	392
CCA	397
cluster	312
ClusterR	331
clValid	321
cubature	45
datasets	151
dbscan	336
energy	162
factoextra	346
fBasics	128
fmsb	81
fMultivar	155
foreign	31
fpc	320
gap	301
ggplot2	346
glmnet	255
gplots	325
graphics	64
HSAUR2	301
Hotelling	198
ICSNP	175
kernlab	293
kohonen	326
lavaan	218
lme4	361
MASS	150
MCMCpack	24
mediation	402
MVA	66

© Springer Nature Switzerland AG 2022
D. Zelterman, *Applied Multivariate Statistics with R*, Statistics for Biology and Health,
https://doi.org/10.1007/978-3-031-13005-2

R Libraries used, cont'd.	
Name	First page cited
mvShapiroTest	162
mvtnorm	38
mvnormtest	195
mvtree	296
nortest	128
OpenImageR	326
psych	195
psychometric	160
quantreg	405
rpart	344
robustbase	264
stats	313
supc	349
TeachingDemos	47
TH.data	232
TSA	390
vars	380

Selected Solutions and Hints

2.1 Some solutions are

```
c(0 : 10 / 10, 2 : 10)
c(seq(0, 1, .1), 2 : 10)
c(seq(0, 1, .1), seq(2, 10))
```

2.3 a.

```
mad <- function(x)
    { mean( abs( x - mean(x) ) ) }
```

2.4 The **R** code

```
> pchisq(1.2, 1) - pchisq(.5, 1)

[1] 0.2061784
```

provides the result.

2.5 All the test scores are very highly correlated with each other. This suggests that any one test score is representative of the whole data from each country. See also Exercise 8.9.

2.10 c. Here are examples of operations resulting in `Inf` and NaN. Notice **R** only produces an error message in the second of these examples but not the third.

```
> 5 / 0

[1] Inf

> sqrt(-3)

[1] NaN
Warning message:
In sqrt(-3) : NaNs produced
```

© Springer Nature Switzerland AG 2022
D. Zelterman, *Applied Multivariate Statistics with R*, Statistics for Biology and Health,
https://doi.org/10.1007/978-3-031-13005-2

```
> 0/0

[1] NaN
```

2.11 A simple solution is

```
spacing(x) <- function(x)  diff(sort(x))
```

Notice this code does not check for empty or a scalar x, situations where spacings are undefined. A somewhat more cryptic definition   including the error checking is

```
spacing <- function(x) if(length(x) > 1) diff(sort(x)) else NA
```

3.7 This **R** program draws and peels away five convex hulls.

```
x <- housing$Apartment          # temporary copies of the data
y <- housing$House
plot(x, y, xlab = "Apartment", ylab = "House",
  pch = 19, col = 2, cex = 1.25)    # initial scatterplot
for (i in 1 : 5)                     # number of onion layers
    {
    ch <- chull(x, y)            # indices of convex hull
    chl <- c(ch, ch[1])          # loop back to the first point
    lines(x[chl], y[chl], type = "l",
       col = 3)                  # draw the layer
    x <- x[ -ch]                 # peel away the layer
    y <- y[ -ch]
    }                            # ... and repeat
```

4.3 If y is a vector of all 1's, then $y'X$ is a vector containing the column sums in X and Xy (for y of a possibly different length) are the row sums in X.

4.6 The matrix inverse is
$$\begin{pmatrix} 1 & -1 \\ -1 & 2 \end{pmatrix}.$$

The eigenvalues are $(3 \pm \sqrt{5})/2$ or approximately 0.382 and 2.618.

5.2 Let U have a uniform distribution between 0 and 1. Then

$$\Pr[\, U \leq p\,] = p$$

for any number p, between zero and one. We also have

$$\Pr[\, U \leq \Phi(z)\,] = \Phi(z)$$

for any real number z and

$$\Pr[\, \Phi^{-1}(U) \leq z\,] = \Phi(z).$$

This shows the distribution of $X = \Phi^{-1}(U)$ has a standard normal distribution.

5.8 Denote the estimate of the mean by $\widehat{\mu}$ and standard deviation by $\widehat{\sigma}$. Use (5.7) to show the endpoints of the k categories with equal expectations are

$$\{-\infty, \quad \widehat{\mu} + \widehat{\sigma}\,\Phi^{-1}(1/k)\}$$
$$\{\widehat{\mu} + \widehat{\sigma}\,\Phi^{-1}(1/k), \quad \widehat{\mu} + \widehat{\sigma}\,\Phi^{-1}(2/k)\}$$
$$\vdots$$
$$\{\widehat{\mu} + \widehat{\sigma}\,\Phi^{-1}((k-1)/(k)), \quad +\infty\}.$$

6.2 a. Figure 6.2 was produced using the following **R** code:

```
corcon <- function(x, y, correl)
  {
    nx <- length(x)
    ny <- length(y)
    z <- matrix(rep(0, nx * ny), nx, ny)
    for (i in 1 : nx)
      {
        for (j in 1 : ny)
          {
              z[i,j] <- dmvnorm(c(x[i], y[j]), c(0, 0),
                  matrix(c(1, correl, correl, 1), 2, 2))
          }
      }
    return(z)
  }

library(mvtnorm)
del <- .05       # how fine the grid
lim <- 3.25      # std normals plotted on +/- lim
par(mfrow = c(2, 4), mar = c(5, 0, 5, 0))   # Four plots across
contour(corcon(seq(-lim, lim, del), seq(-lim, lim, del), -.5),
          xlab = "Corr = -.5",
          drawlabels = FALSE, axes = FALSE, frame = TRUE)
contour(corcon(seq( -lim, lim, del), seq( -lim, lim, del), 0),
          xlab = "Corr = 0",
          drawlabels = FALSE, axes = FALSE, frame = TRUE)
contour(corcon(seq(-lim, lim, del), seq( -lim, lim, del), .5),
          xlab = "Corr = .5",
          drawlabels = FALSE, axes = FALSE, frame = TRUE)
contour(corcon(seq( -lim, lim, del), seq( -lim, lim, del), .9),
          xlab = "Corr = .9",
          drawlabels = FALSE, axes = FALSE, frame = TRUE)
```

b. Again, using the `corcon` function, defined above, Fig. 6.3 was drawn using

```
library(MASS,mvtnorm,graphics)
layout(t(matrix(c(1 : 2, rep(0, 2)), 2, 2)), widths = c(1, 1))

del < .025    # how fine the grid
lim <- 1.25   # std normals plotted on +/- lim
```

```
image(corcon(seq( -lim, lim, del), seq( -lim, lim, del), 0.8),
        axes = FALSE)

del <- .3       # how fine the grid
lim <- 2.7      # std normals plotted on +/- lim
persp(corcon(seq( -lim, lim, del), seq( -lim, lim, del), 0.8),
      axes = FALSE, xlab = "", ylab = "", box = FALSE,
      col = "lightblue", shade = .05)
```

6.3 This program generates bivariate normals and transforms these to the shape of Fig. 6.7:

```
quad <- function(n)
  {
  quad <- NULL
  for (i in 1 : n)
      {
      x <- rnorm(1)
      y <- rnorm(1)
      dia <- sqrt(x ^ 2 + y ^ 2)
      if(dia > rad)      # outside the circle
          {
          if(x > 0) y <-  abs(y)
              else y <- -abs(y)
          if(x < 0) y <- -abs(y)
              else y <-  abs(y)
          }
      if(dia < rad)      # inside the circle
          {
          if(x > 0) y <- -abs(y)
              else y <-  abs(y)
          if(x < 0) y <-  abs(y)
              else y <- -abs(y)
          }
      quad <- rbind(quad, c(x, y))
      }
    quad
  }
```

Some trial and error suggests `rad` should be about 1.83.

6.5 Here is a useful reparameterization and objective function:

```
biv5r <- function(par)  # all five parameter, reparameterized
  {
  sig1 <- exp(par[3])
  sig2 <- exp(par[4])
  rho <- par[5] / sqrt(1 + par[5] ^ 2)
  cov <- rho * sig1 * sig2
  biv5 <- sum(
    -dmvnorm(cancer, mean = c(par[1], par[2]),
        sigma = matrix(c(sig1 ^ 2, cov, cov, sig2 ^ 2), 2, 2),
        log = TRUE) )
```

```
            print(c(par[1 : 2], sig1, sig2, rho, biv5))
            biv5
    }
```

The code

```
    nlm(biv5r, c(45, 45, 7.25, 7.25, 2))
```

then estimates the five parameters without warnings.
The estimated value of par[5] is 2.053445, so the estimate of ρ is

```
    > 2.053445 / sqrt(1 + 2.053445 ^ 2)

    [1] 0.8990582
```

7.5 Consider an election where citizens cast ballots for one of p different candidates. The data is the numbers of votes received by each candidate. Any vote for one candidate means fewer votes for all of the others.

7.7 a. This program calculates energy residuals:

```
msqrt <- function(a)
# finds matrix square root of positive definite matrix
    {
        a.eig <- eigen(a)           # eigenvalues and eigenvectors of x
        if ( min(a.eig$values) < 0) # check for positive definite
            warning("Matrix not positive definite")

        return(a.eig$vectors %*% diag(sqrt(a.eig$values)) %*% t
        (a.eig$vectors))
    }

energy.resid <- function(dat, R=300)
    {
    n <- dim(dat)[1]                # observations
    p <- dim(dat)[2]                # variables
    std <- dat - t(matrix(colMeans(dat), p, n))
    s <- var(dat)
    std <- as.matrix(std)  %*% solve(msqrt(s)) # standardized data
    rand <- matrix(rnorm(p * R), R, p) # independent normal data

    A <- rep(0, n)
    B <- rep(0, n)
    for (i in 1 : n)
        {
          a <- 0
          b <- 0
          for (j in 1 : R) a <- a + sqrt(sum((std[i, ] - rand[j, ])
              ^ 2))
          A[i] <- a / R             # ave dist between data and random
          for (j in 1:n) b <- b + sqrt(sum((std[i, ] - std[j, ]) ^ 2))
          B[i] <- b / (n - 1)       # ave dist between data
        }
    cc <- 0
    for(i in 2 : R)   for (j in 1 : (i - 1))
```

```
                    cc <- cc + sqrt(sum((rand[i, ] - rand[j, ]) ^ 2))
            C <- 2 * cc /(R * (R - 1))          # ave dist between random values

            2 * A - B - C
        }
```

7.9 This program computes the autocorrelation when columns of the data represent sequential years.

```
autocov <- function(data)
              #  Autocorrelation of annual columns in data
        {
        nyears <- dim(data)[2] - 1
        autocov <- NULL
        for (lag in 1 : nyears)
            {
            lagcor <- 0
            for (year in 1 : (nyears - lag + 1))
                lagcor <- lagcor + cor(data[ , year], data[ , year + lag])
            lagcor <- lagcor / (nyears - lag + 1)
            autocov <- c(autocov, lagcor)
            }
        autocov
        }

ac <- autocov(CS)
```

8.7 The academic scores are highly correlated with each other. Further, these have been standardized. (See Exercise 2.5). The loadings of the principal components analysis are almost the same for each test score. This suggests any one score is representative for the whole set of values for each country.

8.12 The biplot for the correlation matrix of the oil consumption data given in Table 8.5 appears here.

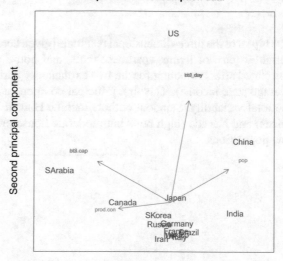

This figure separates low population, oil producing nations (Saudi Arabia and Canada) from high population, oil consuming nations (India and China).

8.14 The plot and code:

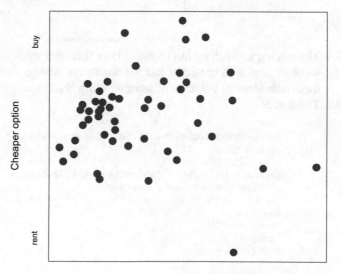

```
pc <- prcomp(housing)$rotation
hres <- -as.matrix(housing) %*% as.matrix(pc)
hres <- hres - t(matrix(colMeans(hres), 2,51))
plot(hres, col = "red", pch = 16, xaxt = "n", xlab = "Cost of living",
```

```
                yaxt = "n", ylab = "Cheaper option", cex.lab = 1.25)
  axis(side = 2, labels = c("rent", "buy"), at = c(-100, 60), tick = F)
```

9.1 The biplot of the three-dimensional residuals (given here) shows all dependent variables (cost of living, apartment rents, and house prices) remain highly correlated after correcting for the two explanatory variables (population and average state income). This first principal component explains over 90% of the total variability. Standout outliers include Hawaii (high rents and house prices) and Nevada (high rents but moderate house prices), both states with low populations.

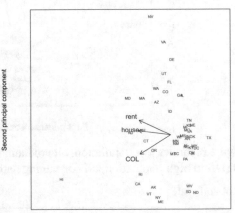

First principal component

9.4 The mining technology has changed over this time span, as the numbers of workers employed in mining and the amount of coal produced. We can't use these data alone as evidence of safer working conditions.

9.5 The **R** code

```
jaw <- read.table(file = "Ramus.txt", header = TRUE,
   row.names = 1)
n <-  dim(jaw)[1]
plot(x = NA, type = "n", xlim = c(8, 9.5),
   ylim = c(min(jaw), max(jaw)),
xlab = "Age", ylab = "Ramus")
age <- c(8., 8.5, 9, 9.5 )
longa <- NULL
longj <- NULL
for (i in 1:n)
   {
    longa <- c(longa, age)
    ramus <- jaw[i,]
    longj <- c(longj, as.double(ramus))
    lines (age, ramus, col = "red")
   }
lines(longa, longj, pch = 16, col = "blue",
   type = "p", cex = .8)
model <- lm(longj ~ longa)
```

```
fit <- model$coefficients[1] + model$coefficients[2] * age
lines ( age, fit, type = "l", col = "green", lwd = 3)
jres <- jaw - fit                    # residuals
sapply(jres, sd)
```

```
    age8    age8_5      age9    age9_5
2.805906  2.897436  2.808309  2.871713
```

produces the spaghetti plot of observed and fitted values:

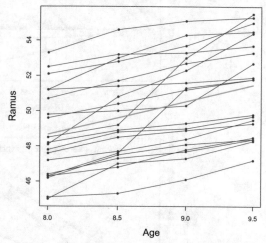

This plot provides good evidence that the variances are constant across ages.

9.10 The **R** code

```
fire <- read.csv(file = "forestfires.csv", header = T)
fire[c(1:3, 515:517),]           # print a few first and last
area <- log(fire$area + 1)       # transform skewed response
expl <- as.matrix(fire[ , -c(3, 4, 13)])  # the explanatory variables
expl[1:3,]                       # check to see if done correctly

fit <- glmnet(x = expl, y = area)
plot(fit, lwd = 2.5, cex.lab = 1.25)
text(c(.165, .23, .23, .125), c(.06, .06, .043, .075), labels= c("wind",
   "rain", "X", "Forest fires using lasso regression"),
   cex = c(1.25, 1.25, 1.5))
fit$beta                         # identify the different lines

fit <- glmnet(x = expl, y = area, alpha = 0)
plot(fit, lwd = 2.5, cex.lab = 1.25)
text(c(.165, .225, .125), c(.06, .06, .075), labels= c("rain", "wind",
        "Forest fires using ridge regression"), cex = c(1.25, 1.25, 1.5))
fit$beta
```

will produce these two figures:

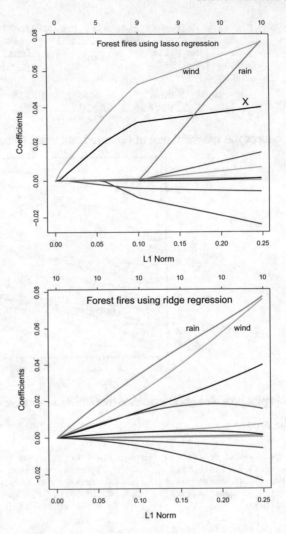

10.16 The **R** code

```
require(mvpart,datasets,graphics)
univ <- mvpart(mpg ~ cyl + disp + am + carb , data = mtcars)
```

produces a regression tree with four leaves:

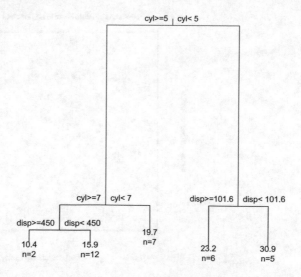

Error : 0.077   CV Error : 0.202   SE : 0.0498

11.6   a. The code for clustering and principal components of the `milk` data

```
library(robustbase)              # library with the milk dataset
milk2 <- milk[ -70 , ]           # omit outlier
colnames(milk2) <- c("dens", "fat", "prot", "casein", "Fdry",
   "Ldry", "drysub", "cheese")# supply new names
                                 # color schemes for K-means
color3  <- rainbow(3)[kmeans(scale(milk2), centers = 3)$
   cluster]
pcm <- princomp(milk2, scores = TRUE)# principal components
plot(pcm$scores[,1], pcm$scores[ , 2], col = color3, pch = 16,
   xlab = "First principal component", xaxt = "n", yaxt = "n",
   ylab = "Second principal component",
   main = "K-means clusters plotted by principal components")
```

produces the figure:

K–means clusters plotted by principal components

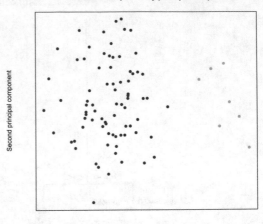

First principal component

11.7 The distribution of X is hypergeometric with probability mass function

$$\Pr[\,X = x\,] = \binom{m}{x}\binom{N-m}{m'-x}\bigg/\binom{N}{m'}$$

defined for

$$\max(0,\, m + m' - N) \leq x \leq \min(m, m').$$

11.9 In the hierarchical cluster

Composition of OAA Title III

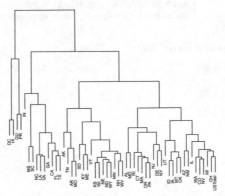

we see DC, Puerto Rico, Guam, and Hawaii cluster together, as do New York, New Jersey, and Delaware. Indiana, Illinois, Alaska, Vermont, and Utah each appear different from all other states.

11.10 b. There are $K = 3$ clusters and the simulation probably alternates between two different pairs of these identified as closest.

11.14 The plot of percent variability explained by cluster size suggests there are two clusters.

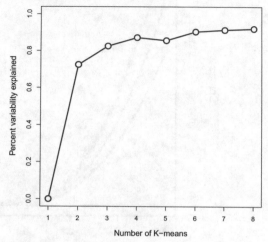

14.14 a. The Poisson devianace can be written as

$$\lambda - x + x \log(x/\lambda) \, .$$

d. The negative binomial deviance can be written as

$$k \, \log\{(\mu + k)/(x + k)\} \, + \, x \log(x/\mu) \, + \, x \, \log\{(\mu + k)/(x + k)\} \, .$$

14.15 b. This is the convexity plot for the Swiss development data. The convexity indicates about the same degree of overdispersion in all parameters.

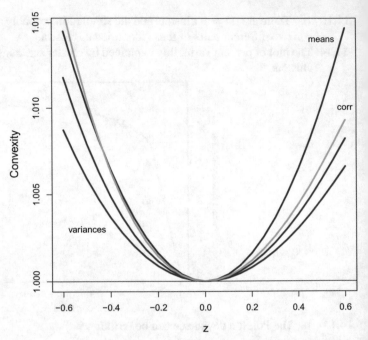

14.16 The leading fundraiser, Bernie Sanders, had far more contributors than would
be expected using the extreme value distribution. The top five fundraisers
appear to be set off from the rest.

14.19
```
brcan <-
read.csv(file = "brcan.csv", header = T) dim(brcan) brcan[c(1 : 3,
283 : 285), ] #  Print some values for Table 15.10

library(mediation)
mediation.model <- glm(degree ~ irrad + nodes + caps,
                       family = binomial, data = brcan)
outcome.model <- glm(recur ~ irrad + degree + nodes + caps,
                     family = binomial, data = brcan)
med.out <- mediate(mediation.model, outcome.model, treat = "irrad",
                   mediator = "degree", robustSE = TRUE, sims = 200)
summary(med.out)
```

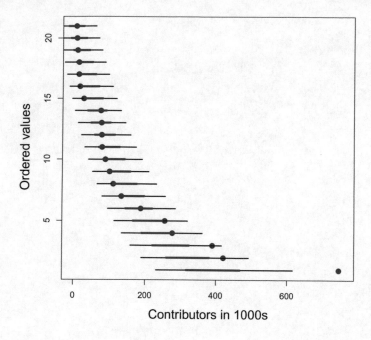

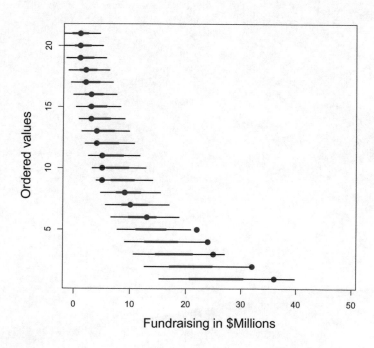

References

Anderson TW (2003). *An Introduction to Multivariate Statistical Analysis.* Wiley. 3rd Edition. Referenced on pages xiii and 14.

Anscombe FJ (1981). *Computing in Statistical Science Through APL.* New York: Springer-Verlag. Referenced on page xiii.

Armstrong JS (1967). Derivation of theory by means of factor analysis or Tom Swift and his electric factor analysis machine. *The American Statistician* **21** 17–21. Referenced on page 217.

Bache K and Lichman M (2013). UCI Machine Learning Repository. Irvine, CA: University of California, School of Information and Computer Science. Referenced on page viii. Available online at: http://archive.ics.uci.edu/ml

Box GEP and Cox DR (1964). An analysis of transformations (with discussions) *Journal of the Royal Statistical Society (B)* **26**: 211-52. Referenced on pages 125.

Bradley RA and Terry ME (1952). Rank analysis of incomplete block designs I: The method of paired comparisons. *Biometrika*, **39**: 324–45. Referenced on page 393.

Chambers JM (1992). *Data for models.* Chapter 3 of *Statistical Models in S.* eds JM Chambers and TJ Hastie, Wadsworth & Brooks/Cole. Referenced on page 77.

Chambers JM, Cleveland WS, Kleiner B, and Tukey JA (1983). *Graphical Methods for Data Analysis.* Chapman and Hall, New York. Referenced on page 87

Chang W (2013). *R Graphics Cookbook* O'Reilly Media, Sebastopol, CA. Available online at: http://books.google.com/books?id=fxL4tu5bzAAC. Referenced on page 87.

Chernoff H (1973). The use of faces to represent points in K-dimensional space graphically. *Journal of the American Statistical Association* **68**: 361–8. https://doi.org/10.2307/2284077. Referenced on page 81.

Cleveland S (1993). *Visualizing Data* Hobart Press, Summit, New Jersey. Referenced on page 87.

Cooley JW, Tukey JW (1965). An algorithm for the machine calculation of complex Fourier series. *Math. Comput.* **19**: 297–301. https://doi.org/10.2307/2003354. Referenced on page 87.

Dempster AP, Laird NM, Rubin DB (1977). Maximum likelihood from incomplete data via the EM algorithm *Journal of the Royal Statistical Society.* Series B **39**: 1–38. Referenced on page 334.

Dunn JC (1973). A fuzzy relative of the ISODATA Process and its use in detecting compact well-separated clusters. *Journal of Cybernetics* **3**: 32–57. Referenced on page 319. https://doi.org/10.1080/01969727308546046.

Elston RC and Grizzle JF (1962). Estimation of time response curves and their confidence bands. *Biometrics* **18**: 148–59. Referenced on page 261.

Everitt B and Hothorn T (2011) *An Introduction to Applied Multivariate Analysis with* R. New York: Springer. Referenced on pages 13 and 66

© Springer Nature Switzerland AG 2022
D. Zelterman, *Applied Multivariate Statistics with R*, Statistics for Biology and Health, https://doi.org/10.1007/978-3-031-13005-2

Fitzmaurice GM and Lipsitz SR (1995). A model for binary time series data with serial odds ratio patterns. *Journal of the Royal Statistical Society Series* C, **44**: 51–61. Referenced on page 362.

Forina M, Leardi R, Armanino C and Lanteri S (1988). *PARVUS: An extendable package of programs for data exploration, classification and correlation* Elsevier, Amsterdam, ISBN 0-444-43012-1. Referenced on page 277.

Friendly M (1999). Extending mosaic displays: Conditional and partial views of categorical data. *Journal of Computational and Graphical Statistics* **8**: 373–395. Referenced on page 356.

Friendly M. (2002). A brief history of the mosaic display. *Journal of Computational and Graphical Statistics* **11**: 89–107. Referenced on page 356.

Gail MH and Gastwirth JL (1978). A scale-free goodness-of-fit test for the exponential distribution based on the Gini statistic. *Journal of the Royal Statistical Society*, Series B, **40**: 350–357. Referenced on page 413.

Goldberg K and Iglewicz B (1992). Bivariate extensions of the boxplot. *Technometrics* **34**:307–20. Referenced on page 66.

Golub GH and Van Loan CF (1983). *Matrix Computations*. Baltimore: The Johns Hopkins University Press. Referenced on page 103.

Hahsler M, Piekenbrock M, Doran D (2019). dbscan: Fast density-based clustering with R. *Journal of Statistical Software* **91**: 1–30. https://doi.org/10.18637/jss.v091.i01. Referenced on page 336.

Hand DJ and Taylor CC (1987). *Multivariate Analysis of Variance and Repeated Measures*. Chapman and Hall. Referenced on page 241.

Hartigan JA and Wong MA (1979). A k-means clustering algorithm. *Applied Statistics* **28**:100–8. Referenced on page 313.

Hotelling H (1935) The most predictable criterion. *Journal of Educational Psychology* **26**: 139–142. Referenced on page 395.

Izenman AJ (2008). *Modern Multivariate Statistical Techniques. Regression, Classification, and Manifold Learning*. Springer. Referenced on page 14.

Jarque CM and Bera AK (1987). A test for normality of observations and regression residuals. *International Statistical Review* **55**: 163–172. JSTOR 1403192. Referenced on page 130.

Jarvis RA and Patrick EA (1973). Clustering using a similarity measure based on shared near neighbors. IEEE Trans. Comput. 22, 11 (November 1973), 1025-1034. https://doi.org/10.1109/T-C.1973.223640. Referenced on page 349.

Johnson RA and Wichern DW (2007). *Applied Multivariate Statistical Analysis* 6th Ed. Prentice Hall, Englewood Cliffs, NJ. Referenced on page 14

Kabacoff RI. (2011). *R in Action. Data Analysis and Graphics with R*. Second edition. Manning Publications. Referenced on page 13.

Krause A and Olson M (1997). *The Basics of S and S-PLUS* New York: Springer. Referenced on page 13.

Lambert D, Roeder K (1995). Overdispersion diagnostics for generalized linear models. *Journal of the American Statistical Association*, **90**: 1225–36. Referenced on page 416.

Lander TA, Oddou-Muratorio S, Prouillet-Leplat H, Klein EK (2011) Reconstruction of a beech population bottleneck using archival demographic information and Bayesian analysis of genetic data. *Molecular Ecology* **20**: 5182–5196. Referenced on page 303. Data available at http://dx.doi.org/10.1111/j.1365-294X.2011.05356.x

Landis, J.R., Miller, M.E., Davis, C.S., and Koch, G.G. (1988). Some general methods for the analysis of categorical data in longitudinal studies. *Statistics in Medicine* **7**:109–37. Referenced on page 353.

Lang S (2010). *Linear Algebra* New York: Springer. Referenced on page 103.

Liang K-Y and Zeger SL. (1986). Longitudinal data analysis using generalized linear models. *Biometrika* **73**: 13–22. Referenced on page 360.

Ljung GM and Box GEP (1978). On a measure of lack of fit in time series models. *Biometrika* **65**: 297–303. Referenced on page 377.

Lumley T (1996). Generalized estimating equations for ordinal data: A note on working correlation structures. *Biometrics* **52**: 354–361. Referenced on page 364.

Mardia KV (1970). Measures of multivariate skewness and kurtosis with applications. *Biometrika* **57**: 519–30. Referenced on page 194.

Mardia KV, Kent JT, Bibby JM. (1979). *Multivariate Analysis*, Academic Press. ISSN 0079-5607. Referenced on page 14.

McFadden D (1974). The measurement of urban travel demand. *Journal of Public Economics* **3**: 303–28. Referenced on page 302.

Mosteller F and Tukey JW (1977). *Data Analysis and Regression: A Second Course in Statistics* Pearson. Referenced on page 72.

Pearl J (2009). *Causality: Models, Reasoning and Inference* Cambridge University Press. Referenced on page 235.

Plackett RL (1981). *The Analysis of Categorical Data*, second edition. London: Charles Griffin. Referenced on page 268.

Rand WM (1971). Objective criteria for the evaluation of clustering methods. *Journal of the American Statistical Association* **66**: 846–50. Referenced on page 320. https://doi.org/10.1080/01621459.1971.10482356

Sarkar D (2008). *Lattice: Multivariate Data Visualization with R*. Springer. http://lmdvr.r-forge.r-project.org/. Referenced on page 87.

Schwager, SJ and Margolin BH (1982). Detection of multivariate normal outliers. *Annals of Statistics* **10**: 943–954. Referenced on page 195.

Shapiro SS, Wilk MB (1965). An analysis of variance test for normality (complete samples). *Biometrika* **52** (3-4): 591–611. https://doi.org/10.1093/biomet/52.3-4.591. JSTOR 2333709 MR205384. Referenced on page 132.

Stanish, W.M., Gillings, D.B., and Koch, G.G.(1978). An application of multivariate ratio methods for the analysis of a longitudinal clinical trial with missing data. *Biometrics* **34**:305–17. Referenced on page 353.

Stigler SM (1994). Citation patterns in the journals of statistics and probability. *Statistical Science* **9**: 94–108. Referenced on page 392.

Sullivan M (2008). *Statistics: Informed Decisions Using Data*, Third Edition. Pearson. Referenced on page 137.

Székely GJ and Rizzo ML (2005). A new test for multivariate normality. *Journal of Multivariate Analysis* **93**: 58–80. https://doi.org/10.1016/j.jmva.2003.12.002. Referenced on page 197.

Takahashi K, Yokota S, Tatsumi N, Fukami T, Yokoi T, and Nakajima M (2013). Cigarette smoking substantially alters plasma microRNA profiles in healthy subjects. *Toxicology and Applied Pharmacology* **272**: 154–160. https://doi.org/10.1016/j.taap.2013.05.018. Referenced on page 313.

Tapia RA and Thompson JR (1978). *Nonparametric Probability Density Estimation*. Baltimore: Johns Hopkins University Press. Referenced on page 129.

Tufte ER (2001). *The Visual Display of Quantitative Information*. Cheshire Press. Referenced on pages 63 and 64.

Tukey JW (1977). *Exploratory Data Analysis* Addison-Wesley. ISBN-13: 978-0201076165. Referenced on page 72.

U.S. Cancer Statistics Working Group. U.S. Cancer Statistics Data Visualizations Tool, based on November 2018 submission data (1999-2016): U.S. Department of Health and Human Services, Centers for Disease Control and Prevention and National Cancer Institute; www.cdc.gov/cancer/dataviz, June 2019. Referenced on page vii.

Venables WN and Ripley BD. *Modern Applied Statistics with S* (Statistics and Computing) New York: Springer. Referenced on page 13.

von Eye A, Bogat GA (2004). Testing the assumption of multivariate normality. *Psychology Science* **46**: 243–258. Referenced on page 195.

Wan H, Larsen LJ (2014). U.S. Census Bureau, American Community Survey Reports, ACS-29, *Older Americans With a Disability: 2008–2012*, U.S. Government Printing Office, Washington, DC, 2014. Referenced on page 200.

Ware JH, Dockery DW, Spiro A III, Speizer FE, and Ferris BG Jr. (1984). Passive smoking, gas cooking and respiratory health in children living in six cities. *American Review of Respiratory Diseases* **129**: 366–74. Referenced on page 366.

Weissman I (1978). Estimation of parameters and large quantiles based on the k largest observations. *Journal of the American Statistical Association* **73**: 812–185. Referenced on page 413.

Wilkinson L (1999) *The Grammar of Graphics*. New York: Springer. Referenced on page 87.

Woolson RF and Clarke WR (1984). Analysis of categorical incomplete longitudinal data. *Journal of the Royal Statistical Society*. Series A. **147**: 87–99. Referenced on page 363.

Zelterman D and Chen C-F (1988). Homogeneity tests against central-mixture alternatives. *Journal of the American Statistical Association* **83**: 179–182. Referenced on page 416.

Zelterman D (1993). A semiparametric bootstrap technique for simulating extreme order statistics. *Journal of the American Statistical Association* **88**: 477–485. Referenced on page 413.

Index

© Springer Nature Switzerland AG 2022
D. Zelterman, *Applied Multivariate Statistics with R*, Statistics for Biology and Health,
https://doi.org/10.1007/978-3-031-13005-2

Printed in the United States
by Baker & Taylor Publisher Services